Applied Nutrition
Livestock, Poultry, Rabbits and
Laboratory Animals

Applied Nutrition
Livestock, Poultry, Rabbits and Laboratory Animals
Third Edition

DV Reddy

BVSc, MVSc, PhD

Professor and Head
Department of Animal Nutrition
Rajiv Gandhi College of Veterinary and
Animal Sciences, Pondicherry

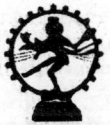

Oxford & IBH Publishing Co. Pvt. Ltd.
New Delhi
(A Unit of CBS Publishers & Distributors Pvt Ltd)

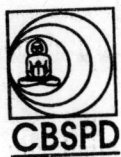

CBSPD

CBS Publishers & Distributors Pvt Ltd

New Delhi • Bengaluru • Chennai • Kochi • Kolkata • Lucknow • Mumbai
Hyderabad • Jharkhand • Nagpur • Patna • Pune • Uttarakhand

Applied Nutrition
Livestock, Poultry, Rabbits and
Laboratory Animals

Third Edition

ISBN-13: 978-81-204-1784-7
ISBN-10: 81-204-1784-4

OXFORD & IBH
New Delhi
(A Unit of CBS Publishers & Distributors Pvt Ltd)

Published by **Satish Kumar Jain** and produced by **Varun Jain** for

CBS Publishers & Distributors Pvt Ltd
4819/XI Prahlad Street, 24 Ansari Road, Daryaganj, New Delhi 110 002, India.
Ph: 011-23266838, 23289259   Website: www.cbspd.com
                                                              e-mail: delhi@cbspd.com
Corporate Office: 204 FIE, Industrial Area, Patparganj, Delhi 110 092
Ph: 011-4934 4934   Fax: 011-4934 4935
                                        e-mail: publishing@cbspd.com; publicity@cbspd.com

Branches

- **Bengaluru:** Seema House 2975, 17th Cross, KR Road, Banasankari 2nd Stage, Bengaluru 560 070, Karnataka, India
  Ph: +91-80-26771678/79   Fax: +91-80-26771680   e-mail: bangalore@cbspd.com
- **Chennai:** 18/8B, Subbarayan Street, Shenoy Nagar, Chennai 600 030, Tamil Nadu, India
  Ph: +91-44-42032115, 26681266   e-mail: chennai@cbspd.com
- **Kochi:** 42/1325, 1326, Power House Road, Opp KSEB, Power House, Ernakulum Kochi 682 018, Kerala, India
  Ph: +91-484-4059061-65,67   Fax: +91-484-4059065   e-mail: kochi@cbspd.com
- **Kolkata:** 147, Hind Ceramics Compound, 1st Floor, Nilgunj Road, Belghoria, Kolkata-700056, West Bengal, India
  Ph: +033-25633055, 033-25633056   e-mail: kolkata@cbspd.com
- **Lucknow:** Basement, Khushnuma Complex, 7 Meerabai Marg (Behind Jawahar Bhawan), Lucknow-226001, UP, India
  Ph: +0522-4000032   e-mail: tiwari.lucknow@cbspd.com
- **Mumbai:** PWD Shed, Gala no 25/26, Ramchandra Bhatt Marg, Next to JJ Hospital Gate no. 2, Opp. Union Bank of India, Noorbaug, Mumbai-400009, Maharashtra, India
  Ph: 022-66661880/89   e-mail: mumbai@cbspd.com

Representatives

- Hyderabad   0-9885175004   • Jharkhand   0-9811541605   • Nagpur   0-8692091830
- Patna   0-9334159340   • Pune   0-9664372571   • Uttarakhand   0-9716462459

Printed at Chaman Enterprises, Daryaganj, New Delhi, India

Preface to the Third Edition

The third edition consists of 15 chapters. With the publication of textbook *Applied Nutrition: Cats Dogs Wild animals & Birds* in 2014, chapters on Cat and Dog nutrition, therapeutic diets, and preservation of foods are omitted in this edition. This edition updates the requirements of cattle, buffaloes, sheep, goats, poultry, pigs, horses and rabbits based on recent research and a need to consider higher levels of productivity by larger and improved genotypes. BIS specifications, ICAR (2013) requirements and NRC requirements have been updated.

New information has been added in several chapters for quick grasp, comprehension and to make the textbook reader-friendly. Text is enriched with flow charts and illustrations. These include conduct of metabolism trial and example on calculation of digestibility, illustrations of ruminant stomach, gastrointestinal tract of horse, equine stomach and avian digestive tract and flow charts depicting the occurrences in the rumen. All these efforts have been made to meet the objective: "Complete information in a comprehensible way".

No one person can write a book on Applied Animal Nutrition (dealing with feeding of domestic ruminants, poultry, pigs, horses, rabbits and laboratory animals) and claim both expertise and original thoughts in all the areas. The same applies to me. When and where possible, I have provided pertinent references. During my 33 years of service as a teacher / researcher / extension worker at various institutions and at various levels to deliver to diversified audience, I have developed the habit of making notes while reading or attending professional meetings. Indeed even as a UG student my evenings are spent in library on week days. This habit of documentation as a way of life helped me to author the book.

I am indebted to my students: to my undergraduates who have shared in my experiments with nutrition syllabuses and my postgraduates who motivated me to deliver on contemporary thoughts on the subject. For the same reasons I am indebted to my colleague teachers / researchers / extension workers in several institutions spread over the Indian Union. I give my heartfelt thanks. I thank my colleague teachers in the department Dr. C.M.Tiwari and Dr.D.Uma Maheswari for their feedback.

I extend my sincere appreciation to Dr.N.Elanchezhian (a colleague in the department) for the balanced diet charts in the chapter on Poultry Nutrition (including those in the Appendix) and Dr.R.Ganesan (Dept of AGB) for updates on experimental designs in the chapter 1. I am thankful to the publishers for meticulous planning and publication of the book. Above all, I thank God for His guidance and inspiration.

December 2014   **Duvvuru Venka Reddy**

Preface to the Second Edition

Response to Feedback Request and Action Taken

Response to my request letters for feedback by post as well as by email had been quite substantial and satisfying, from all Veterinary Colleges and majority Animal and Veterinary Research Institutes of India. I am extremely grateful to all those of my colleagues and students who have offered numerous helpful suggestions. Accordingly, Horse Nutrition has been added (chapter 10), Rabbit Nutrition (chapter 16) has been thoroughly revised, and new useful information has been provided in Appendix II and in several chapters in an effort to make a more complete text on Applied Nutrition. I take this opportunity to express my gratitude to the publishers for meticulous planning and intelligent publishing of the books.

June 2009   **Duvvuru Venka Reddy**

Preface to the First Edition

There are several textbooks on Animal Nutrition and Feeding written by eminent teachers and scientists. But no single textbook caters the needs of undergraduate students of Veterinary Science by providing all the needed information comprehensively on Animal Nutrition subject at a single source. As per the Veterinary Council of India (Minimum Standards of Veterinary Education Degree Course-BVSC & AH) Regulations, 1993, Animal Nutrition courses encompass principles of animal nutrition, evaluation of feedstuffs and feed technology and Applied nutrition covering feeding of livestock, poultry, human beings, pet, rabbit and laboratory animals. The examination system comprises an internal assessment (50%) at the end of each semester and an external assessment (50%) conducted by an annual board appointed by the university at the end of the academic year. The new syllabus and the examination system make the student and the teacher as well, to run to different sources for procuring the needed information for each of the four Animal nutrition courses (ANN 211, ANN 212, ANN 221 and ANN 222). Being in the teaching line since 1981 and specifically teaching Animal Nutrition as per the new syllabus since its introduction from 1995, I have prepared the manuscript. It will be published as two books: 1. Principles of Animal Nutrition and Feed Technology and 2. Applied Nutrition (Livestock, Poultry, Human, Pet, Rabbit and Laboratory Animal Nutrition).

Each textbook consists of two sections (Part I & II) and thus the four sections correspond to the four courses. Each section provides a structured approach to learning by covering all the topics in a uniform, systematic format. This (section – or) course-wise topic-led organization is a distinct advantage of these books since they meet the needs of the students for each course of Animal Nutrition Semester-wise. Some of the topics have been detailed beyond the syllabus level to enlarge the knowledge of the readers because of their importance in applied feeding practice, for example feed additives. These books are designed to give students rapid, easy access to all the material in a course wise format which benefits them prepare for the internal examinations and external examinations economically and ensure exploit their potential to a greater extent. The topics are detailed in a straightforward and hopefully lucid manner. "Complete information in a comprehensible way" is the watchword of the books.

A list of suggested reference books are given at the end of the textbooks. Scientific names of food and fodder crops, popular varieties of fodder crops, metabolic body size figures for body weights, very useful conversion factors and others are furnished in the appendix.

These textbooks are also useful to teachers and scientists of department of Animal Nutrition, personnel of feed industry involved in feed manufacturing and marketing, postgraduate students of Animal Sciences i.e. Animal Nutrition, Avian Production and Management, Livestock Production and Management and Animal Husbandry Extension. Further, they are useful to field veterinarians, extension workers of departments of Animal Husbandry and Dairying and Rural Development, Progressive Animal farmers and Animal lovers. I take this occasion to express my gratefulness to Dr. K.V.S. Reddy, a modesty personified, for providing moral support from time to time. I appreciate the contribution of my wife, Prasuna and children, Amar and Vamsee for providing me cheerful environment and allowing me to spend many hours with drafts of manuscripts rather than with them. Above all I thank God for His guidance and inspiration.

February 2001   **Duvvuru Venka Reddy**

Suggested Reference Books

1. **Animal Nutrition**
   by L.A. Maynard, J.K. Loosli, H.F. Hintz and R.G. Warner, 7th edition, 1979.

2. **Animal Nutrition**
   by P. McDonald, R.A. EDWARDS AND J.F.D. GREENHALGH, 5th edition, 1995.

3. **Feeds and Principles of Animal Nutrition**
   (Revised edition of Animal Nutrition) by G.C. Banerjee, 1st edition, 1988. Reprint 1998, 1999.

4. **Vitamins in Animal Nutrition** (Comparative Aspects to Human Nutrition) by L.R. McDowell, 1st edition, 1989.

5. **Minerals in Animal and Human Nutrition**
   by L.R. McDowell, 1st edition, 1992.

6. **Animal Nutrition**
   by J.W. Lassiter and H.M. Edwards, Jr. 1st edition, 1982.

7. **Trace Elements in Human and Animal Nutrition**
   by E.J. Underwood, 4th edition 1977, 5th edition by Walter Mertz, 1987.

8. **The Mineral Nutrition of Livestock**
   by E.J. Underwood and N.F. Suttle, 3rd edition, 1999.

9. **The Rumen and its Microbes**
   by R.E. Hungate, Ist edition, 1966.

10. **Advanced Animal Nutrition for Developing Countries**
    edited by U.B. Singh, 1st edition, 1987.

11. Advances in Dairy Animal Production
by V.D. Mudgal , K.K. Singhal and D.D. Sharma, 1st edition, 1995. 2nd edition 2003

12. Commercial Poultry Nutrition
by S. Leeson and J.D. Summers, 1st Indian reprint, 1993.

13. Applied Animal Nutrition
by E.W. Crampton and L.E. Harris, 2nd edition, 1968.

14. Livestock Feeding
by S.N. Ray; 1st edition, 1978.

15. Animal Nutrition in the Tropics
by S.K. Ranjhan, 4th edition, 1997.

16. Agroindustrial Byproducts and Nonconventional Feeds for Livestock Feeding
by S.K. Ranjhan, 1st edition, 1990.

17. Chemical Composition and Nutritive Value of Indian Feeds and Feeding of Farm Animals
by S.K. Ranjhan, 1st edition, 1991.

18. Nutritive Value of Indian Cattle Feeds and Feeding of Animals
by K.C. Sen, S.N. Ray and S.K. Ranjhan, 6th edition, 1978.

19. Textbook of Feed Processing Technology
by N.N. Pathak, 1st edition, 1997.

20. Nutrient Requirements of Livestock and Poultry
by S.K. Ranjhan, 2nd revised edition, 1998.

21. Feeding of Poultry
by B. Panda, V.R. Reddy, V.R. Sadagopan and A.K. Shrivastav, 1st edition, 1984.

22. Dictionary of Animal Nutrition and Feed Technology
by K.K. Singhal, 1st edition, 1992.

23. Clinical Nutrition of the Dog and Cat
by J.W. Simpson, R.S. Anderson and P.J. Markwell, 1st edition, 1993.

24. The Waltham Book of Clinical Nutrition of the Dog and Cat
by J.M. Wills and K.W. Simpson, 1st edition, 1994.

25. Nutritive Value of Indian Foods
by National Institute of Nutrition, Indian Council of Medical Research, 1989.

26. **Nonconventional Feed Resources and Fibrous Agricultural Residues - Strategies For Expanded Utilization**
   Proceedings of a Consultation held in Hisar, India, 21-29 March 1988, Edited by C. Devendra, IDRC and ICAR.

27. **AFRC (1993) Energy and Protein Requirements of Ruminants**
   An advisory manual prepared by the AFRC Technical Committee on Responses to Nutrients. CAB International, Wallingford, U.K.

28. **Small Ruminant Production in India By the year 2000 - Strategies for development**
   Proceedings of the National Seminar held in Tirupati (AP), India, 13-17 November 1990, Edited by G.V. Raghavan, M.R. Reddy and N. Krishna, APAU, ICAR and IDRC.

29. **Small Ruminant Production and Post-Production Systems - Current Status and Development**
   Proceedings' of the workshop held at CLRI, Chennai, India, 4-6 December 1996, Edited by N. Krishna, A. Subbarama Naidu and D. Chandramouli, CLRI, ANGRAU, IDRC.

30. **Principles of Animal Nutrition and Feed Technology 2nd edition 2010** (ISBN 978-81-204-1752-6, xx plus 431 pages) by D.V. Reddy.

31. **Advanced Animal Nutrition 2011** (ISBN 978-81-204-1756-4, x plus 507 pages) by D.V. Reddy.

32. **Applied Nutrition: Cats, Dogs, Wild Animals and Birds 2014** (ISBN 978-81-204-1774-8, xv plus 285 pages) by D.V. Reddy.

33. **Fodder Production and Grassland Management 2nd edition 2014** (ISBN 978-81-204-1772-4, 200 pages) by D.V. Reddy.

Contents

Applied Nutrition I
(Ruminants)

Applied Nutrition II
(Non-ruminants, Poultry, Rabbits and Laboratory Animals)

1

Introduction to Feeding of Livestock — Importance of Scientific Feeding — Feeding Experiments

INTRODUCTION

We have studied the different nutrients which are required by the animal body and the metabolic changes which they undergo in serving its (the body's) various functions.

A knowledge of the quantitative needs of the body for these nutrients and of the relative value of feeds as sources of them is the basis of scientific feeding. This knowledge has been gained gradually by means of research and experience over many years. An understanding of the methods by which it has been attained and which are still being employed to augment it is essential for the student of nutrition.

Feeding Experiments

Trial and experience were the means by which the art of feeding animals was originally developed. A feeding trial with the species in question still remains the most useful method of obtaining results which have a direct application to feeding practice. Minimum number of animals per group should be 4. Completely Randomized Design (CRD) or Randomised Block Design (RBD) may be followed.

1. *Comparative feeding trials:* A feeding trial, in its simplest form, is a record of the results produced in terms of growth, milk production, or other function from a given feed or ration. Two or more rations may be compared with each other on this basis. In case of two rations 't' test is used while in case of three or more rations 'analysis of variance' test is applied to analyse the data-feed consumed per day, average daily gain (ADG), feed consumed per kg gain (feed efficiency), etc. for statistical significance. A comparison was made between fish meal and linseed meal as protein supplement for swine (Maynard *et al.*, 1979). This shows that fish meal is a better protein supplement for swine than linseed meal. But it tells nothing as to why the fish meal was better. Is it due to higher per cent of protein, or higher biological value of protein or larger amount of calcium supplied by FM or presence of certain vitamins?

Comparison of Fish Meal with Linseed Meal as Protein Supplement for Swine.

	ADG, kg	Feed for 100 kg gain, kg
Ration 1		
200 kg corn, 100 kg wheat middlings	0.5	390
75 kg fish meal (FM)		
Ration 2		
200 kg corn, 100 kg wheat middlings	0.32	440
75 kg linseed meal		

It is important to know the specific nutritive quality which makes one feed better than another. For example, if the superiority of FM ration is due to the extra calcium, the addition of ground limestone to the linseed meal ration would be cheap. The comparison of two feeds with respect to a specific nutrient such as Ca, or protein requires that all other nutritive factors be held alike and adequate in the two rations. However, this can never be achieved absolutely. But feeding trials can be set up to get the specific information desired.

2. *Feeding trials with laboratory animals:* Today many of the problems of nutrition are being studied with small animals, such as rat. The processes of growth, reproduction and lactation can be effectively investigated.

Advantages

(i) Much small cost in terms of animals, feed and labour and the much shorter time involved for a given experiment, in view of the short lifecycle of the lab animal.

(ii) The influence of individual variability (it is a seriously disturbing factor in large animal experimentation) can be reduced to a minimum by the use of animals of similar genetic and nutritional history, by using large number of animals and by close environmental control.

(iii) Slaughter for chemical and histological examinations, a desirable feature of many feeding trials, presents little difficulty with small animals, compared with the economic and other considerations involved in the case of farm animals.

The results obtained in feeding trials with small animals, however, cannot be considered to have direct application to the various species of farm animals, because of the differences in physiology and other considerations. Even here studies with small animals serve as pilot experiments, by means of which much preliminary information can be obtained more quickly and at much less cost. Final test can be done with the large animals.

3. *The purified diet method:* Purified diets were used in conducting feeding trials with lab animals. Purified diets consist of purified sources of the various nutrients. For example, *protein* is supplied as casein, purified soybean protein, or urea; *carbohydrates* as starch, glucose, or sucrose; *fat* as lard or some oil; *minerals* as chemically pure salts and *vitamins* as pure crystalline compounds. Such a diet makes it possible to include or withdraw a given nutrient with a minimum of disturbance of any of the other nutrient relations.

In 1816, Magendie fed diets of pure sugar and of pure fat to dogs to ascertain whether or not N was required in the food. Later J.B. Boussingault, the famous French chemist carried on nutrition studies with various species, involving the use of diets consisting in part of purified nutrients. Later McCollum and Davis and Osborne and Mendel used this method.

Purified diet method became responsible for much of our modern knowledge of nutrition, including the physiology of the vitamins, the establishment of differences in protein quality and more exact information regarding many of the minerals. Studies of the role of an element needed by the body in small amounts can be effectively carried out only with basal diets which may be freed from it and to which it may be added in known amounts. This is only possible with purified diets, because a diet cannot be prepared from natural foods which will be free from the element in question.

Limitations of the Purified diet Method

1. The ingredients of these diets cannot be considered pure in the absolute sense. For example, starch cannot be entirely freed from mineral elements. Some of the vitamins were identified as "impurities".

2. Some of the constituents, notably protein, in purified diets may be altered from their natural state in the process of purification.
3. The kind of pure carbohydrate used affects the significance of the results in the case of certain vitamins because of the effects of various carbohydrates on vitamin synthesis in the alimentary tract.
4. All the nutrient requirements of the species should be known to prepare a completely successful purified diet.
5. The diet must be of suitable physical nature and sufficiently palatable so that it will be consumed as per the need.

The method has been developed to its highest degree of usefulness in the case of rat and chick because of the lesser problem involved in preparing purified nutrients on a small scale and many years of experiments with these species. As regards farm animals, the use of purified diets has contributed greatly to the modern knowledge of poultry nutrition. Other applications of the method have made important contributions to our knowledge of the nutritional needs of lambs, sheep, cattle and pigs.

4. *Germfree Technique:* Contributions of intestinal organisms to the nutrition of the host complicate the interpretation of data obtained in feeding trials on dietary requirements of various vitamins. Thus, the nutrition scientist has a special interest to obtain germfree animals at birth and to rear them in an uncontaminated environment thereafter. Germfree means free of contamination by bacteria, yeasts, moulds, fungi, protozoa and parasites in general, that is, free of all other life.

The newborns are obtained by caesarean section and reared in specially designed apparatus by appropriate techniques using sterilized diets, etc. Success has been reported with rats, rabbits, hamsters, mice, chickens, turkeys and monkeys. Techniques have been developed for obtaining "specific pathogen-free" (SPF) baby pigs by hysterectomy. These were used for nutrition experiments.

5. *Group feeding versus Individual feeding:* Feed records are a desirable feature of all feeding trials. In many feeding experiments, particularly those with farm animals, the animals have been fed as a group. This is the simplest procedure from the standpoint of equipment needed and labour cost. But in many experiments it introduces complications in the interpretation of results.

Such complications arise when there is a wide variability in the individual behaviour within the group, as to its production, feed consumption, etc. The difficulty is increased when an animal, owing to accident or other unavoidable cause, has to be removed from the lot. The performance of the animal can be eliminated from consideration, but the food which it ate cannot.

Individual feeding eliminates these disadvantages. It makes possible the correlation of individual performance record with the feed consumption. It preserves the identity of the individual. Certain species which are fed together may consume somewhat less than when fed individually. This may be due to "competition in the feed lot". Individual records are highly desirable in studies where only small differences are to be expected and where quantitative data are of special importance.

Individual records are much more useful from the standpoint of statistical treatment.

6. Controlled versus Ad Libitum feeding: Ad libitum feeding is the most commonly used procedure in farm animal investigations and gives unbiased results for direct practical application. In growth trials, *ad libitum* feeding is to be given. Feed per kg gain can be calculated.

Ad libitum feeding method does not provide the controlled conditions required for certain purposes, for example, the determination of digestibility. Osborne and Mendel from their studies of protein quality recognized that *ad libitum* feeding frequently gave rise to variable results. Thus in many instances there is an advantage in using some system of controlled feeding. Food intake was adjusted in accordance with increase in weight. In digestion and metabolism trials controlled feeding is followed; 90% of feed intake is offered.

7. Equalized Paired feeding or Paired feeding: Feed intakes are completely controlled. In this method of comparing two rations the animals are fed alike in a preliminary period. Then animals are selected by pairs and are kept on ration A and ration B and are fed same quantity of feed limiting the intakes of both to that of the animal consuming the lesser amount.

The two animals of the pair are similar in size, age and previous history. But such equalities are not essential from pair to pair. The equalization of feed intake is also limited to within the pair. Minimum of four pairs of animals are to be used to carry out statistical analysis. e.g. Dicalcium phosphate, A; Bone meal, B are compared as sources of phosphorus for bone growth (in rats). When it is desired to compare three rations at the same time, the animals can be selected in trios. This may involve complications in comparing more than three rations.

Limitations

1. The faster-growing animal is penalized because of restricted feeding.
   As the animal on the superior ration increases in weight over its mate,

its maintenance requirement becomes greater than that of its mate. Under these conditions, an equal feed intake for both means that the larger animal must be using a larger proportion for maintenance and less remains for growth promotion. That is how the faster-growing animal is penalized.

2. The frequent effect of a nutritionally deficient ration is to decrease feed consumption. By limiting feed intake the full effect of the better ration cannot express itself.

3. The method is not suitable for finding out how much superior one ration is to another for growth. Lactation studies which adjust the feed of each animal on the basis of body weight and production represent a special type of controlled-feeding experiment.

Lucas (1943) designed an equalized feeding system which reduced the variability of responses of lactating cows that are fed individually.

8. Slaughter experiments: Relative value of the two mineral supplements was measured in terms of calcium and P content of bones because the growth of the animals as a whole would not have given definite information as to bone development. Such a procedure, which involves the killing of the animals and the analysis of certain specific tissues or of the body as a whole, is commonly referred to as a slaughter experiment.

In many feeding trials, it is desirable to obtain more specific information regarding the effect of a given ration than is furnished by the common measures of weight and size. For example, in studies of the optimum energy and protein requirements for growth, it is important to know the specific effect of the ration in terms of the composition of the tissue formed, since the increase in the body weight as a whole may be due to water, fat, minerals as well as protein, the relations of which may vary. Lawes and Gilbert have used this slaughter method.

To study the effect of a given diet on changes in body composition a group of like animals are selected and a part of them are slaughtered and analyzed at the start of the experiment. The others are fed different experimental diets for a given period and then slaughtered and analyzed. The difference in their composition from that of the animals killed at the start reveals the effect of the diet fed.

Limitations

1. It requires much more time and labour than is involved in merely weighing feed and animals.

2. Difficult problems are presented in the selection of representative samples of tissues and in their preparation for analysis. Similarly

utmost care has to be taken in taking truly representative sample of the carcass after thorough mixing of minced carcass. The author conducted these experiments in pigs and sheep in a research project on prediction of body composition of live meat animals using isotope techniques.

9. Experimental designs: The statistician refers to those feeding trials which are set up in such a way as to allow statistical analysis as experimental designs e.g. CRD and RBD. In addition, there are certain specific designs with which the student should be familiar.

1. **Factorial experiments:** Two factors:

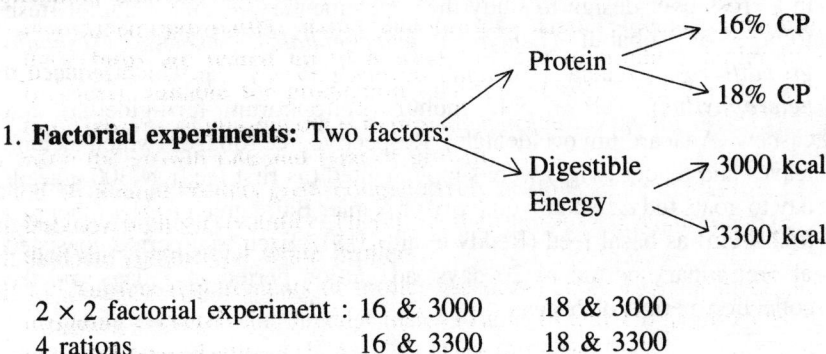

2 × 2 factorial experiment : 16 & 3000   18 & 3000
4 rations   16 & 3300   18 & 3300

2. **Latin square design (LSD):** In a 4 × 4 LSD four experimental rations ($\tau 1$, $\tau 2$, $\tau 3$ and $\tau 4$) can be evaluated using four animals (A, B, C and D) in four periods (preliminary period, 14 days and collection period, 7 days) for their digestibility and nutrient balance. Animals are shifted from one ration to another and at the end of four periods data from four animals are available for each ration.

Rations

	$\tau 1$	$\tau 2$	$\tau 3$	$\tau 4$
1	A	B	C	D
2	B	C	D	A
3	C	D	A	B
4	D	A	B	C

Periods (left of rows 1–4)

3. **Cross-over design:** Cross-over design or change-over design is a special class of experimental design in which one group of experimental animals receives different treatments during the different time periods, i.e., the group of animals crossover from one treatment to another treatment. This facilitates conduct of multi-treatment animal experiments and statistical analysis of the data with the availability of only 4 to 6 animals. Cross-over experimental design allows for an increase in precision when less variability is expected within animals than between animals.

Example of cross-over experimental design: Six metabolism trials were conducted using four male goats (local nondescript breed; BW 13.5 kg) in a cross-over design to study the supplementary feeding value of fresh foliage of subabul (*Leucaena leucocephala*), sesbania (*Sesbania grandiflora*), acacia (*Acacia auriculiformis*), jack (*Artocarpus heterophyllus*), yellow gold mohur (Peltophorum ferrugineum) and cashew (Anacardium occidentale). Respective tree foliages (which include leaves and tender twigs) were supplemented (as first feed) @ 300 g/head/day to goats fed *ad libitum* quantity of Napier Bajra green fodder (chopped to 2-4 cm) as basal feed (Reddy et al., 2009). Each trial period consisted of preliminary period of 20 days, adaptation period of 3 days and the collection period of 5 days.

2

Evaluation of Feeds by Digestion Experiments

History of Digestion Experiments

The digestion experiments were started almost at the same time when the feedstuffs were being analysed chemically at the Weende experiment station, Germany. Actually the work on losses of nutrients in the faeces was conducted even before 1860 to calculate the TDN. Schneider and Flatt (1975) recorded the results of more than 3000 publications.

In India, ICAR published the results of over 430 digestion trials conducted with the Indian feeds and fodders at different research stations (Sen, Ray and Ranjhan, 1978).

Measurement of Digestibility Coefficients

Chemical composition of feeds and fodders gives only the potential value of a feed and it does not give the actual nutritive value of the feedstuffs until the nutrients lost in faeces, urine, gases, etc. from the animal during digestion, absorption and metabolism are also taken into consideration. Major portion of the nutrients are excreted in faeces because of being not digested in the alimentary tract. Therefore, the first consideration is digestibility of the feed.

The digestibility of a feedstuff is defined as that portion of feed or of any single nutrient of feed which is not recovered in faeces or in other words the portion which is acted upon by the microbes and digestive enzymes in the digestive tract and is absorbed by the system. When the digestibility is expressed in percentage it is known as digestibility coefficient.

$$\text{Dig. coe. of a nutrient} = \frac{\begin{array}{c}\text{Amount of the}\\\text{nutrient in}\\\text{feed eaten}\end{array} - \begin{array}{c}\text{Amount of the}\\\text{nutrient in}\\\text{faeces}\end{array}}{\begin{array}{c}\text{Amount of the nutrient in}\\\text{feed eaten}\end{array}} \times 100$$

Example 1: A bullock consumed 10 kg grass hay and excreted 4 kg of dung dry matter. Moisture content of hay was 10%. Calculate the dig. coe. of DM of grass hay. (This illustrates the determination of digestibility of feeds by direct method).

Solution: Grass hay consumed = 10 kg;   Moisture = 10%
                                                    Dry matter = 90%

DM of grass hay consumed = $10 \times 0.9 = 9$ kg

Dung DM excreted = 4 kg

Dig. coe. of DM $= \dfrac{9.0 - 4.0}{9.0} \times 100 = 55.6$

The digestibility coefficient determined is apparent since the faeces/dung contain metabolic (mucosal debris, unspent enzymes, undigested microorganisms) as well as undigested feed.

Say, in the aforementioned example,

Dung DM excreted = 3.7 kg from feed + 0.3 kg from body.

Then true dig. coe. of DM $= \dfrac{9.0 - 3.7}{9} \times 100 = 58.9$

$$\text{Apparent digestibilty (\%)} = \frac{\begin{array}{c}\text{Amount}\\\text{consumed}\end{array} - \begin{array}{c}\text{Faecal}\\\text{excretion}\end{array}}{\text{Amount consumed}} \times 100$$

$$\text{True digestibility (\%)} = \frac{\begin{array}{c}\text{Amount}\\\text{consumed}\end{array} - \left\{\begin{array}{c}\text{Total}\\\text{faecal}-\\\text{excretion}\end{array} \begin{array}{c}\text{Metabolic}\\\text{losses}\end{array}\right\}}{\text{Amount consumed}} \times 100$$

Thus the apparent digestibility of feed is less than the true digestibility. The losses of the ingested carbohydrates as methane and carbon dioxide are also accounted in digestibility. So digestibility of carbohydrates is overestimated. Digestibility coefficients are estimated for all organic nutrients. For ash or minerals, digestibility is not determined because 1. it does not contribute to the energy content of the feed, and 2. most of the absorbed minerals are excreted through the gut. The actually digested or available minerals can be determined by using isotopes (labelled minerals).

Methods of Determining Digestibility

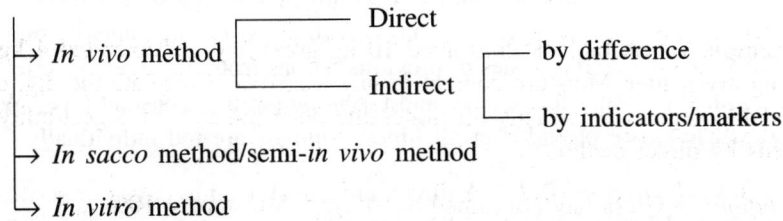

IN VIVO DETERMINATION OF DIGESTIBILITY

Digestion and Metabolism Trials

A digestion trial involves a record of the nutrients consumed and of the nutrients voided in faeces. Digestion trial is carried out to evaluate the utilization of a feedstuff i.e. its nutrients by the animal and to quantitate the intake of digestible nutrients. In conventional digestion studies animals are either confined in a cage or stall to facilitate collection of faeces and/or urine (Metabolism trial). A metabolism trial is conducted to calculate balance of nutrients retained in the body which requires quantitative collection of urine and milk, in case of a milch animal, besides the faeces.

Example: Nitrogen (N) balance, mineral balance, etc.
Nitrogen balance = N intake - N outgo in faeces, urine and milk

Measurement of Digestibility by Conventional Method: Norms Adopted in Conducting Digestion and Metabolism Trials

1. *Selection of animals:* The animals should be of the same breed, sex, age and body weight. Generally a minimum of four adult animals are needed. Animals should be healthy and free from parasitism. Male animals are preferred to females because it is easier to collect faeces and urine separately with the male.

2. *Preliminary Period:* The test feed has to be fed in constant daily amounts, as per the requirement of the animal, for an extended period. This is called as preliminary period. The purpose is to make the gastrointestinal

tract free of any indigestible material coming from the feed consumed prior to the start of the digestion trial. In monogastric animals such as pig, digestion and evacuation are usually complete in 24 hours after the test feed is ingested. In ruminants eating a roughage ration, the last residues may not be voided until 150 to 200 hrs (6-8 days) have elapsed, though 95% are usually voided within 140 hrs. So a preliminary period of 2-3 days (some times 3-5 days) in pigs and 7-14 days (8-10 days) in ruminants is followed to eliminate the feed residues of previous rations from the digestive tract and to stabilize the daily feed intake and faecal output to a constant level. Water and salt licks are provided at all times. Animals are fed individually.

3. *Collection Period:* Animals are transferred to cages or stalls and a 2-3 day adaptation period is allowed for their acclimatisation. This follows collection period of 7-10 days duration; A 5-7 day collection period is mostly followed. In general, the longer the period of collection the more accurate the results provided the stated amount of feed continues to be consumed regularly and completely, since the effect of periodic fluctuations is minimized. Water and salt licks are provided at all times. Quantitative collection of faeces (and/urine) is done. Representative samples of feed offered, feed leftovers and faeces voided are preserved and analysed for nutrient composition.

4. *Test feed and feeding management:* The test feed should not be deficient in the nutrients because a deficiency of some of them may affect digestion process. The test feed should be fed at the level required for meeting the requirements of the animals. Normally 90% of the actual feed intake, as measured during the previous week, is offered.

Apparatus and Equipment Required and their Preparation

  (a) Buckets with lid;
  (b) Faeces bags;
  (c) Metabolic cage/stall optional;
  (d) Balance to weigh feed and faeces accurately up to a gram;
  (e) Polythene covers for preservation of faecal samples in the deep freeze. Polythene covers for storage of feeds offered, leftovers collected.

All the equipments are to be cleaned and kept ready. Animals are to be washed. The shed should be well-ventilated and free from flies and mosquitoes. Once the animals are kept in cages or stalls the comfort of the animals should be taken care of. Avoid tight harnessing the animals.

Things to be done during the Collection Period

1. Feeds offered, feed leftovers, faeces/dung voided are to be recorded daily for each animal.
2. Representative samples of feeds offered, feed leftovers and faeces (2-10%) voided daily are to be collected and composited during the collection period. Faeces are preserved in deep freeze.
3. At the end of the collection period, dry matter of the samples (feed and faeces) is estimated and the remaining sample is dried at 65°C for the analysis of other nutrients.
4. If the feed under test is a green fodder, dry matter has to be determined daily for the fodder offered and refusals, if any on the subsequent day.

From the above data, dry matter offered and dry matter leftover is calculated to arrive at dry matter consumed by each animal per day; dry matter of dung voided is also calculated.

CALCULATION OF DIGESTIBILITY COEFFICIENTS BY DIRECT METHOD

A bullock was fed 10 kg hay per day and given water to drink. Over the experimental period the animal excreted on an average: 15 kg wet faeces per day. Calculate the digestibility coefficients of organic nutrients.

The analysis and calculations are shown below

Constituent	Composition %		Actual amounts in		Amount digested and absorbed kg	Digestibility coefficient
	Hay	Faeces	10 kg hay	15 kg faeces		
O.M	79.5	18.6	7.95	2.79	5.16	64.9
C.P	9.7	2.6	0.97	0.39	0.58	59.8
E.E	2.5	0.8	0.25	0.12	0.13	52.0
C.F	26.3	6.4	2.63	0.96	1.67	63.5
N.F.E	41.0	8.8	4.10	1.32	2.78	67.8

The calculation for organic matter (O.M.) digestibility coefficient is illustrated here.

10 kg. hay contain 10 × 79.5 ÷ 100 = 7.95 kg organic matter.

15 kg. faeces contain 15 × 18.6 ÷ 100 = 2.79 kg organic matter

Digestibility Coefficient of ORGANIC MATTER

$$\frac{7.95 - 2.79}{7.95} \times 100 = \frac{5.16}{7.95} \times 100 = 64.9\%$$

The digestibility coefficients of CP, EE, CF and NFE are calculated in the similar way.

Direct determination of digestibility of individual feed may be done if it provides a satisfactory ration for the test period when fed alone. **Examples**: Maintenance type fodders such as green maize, green oats and their hays and productive type fodders such as legume fodders and hays (Example 1, Table 1).

TABLE 1. Procedure for Determining the Digestion Coefficient for Protein in Alfalfa Hay.

Information	Example	How determined
1. Feed consumed	8 kg DM	Measure feed consumed per day during digestion trial; Multiply with DM of feed
2. Feed composition	20 % CP	Proximate analysis on DMB
3. Nutrient intake	1.6 kg protein	$8.0 \times 0.2 = 1.6$
4. Faecal excretion	2.9 kg DM	Faecal collection during collection period per day; Multiply with DM of faeces
5. Faecal composition	13.8% CP	Proximate analysis on DMB
6. Nutrient excretion	0.4 kg protein	$2.9 \times 0.138 = 0.4$
7. Digestible nutrient	1.2 kg protein	$1.6 - 0.4 = 1.2$
8. Digestion coefficient, %	75	$(1.2 \div 1.6) \times 100 = 75$

Some feeds, however, can not be fed alone as they do not supply the bulk and therefore their digestibility coefficients can not be determined directly. **Examples:** Concentrates (oilseed cakes, cereal grains, concentrate mixture). Similarly, non-maintenance type of roughages like straw, stovers, dried grasses, etc. do not supply the required amount of nutrients and so they can not be fed alone to the experimental animals. In aforementioned cases digestibility is determined by indirect methods.

Indirect Method of Determining the Digestibility: Digestibility by Difference

Here two or more digestion trials are conducted. In the first trial, a basal maintenance type fodder is fed and the digestibility of nutrients is determined. In the second trial basal maintenance type fodder and the test feed (concentrate feed e.g. oilseed cake) are fed together. Digestibility of nutrients of the test feed (oilseed cake) is calculated by difference on the assumption that the nutrients in the original basal roughage have the same digestibility. In case of determining the digestibility coefficients of poor quality roughage (non-maintenance type), three digestion trials are conducted. In the third trial the test forage (non-maintenance type) is fed along with a concentrate feed (oilseed cake) and the digestibility of nutrients of the test forage is determined.

Calculation of Digestibility Coefficients by Indirect Method

Example

A cow was fed 4.5 kg of hay and 1.4 kg of cottonseed daily. The daily average output of the faeces on the combined ration was 10 kg. **Calculate the digestibility coefficients of the cottonseed**. (Digestibility of grass hay was determined in the first digestion trial. Hay and cottonseed were fed in the 2nd digestion trial. Digestibility of cottonseed has to be calculated by indirect method with the help of digestibility by difference.)

Calculation of CP Digestibility is shown here as an example in stepwise sequence.

- Note down the composition of hay, cottonseed and faeces for CP: 4.8%, 18.2% and 2%.

- Calculate the intake and outgo

4.5 kg hay contains $4.5 \times 4.8 \div 100 = 0.22$ kg CP;

1.4 kg cottonseed contains $1.4 \times 18.2 \div 100 = 0.25$ kg CP;

Total intake = 0.47 kg

10 kg dung contains $10 \times 2 \div 100 = 0.20$ kg CP

Total digested = $0.47 - 0.20 = 0.27$ kg

From the first trial data, digestibility of CP of hay was known as 43%.

Hence the digested CRUDE PROTEIN from hay $0.22 \times 43 \div 100 = 0.09$ kg CP.

Therefore, digested CP from cottonseed = $0.27 - 0.09 = 0.18$

Digestibility coefficient (DC) of CP of cottonseed = CP digested ÷ CP intake × 100 = $0.18 \div 0.25 \times 100 = 72$

Digestible crude protein = $18.2 \times 0.72 = 13.1\%$.

The analysis and calculation of digestibility coefficients of cottonseed are shown below columnwise:

		E.E	C.F	C.P	NFE
1.	% Composition of hay	1.1	37	4.8	46.4
2.	% Composition of cotton seed	18.4	25	18.2	27.5
3.	% Composition of faeces combined ration	0.50	7	2	9.7
4.	D.C of basal hay	70.0	65	43	62
5.	4.5 kg of hay contains	0.05	1.67	0.22	2.1
6.	1.4 kg of cottonseed contains	0.26	0.35	0.25	0.39
7.	10 kg of the dung contains	0.05	0.70	0.20	0.97
8.	Digested nutrients from hay	0.04	1.10	0.09	1.30
9.	Undigested Nutrients from hay (5-8)	0.01	0.57	0.13	0.8
10.	Undigested nutrients from cotton seed (7-9)	0.04	0.13	0.07	0.17
11.	Digested from cottonseed (6 - 10)	0.22	0.22	0.18	0.22
12.	D.C of cotton seed	85	63	72	56.4
13.	% Digestible Nutrients in cotton seed.	15.64	15.8	13.1	15.51

From the digestible nutrients furnished in the table, the TDN of cotton seed can be calculated.

Calculation of nutritive value in terms of DCP and TDN: some examples

Example 1: Digestibility of nutrients of a dried grass by a dairy cow

During a digestion trial a dairy cow consumed 44.684 kg dry matter and voided 11.609 kg dry matter. Calculate the digestibility coefficients of organic nutrients and DCP and TDN of the grass.

Chemical composition (%) of grass and dung are as follows: CP 22.86, 22.04; CF 18.47, 18.59; NFE 46.60, 34.82; EE 3.80, 6.74.

	Crude Protein	Carbohydrates		Ether extract
		Fibre	NFE	
Intake of 44,684 g dry matter contain, g				
Output of 11,609 g faecal dry matter contain. g				
Digested nutrients, g				
Digestibility of nutrients, %				

Example 2: Calculation of DCP and TDN

Organic Nutrient	Total nutrients in 100 kg, kg	Digestibility of nutrients, %	Digestible nutrients, kg
Crude protein	20.11	75.0	15.08
Crude fibre	16.25	73.9	12.01
Nitrogen free extract	40.99	80.6	33.03
Ether extract	3.34	53.9	(1.80 × 2.25) = 4.05
Total digestible nutrients			64.17

Associative Effect of Feeds

Calculation of digestibility coefficients by the difference method may not be very correct since the addition of oilseed cake to the basal diet may influence the digestibility of the basal diet. But the credit is given to the supplement i.e. oilseed cake assuming that the digestibility would remain the same when the basal diet was fed alone. The effect of supplement e.g., oilseed cake on the digestibility of the basal roughage is known as associative effect of feeds.

This method has a major flaw because feeds interact with each other, especially during fermentation in the rumen. This effect, associative digestibility, is caused by the extent or rate of digestion of one ingredient being either enhanced or inhibited by the presence of constituents in the other feed. For example, groundnut meal, which is rich in ruminally available nitrogen, will improve the digestion of a low-quality, low nitrogen forage such as rice straw.

On the other hand, increased amounts of readily fermentable carbohydrates (barley or wheat grains) will reduce the extent of fibre digestion in low-quality forages. Economides (1998; Livestock Production Science, 55, 89-97) has reported data which illustrate these points very well.

Digestibility Determination in Poultry

Determination of digestibility of organic nutrients in poultry is little complicated since the nutrients are excreted from a single opening, the cloaca. There are two ways by which digestibility of nutrients can be determined in poultry. One is the surgical means where faeces and urine are voided separately. The second method is by chemical means through which urine nitrogen and faeces nitrogen can be separated. In the urine the nitrogenous compound is uric acid and ammonia whereas in faeces mostly protein (true protein) is excreted.

Indicator Method of Determining Digestibility

The conduct of a digestion trial is obviously a laborious and time-consuming procedure. There is an indirect method using 'inert reference substance' as an indicator/marker. This method is useful when we cannot make total faecal collections.

The ideal specifications of an indicator/marker are
1. It should be totally indigestible and unabsorbable.
2. It should not have any pharmacological action on the digestive tract. It should be inert to the digestive system.

3. It must mix intimately with and remain uniformly distributed in the digesta.
4. It should pass through the tract at a uniform rate and should be voided entirely.
5. It can readily be determined chemically, and
6. Preferably be a natural constituent of the feed under test.

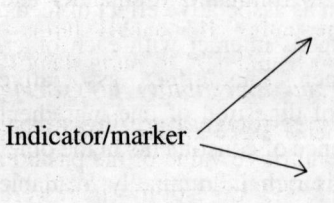

Indicator/marker

Internal or natural indicator i.e. component of a feed. e.g. Lignin, Silica, Acid Insoluble Ash, n-alkanes

External marker e.g. chromic sesquioxide (chrome green or chromic oxide, $Cr_2 O_3$), magnesium ferrite, carmine red, chromium mordanted plant fibre, lanthanum and ytterbium chloride
Radioactive isotopes- [51] Cr - EDTA and [144] Ce; rare earth elements-cerium (Ce), Ytterbium (Yb), Samarium (Sm);

Internal indicators such as silica, AIA and lignin are indigestible and can easily be determined. Chromic oxide is the most commonly used marker for digestion trials with avians, swine and carnivorous species. In herbivorous animals, it may not yield accurate result. Nowadays it is common to find the term 'marker' more in use rather than 'indicator'.

The digestibility of a nutrient is calculated by estimating the concentration of the indicator/marker in feed and faeces and that of the nutrient in the feed and faeces without the quantitative collection of total faeces and measuring the feed consumption.

$$\text{Dig. coe. of a nutrient} = 100 - \left(100 \times \frac{\% \text{ indicator in feed}}{\% \text{ indicator in faeces}} \times \frac{\% \text{ nutrient in in the faeces}}{\% \text{ nutrient in the feed}}\right)$$

The assumption here is that the reference material is excreted uniformly and therefore a small amount of faeces collected at any time during 24 hrs should be sufficient to provide the amount of nutrient per unit of indicator (reference material). But in most of the external markers diurnal variation has been reported and chromic oxide, for example, was recovered only 94%. Hence the formula has been changed (Lucas, 1952) to

$$\text{Dig. coe. of nutrient} = 100 - \left(100 \times \dfrac{\dfrac{\% \text{ recovery of indicator}}{\% \text{ indicator in faeces}} \times \dfrac{\% \text{ indicator in feed}}{}}{} \times \dfrac{\% \text{ nutrient in faeces}}{\% \text{ nutrient in feed}}\right)$$

This method has been applied successfully in horses, swine, chickens, rabbits, foxes, minks, men, etc., in addition to ruminants (Schneider and Flatt, 1975).

Measurement of pasture consumption and digestibility in grazing animals: It is essential to know the quantity of forage a grazing animal consumes from the pasture or a range and the nutritive value of the pasture. So initially pasture grasses were harvested and digestion trials were conducted in the stall. This method was not correct since the grazing animals have a tendency of selective grazing. Subsequently the grazing animals were harnessed with faeces bags and faeces voided in 24 hrs was determined. This can provide total dry matter voided. Pasture grasses were harvested and fed in the stalls to determine digestibility coefficients. From these two figures the total dry matter intake (DMI) of the animals was calculated.

Limitations: It is difficult to obtain, the representative sample of forage actually eaten by the grazing animal and quantitative collection of faeces by faeces bag. Therefore markers have been used both for determination of digestibility of the pasture herbage and the DMI through grazing. Digestibility can be determined through use of an internal indicator. Faecal output is measured concurrently by using an external marker and intake is calculated as follows.

Normally chromic oxide is fed in a capsule to the grazing animals and then number of grab samples of faeces are taken at different time intervals to determine the average concentration of the indicator per unit weight of faeces.

$$\text{Faecal DM output (Dry matter voided per day)} = \dfrac{\text{Marker consumed(g/d)}}{\text{Marker concentration in faeces(g/g DM)}}$$

$$\text{DM intake} = \text{Faecal DM output} \times \dfrac{100}{\% \text{ indigestibility of DM}}$$

Determination of pasture consumption and digestibility coefficients by indicator method: Estimation of total faeces by grab samples [Santra et al., Small Ruminant Research, 44(2002) 37–45]

After nine weeks of the feeding trail, a digestion trial by indicator method was conducted on six range-managed lambs. Diet samples of pasture vegetation consumed by the lambs were collected by mouth grab sampling for seven consecutive days. Diet samples were collected daily by the operators by snatching 60-70 bites before swallowing from the mouth of each lamb.

Faeces collection by grab sampling is a process of removing part of faecal sample from rectum manually. Total faeces output for a grazing animal can be determined by feeding a quantitative amount of an external indicator to the animal and collecting grab samples of faeces.

Chromic oxide is the best external indicator for this purpose. Blank samples containing faeces without chromic oxide should be run to correct for naturally occurring materials.

Administration of Chromic Oxide

The required dose of chromic oxide (10 g) is impregnated on cellulose or paper, and enclosed it in a gelatin capsule and administered to the experimental animals. The preliminary period should be at least 10 days and collection period should be 7 days. Collect at least 50 grab samples of faeces from each animal. To overcome diurnal variation, collect randomly in the pasture or pen. If more than one animal is in a pasture, coloured polyethylene particles may be administered to the animals so that the faeces may be distinguished from one animal to another. Diets and faeces samples of individual lambs were dried separately at 60°C. Chromic oxide was estimated in the diet and faeces samples.

% Composition on DMB	Lignin	Protein	Chromic oxide
Forage	13.0	7.7	--------
Faeces	22.6	6.0	1.15

$$\text{Faecal dry matter voided} = \frac{\text{Amount of external indicator fed}}{\text{External indicator in dry faeces}}$$

$$= \frac{10}{0.0115} = 870 \text{ g}$$

$$\text{Dry matter intake} = \frac{\text{Faecal dry matter voided} \times \% \text{ lignin in faeces}}{\% \text{ lignin in forage}}$$

$$= \frac{870 \times 22.6}{13.0} = 1512 \text{ g}$$

Dry matter intake is also calculated as follows.

$$\text{Digestibility (apparent) of DM} = 100 - \left\{ 100 \times \frac{13.0}{22.6} \times \frac{100}{100} \right\}$$

$$= 100 - 100 \times 0.575 \times 1 = 42.5$$

$$\text{Dry matter intake} = \frac{\text{Faecal dry matter output} \times 100}{\% \text{ indigestibility of DM}}$$

$$= 870 \times 100 \div 57.5 = 1513 \text{ g}$$

$$\text{Apparent digestibility coefficient of CP} = 100 - \left\{ 100 \times \frac{13.0}{22.6} \times \frac{6.0}{7.7} \right\}$$

$$= 100 - 100 \times 0.575 \times 0.779$$
$$= 100 - 44.81 = 55.19$$

Example 2: A grazing animal was fed 2g of Cr_2O_3 in a capsule per day. Find out the forage intake and its DM digestibility. The data is as follows:

	DM	Lignin (Internal indicator)	Cr_2O_3 (External marker)
		% composition	
Forage	20	0.05	—
Faeces	15	0.10	0.1

Solution

Daily DM voided in faeces, g/day

$$= \frac{\text{Amount of } Cr_2O_3 \text{ fed daily}}{\text{g of } Cr_2O_3 \text{ per g of faeces}} = \frac{2}{0.001} = 2000 \text{ g}$$

$$\text{DM dig. coe. of forage} = 100 - \left(100 \times \frac{0.05}{0.10} \times \frac{15}{20} \right)$$

$$= 100 - 37.5$$
$$= 62.5$$

$$\text{DM intake} = \frac{\text{DM voided}}{\% \text{ of DM indigestibility}} \times 100$$

$$= \frac{2000}{37.5} \times 100$$

$$= 5333 \text{ g}$$

$$\text{Fresh forage intake} = \frac{5333}{20} \times 100$$

$$= 26.665 \text{ g/day}$$
$$= 26.665 \text{ kg/day}$$

Uses of Markers

1. Measurement of digestibility coefficients without total faecal collection
2. Measurement of herbage intake in grazing animals
3. Markers are also used for quantifying rate of passage and extent of digestion in different segments of the gut. Rare earths (lanthanam, samarium, cerium, ytterbium and dysprosium) may be used as reliable markers of particulate phase of digesta. Polyethylene glycol (PEG), chromium EDTA and cobalt EDTA are liquid phase markers in ruminant studies.

Problems

1. Assume in a digestion trial for a steer, it was fed 7 kg of alfalfa hay daily yielding the following results.

	Weight kg	Water g	Ash g	N g	CF g	EE g
Hay	7	634	560	172	2000	133
Faeces	13	10,487	235	50	1101	93

   (i) Calculate the percentage of CP, CF, EE and NFE.

   (ii) Calculate TDN. (Solutions: 1. 15.4, 28.6, 1.9, 37.1% 2. 51.1%)

2. Suppose that the caloric values of various heat losses in the above digestion trial were 15.4 Mcal for the faeces, 1.4 Mcal for the gases, 1.3 Mcal for the Urine, and 3.9 Mcal for the HI While GE in the 7 kg feed was 30.8 Mcal.
   Calculate the GE, DE, ME and net energy of the alfalfa hay.
   (Solution: GE 4400; DE 2200; ME 1814 and NE 1257 Kcal/kg hay).

3. A sheep consumed 1.05 kg of cowpea hay (moisture 11%) and voided 0.78 kg of faeces (moisture 59%). Calculate the apparent digestibility of DM of cowpea hay. ADF of hay and faeces are 37% and 45% (on DMB) respectively. Calculate the digestibility of ADF of the cowpea hay (Solutions: 57.5%, 48.4%).

4. A sheep consumed 1.2 kg of hay DM per day. The AIA content of the hay is 1.6% and faeces is 3.3% on DMB. Calculate the DM digestibility of hay (Assume that dietary AIA is excreted quantitatively). If the CP content of the hay is 9.5% and that of faeces 7.7% (on DMB), calculate the digestibility of CP of the hay (Solutions: 51.5%; 60.7%).

5. Calculate the apparent DM digestibility and DM intake of a steer grazing on a pasture. AIA content of the material consumed is 1.8% of DM and that of the faeces is 4.2% on DMB. The steer was dosed twice daily with a bolus containing 8 g of chromic oxide (16 g per day). Chromic oxide content of the faeces was 0.51%. (Solutions: Faecal output = 3.14 kg/d; DM digestibility = 57.1%; DM intake = 7.32 kg/d).

Laboratory Method of Determining Digestibility

In vivo determination of digestibility in the animal requires a minimum of four animals and a large quantity of the feed sample, and daily record for intake of feed and outgo of faeces are to be determined. This requires metabolic cages or metabolism stalls and other accessories. This proce-dure is not only costly but also very laborious. Various techniques have been used to determine the digestibility of feeds without feeding them to the animals.

1. Digestibility of feeds and total digestible nutrients (TDN) can be calculated from chemical composition with the help of regression equations
2. Semi - *in vivo* technique/*In Sacco* method
3. *In vitro* technique

Semi - *in vivo* Technique

Digestibility/Degradability of feeds in the rumen can be determined by keeping the feed sample in bags which are immersed in rumen contents of rumen fistulated animals. The bag is made of nylon, dacron or silk cloth which is indigestible (Natural fibre is made of cellulose and is digested by cellulolytic bacteria in the rumen) and should be of very fine mesh so that the test feed particles should not pass out of the bag undegraded but at the same time it should allow the rumen microbes to enter into the bag and act on the test feed. The bags, on removal at different time intervals are washed till the wash water is clear and dried at 60°C for 48 hrs. The per cent disappearance of dry matter, nitrogen/crude protein, different fibre fractions, etc. are determined. This technique is called *in sacco* or *in situ* or *semi in vivo* technique.

Applications of the Technique

1. This technique provides a powerful tool for initial evaluation of feedstuffs, and is useful in screening, rapidly, large number of samples developed in forage breeding experiments.
2. This technique is helpful to understand the rumen processes. It is possible to vary the factors within the bag or within the rumen. The animal can be fed a constant diet, and the effect of (treated straw over untreated straw, or hay or complete diet) manipulating the feedstuff incubated in the bag on its degradation kinetics can be studied. Alternatively, the conditions within the rumen i.e. rumen environment, can be varied (by adding catalytic amounts of supplement to the basal diet to supply the nutrients to the rumen microbes) and a standard material incubated in the bag in order to study the effect of rumen environment on the rate of degradation.
3. Degradation of protein supplements: A test protein supplement was incubated in the rumen. Data of losses of protein was obtained at different time intervals *viz.* 3, 6, 9, 15 and 25 h after incubation. The per cent of material degraded 'p' after time 't' hours may be described by the equation $p = a + b (1 - e^{-ct})$. The effective rumen degradability (P) of the protein can then be calculated from the equation.

$$P = a + \frac{bc}{(c + k)}$$

where, a = water soluble N,
b = potentially degradable
c = fractional rate of degradation of feed N per hour
t = time

The constants a, b and c were calculated by an iterative least squares procedure with the help of a computer (Orskov *et al.*, 1980) and 'k' was the turnover rate of rumen digesta. *In sacco* technique has the advantage of giving a very rapid estimate of the rate, and extent, of the degradation of the feedstuff in the functioning rumen, without necessitating any procedure more complicated than simple weighing. Effective rumen degradability of protein of some feed supplements are presented in Table 2.

Limitations

The technique has certain inherent limitations. The test feed in the bag is not subjected to the total ruminal experience, i.e., mastication, rumination and passage. What is actually measured is the breakdown of material to a size

TABLE 2. Effective Degradabiliy of Protein of some Feed Supplements at Rumen out Flow Rate of 0.05/h.

Feed Supplement	Effective rumen Protein degradability %
Wheat bran	84.5; 67.2
Cottonseed cake	59.3
Silk cottonseed cake	77.6
Groundnut cake	78.4, 70.2
Gingelly oilcake/Til cake	67.0
Linseed cake	42.4
Mustard cake	84.1
Nigerseed cake	76.7
Safflowerseed cake	60.9
Sunflowerseed cake	46.1
Fish meal A	39.9
Fish meal B	70.2
Fish meal C	52.7
Fish meal	58.9
Meat meal A	40.6
Meat meal B	39.1
Meat meal C	73.6

small enough to leave the bag and not necessarily a complete degradation to simple chemical compounds.

Calculation of Dry Matter Disappearance at Each Incubation Time

Weight of empty bag + marble $\quad$ $W_1 = 6.127$ g

W_1 + test sample $\quad$ $W_2 = 9.184$ g

Weight of test sample (W_2-W_1) $\quad = 3.057$ g

Weight of test sample dry matter $\quad = A = 3.057 \times 0.915 = 2.797$ g

Weight of bag + marble + sample residue after incubation and drying $W_3 = 7.039$ g

Test sample residue dry matter weight $(W_3-W_1) = B = 0.912$ g

$$\% \text{ DM disappearance} = \frac{A - B}{A} \times 100 = \frac{2.797 - 0.912}{2.792} \times 100 = 67.4$$

Factors that Affect the Degradability

The factors known to affect the degradability results obtained with the *in sacco* technique are particle size of the test feed, bag porosity, sample size to bag surface ratio, diet of the animal, bags per animal, animal species, number of animals, number of replicate bags per animal per incubation time, positioning of bags in the rumen, incubation length, timing of bag introduction in the rumen and preruminal soaking. Particle size of test feed, bag porosity and sample size to bag surface ratio are important parameters for among the laboratory comparisons of the degradability results of a feedstuff. These factors are described here.

Particle size: Since the test feed kept in the bag has no chance neither for mastication nor for rumination, microbial fermentation and detrition by ruminal activity are the only means by which particle reduction occurs. Generally, longer and coarser materials are associated with slower rates of digestion and greater variation while finely ground materials are subjected to greater mechanical losses from the bags (assumed to be associated with the rapidly degradable and readily available fraction) but variation is more controlled. The test feed sample should be ground through 1 or 2 mm screen and then remove the finer feed particles.

Bag porosity: The appropriate porosity is a compromise between limiting the influx of rumen feed particles and allowing the influx of microbial populations to degrade the test feed while at the same time limiting the efflux of undegradable feed particles. A porosity of 40 to 60 µm has been found to be optimum.

Sample size to bag surface ratio: The optimum sample size is that which provides enough residues at the end of extended rumen incubation for chemical analysis without over-filling the bag so as to delay bacterial attachment, increase lag time, and underestimate digestion rates. The amount of sample to be incubated will also depend on the bulk density of the prepared sample. For a bag of 14×9 cm (when laid flat) size, it has been recommended about 2 g straw, 3 g good hay, 5 g concentrate feed (air dry ground) and 10-15 g fresh herbage (chopped) sample. A range of 10 to 20 mg/cm^2, of sample size to bag surface area ratio should be the criterion for most forage and concentrate type ingredients.

Three rumen fistulated animals are required at least. Feeding them at maintenance may be more useful in comparing results between laboratories. Basal diet should contain small amounts of a wide range of ingredients to establish a diverse microbial population apart from the test feed sample. The incubation times may be 3, 6, 9, 12, 18, 24, 48, 72 h........ 120 h, which are to be chosen depending on type of the test feed sample and the nutrient under study. At each incubation interval measurements are to be done in duplicate bags.

In Vitro Digestibility Technique

Digestibility of feeds can be estimated in the laboratory by using *in vitro* rumen fermentation methods. This method is used to rapidly screen large number of forage samples in plant breeding experiments for ranking them in the initial stages of developing quality fodder. This is also useful in evaluation of newer feedstuffs such as unconventional feeds.

The *in vitro* techniques developed and modified so far could be discussed under two main heads.

a. One-stage technique: The principle involved is that rumen microbial digestion of animal is simulated in laboratory where the feedstuff is incubated with rumen liquor at 39°C under anaerobic conditions in an artificial rumen. This technique involves the test feed sample, artificial saliva and the rumen inoculum. This mixture is placed under anaerobic conditions and incubated at 39°C a specified period. After incubation, the samples are removed and the disappearance of dry matter (IVDMD) or organic matter (IVOMD) is determined and expressed on per cent basis.

b. Two-stage technique: First stage simulates the digestive process in the rumen. The residue left after the first stage is further treated with acid-pepsin solution (Tilley and Terry 1963) or with neutral detergent solution (Van Soest *et al.*, 1966).

The acid-pepsin digestion (2nd stage) stage simulates the *in vivo* breakdown of feed and microbial protein by the digestive enzymes of the lower gut. The 2nd stage procedure with neutral detergent solution estimates the true digestibility rather than the apparent digestibility of test forage sample because neutral detergent solubilises bacterial cell wall and other endogenous products.

VIVAR Technique: An *in vivo* artificial rumen (VIVAR) was developed for studying nutrient utilization by rumen microorganisms under controlled conditions of rumen. The VIVAR tube is made up of stainless steel or glass and fitted with the semipermeable membranes. The rumen microflora pass through the semipermeable membrane and degrade feed sample present inside the VIVAR tube, but the sample particles can not move outside. After completion of the fermentation period, VIVAR tube is removed. The DM disappearance may be recorded by difference in weight of the sample and the residue left in VIVAR tube.

Rusitec: The continuous culture fermenter, such as "Rusitec" has become popular. It can be a partial substitute for *in vivo* animal experimentation. This 'rumen simulation technique' was first designed and developed in 1977 by

J.W. Czerkawski and G. Breckenridge, at the Hannah Research Institute, Scotland for simulating rumen fermentation in the laboratory. This has been remodeled by Dr. V. Balakrishnan of Madras Veterinary College, Chennai and marketed by Eaga Tools & Instruments, Chennai, Tamil Nadu.

Gas Production

Carbon dioxide and methane are produced in stoichiometric amounts to the amount of organic matter fermented by rumen microorganisms. This implies that measurements of gas production can be used to estimate organic matter fermentation by rumen microorganisms. However, there were some significant plumbing problems to overcome before this method became practicable. These have now been successfully overcome, and gas production (i.e. the volume of gas produced per unit time) is now frequently used to investigate the nutritional properties of feeds. It was observed that the volume of gas produced is a sure reflection of short chain fatty acid (VFAs and others) production in the rumen. *In vitro* gas production method was developed by K.H. Menke (a German scientist) and his coworkers in 1979 initially and later standardized (Menke and Steingass, 1988).

Factors Affecting the Digestibility of Feedstuffs

A large number of factors affect the digestibility of nutrients. These can be broadly grouped into as follows. **A. Animal factors B. Plant factors C. Feed preparation**.

A. a. Species of the animal: Roughages high in crude fibre are better digested by ruminants than by nonruminants due to the pre-gastric fermentative digestion that occurs in the former. In several nonruminants post-gastric fermentative digestion occurs which helps in digestion of crude fibre. Pre-gastric fermentative digestion is highly efficient since the nutrients released are digested and absorbed in stomach and small intestine. The ruminant is more efficient in the digestion of high-fibre, low-protein forage; the simple-stomached pig is more efficient in digestion of high-protein, low-fibre feedstuffs.

b. Age of the animal: Very young or very old animals are usually less efficient in their digestion of feeds. The young ruminants can neither eat nor digest roughage until their digestive tracts, specially their rumens are developed. After 6 months of age there appears to be no difference in the digestibility of the ration in the calf and adult dry animal. In newly born piglets, development of digestive enzyme system takes place gradually. Digestibility of fat in chickens is higher in adults than in young chicks.

In case of old animals their ability to digest feed is often impaired by poor teeth, which makes adequate chewing of their feed very difficult. Declining health may further adversely affect digestibility at an advance age.

    c. Work: Light exercise/work seems to improve digestibility of feeds while heavy exercise/work depresses it.

    d. Individuality: Individual variation of as much as 25% has been observed in the digestive ability of the same feed among animals. However, most animals have shown variation of about 4-5%.

    e. Level of feeding: Generally, higher level of feeding results in faster rate of passage of the digesta through the alimentary canal. At higher level of feed intake the digestibility of DM and of various nutrients falls due to less retention time in the alimentary canal. Such effect is more significant in the case of ruminants, but has been observed in swine as well.

    B. Plant factors-*Chemical composition of feed:* Generally grains are well utilized by all class of livestock. The digestibility of the forage is closely related to its chemical composition. The chemical composition of the forage is affected by a number of factors like soil composition, manuring and fertilization, water supply, stage of maturity of the plant, frequency of cutting, variety and strain of the plant, climate, etc., the predominant factor being the stage of maturity when cut. Differences among varieties within the same species may be due to the physical composition of the plant i.e. leaf to stem ratio, soil fertility, etc. Early-cut fodder has higher digestibility than late-cut. The protein, minerals and vitamins decrease while crude fibre increase as the plant matures.

    Feeds higher in protein content give higher apparent digestibility for the consumed protein. That is, the apparent digestibility of protein is higher at higher dietary protein levels because MFN output depends on the amount of feed consumed and not on the amount of protein consumption and so at higher protein intake levels the MFN excretion becomes a smaller fraction of the protein intake. At lower dietary protein levels lower apparent digestibility of protein has been obtained.

C. Preparation of Feed

    a. Particle size of the feed: Grinding of grain and other feed help to improve digestibility in young piglets with undeveloped teeth and in old animals with impaired teeth. In general grinding increases digestibility because of increased surface area for enzymatic action and disruption of grain coat. If grain or any other feed is ground to a fine particle size, the feed is less palatable and digestible. If particle size is less than 600 μ, pigs may suffer from gastric ulcers. If roughages are ground to fine grinding, digestibility of fibre is decreased while total consumption is increased due to increased rate of passage. Rumen fermentation pattern is also changed due to fine grinding of feed.

b. *Soaking* of grains and feed in water before feeding generally increases digestibility.

c. *Processing of grains/feed:* Processing is done to increase palatability, digestibility and thereby feed intake. Boiling, steam processing, micronization, pelleting, extrusion cooking improve their digestibility. However some processing methods depress digestibility due to increased DM consumption and the eventual faster rate of passage. This is more conspicuous in pelleting of roughages where digestibility of DM and crude fibre decreases. Digestibility of nutrients falls due to less retention time in the gastrointestinal tract.

d. *Nutrient content in the ration/Ration composition:*

(i) *Protein level:* When several feeds are fed in a ration, one feed may influence the digestibility of the other. This 'associative effect' of feeds on one another's digestibility is more evident in the case of ruminants when the addition of a protein or NPN compound to a low protein ration increases the microbial digestion of the crude fibre by stimulating the growth of microorganisms in the rumen. Thus, as the dietary protein level increases, the digestibility of all the nutrients increase. Similarly, as the dietary protein level is lowered, the digestibility of all the nutrients decrease.

(ii) *Carbohydrates:* The nature and level of dietary carbohydrates affect the digestibility of all nutrients present in the diet. In ruminants, excessive levels of soluble carbohydrates (e.g. molasses 7% and above) result in lower microbial breakdown of crude fibre. It tends to depress not only the digestibility of cellulose, hemicellulose, etc. but of the other nutrients also. High crude fibre content of mixed diets decreases their digestibility. The higher the percentage of crude fibre in a ration, the lower is the digestibility of DM and all other nutrients.

(iii) *Lipids:* Addition of oil or fat in a diet increases the digestibility coefficient of ether extract, as such fats have higher digestibility than other constituents of the ether extract. Higher levels of fat in the diets generally reduce the digestibility of other nutrients, particularly of dietary fibre.

(iv) *Minerals:* In the diets of pigs and poultry, mineral content does not seem to influence the digestibility of other dietary constituents while mineral deficiency produces more severe deficiency symptoms in their body. Deficiency of minerals in herbivorous animals limits the growth of microorganisms and this will reduce the digestibility of crude fibre and of other nutrients as well. Adequate amount of salt and water tend to improve digestibility.

Factors Affecting the TDN Value of a Feed

1. The per cent of DM: The more water present in a feed, the less there is of other nutrients and lower the TDN value.
2. The digestibility of DM: Unless the DM of a feed is digestible, it has no TDN value. e.g. Mineral oil has a high gross energy value, but it can not be digested and so has no DE or TDN value.
3. The amount of mineral matter in the DM: The more mineral matter a feed contains, the lower will be organic matter and its TDN value.
4. The digestibility of fat in the DM: The more digestible fat a feed contains, the greater will be the TDN value. (Look for an account of TDN in *Principles of Animal Nutrition and Feed Technology*).

$$TDN = DCP + (DEE \times 2.25) + DCF + DNFE$$

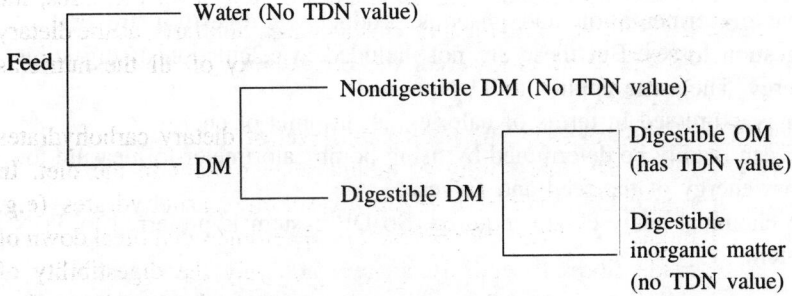

Weaknesses of the TDN System

* It is based on proximate analysis of the feed. Proximate analysis does not partition feed into well defined chemical constituents. Almost all proximate principles are composed of more than one chemical compound. The supposedly highly digestible NFE contain part of hemicellulose and lignin while crude fibre residue contains all the original cellulose, variable proportions of the hemicellulose and small, though again, variable portion of the lignin. That is why the assumption about high digestibility of NFE

and low digestibility of CF is always not true and for some feeds crude fibre is as digestible as NFE.

* The factor, 2.25 used in case of fat to equalise its high energy content with that of carbohydrate and protein is not always a constant. It is also based on human and dog experimental data. The ether extract of various feeds differ in the true fat content.
* It does not measure energy in energy units.
* It does not measure all losses from the body; losses due to GPD, HF are not included.
* It attempts to measure what feeds 'contain' rather than what they 'accomplish' or produce.
* It overestimates the energy value of forages in relation to concentrates.
* The term TDN implies that digestion losses only are taken into account. But actually this is not the case. To put protein on an equivalent carbohydrate basis, as was done for fat, digestible protein should have been multiplied by a factor namely, 1.3 (5.20/4 = 1.3). But this is not being done. That is how calculation of TDN took account of urine as well as digestion losses. Actually, as calculated, it is a measure similar to ME for those species having no gaseous losses. Thus TDN does not mean what it implies.

TDN Versus Digestive Energy

* Heat of fermentation and gaseous products of digestion are part of digestion losses. But these are not included in calculation of digestible energy. The same applies to TDN as well.
* DE is expressed in terms of calories i.e. in units of energy.
* DE can readily be determined by using bomb calorimeter to measure the gross energy of the feed and faeces.
* No chemical analyses are required. So DE system is preferred to TDN system.

Factors Affecting the Metabolizable Energy Value of Feeds

1. Main factors that affect the metabolizable energy value of a feed are those which influence its digestibility.
2. ME value of a feed will obviously vary according to the species of animal to which it is given, or more specifically, to the type of digestion to which it is subjected. Fermentative digestion incurs losses of energy as methane. A disadvantage of the intervention of microorganisms in digestion is an increase in the losses of energy in

either urine (as the breakdown products of the nucleic acids of bacteria that have been digested and absorbed) or faeces (as microorganisms grown in the hindgut are not digested).

In general, losses of energy in methane and in urine are greater for ruminants than for nonruminants. So feeds such as concentrates, that are digested to the same extent in ruminants and nonruminants, will have higher ME value for nonruminants.

3. The ME value of a feed will vary according to whether the amino acids it supplies are retained by the animal for protein synthesis or are deaminated and their nitrogen excreted in the urine as urea/uric acid. For this reason, ME values are sometimes corrected to zero nitrogen balance.

4. Preparation of feed: For ruminants the grinding and pelleting of roughages leads to an increase in faecal losses of energy, but this may be partly offset by a reduction in methane production.

   For poultry the grinding of cereals has no consistent effect on ME values.

5. Increases in the level of feeding of ruminants may cause an appreciable reduction in the digestibility of their feed, and hence in its, ME value.

   For finely ground roughages and for mixed roughage and concentrate diets, ME value is reduced by increases in level of feeding.

6. The end-products of rumen fermentation influence the value of ME: High concentrate, low roughage rations increase propionic and butyric acids and lower the acetic acid in the rumen contents; methane production is also reduced.

3

Methods Adopted for Arriving at Nutrient Requirements of Livestock and Poultry; Energy and Protein Requirements for Maintenance, Production and Reproduction, Requirement for Minerals and Vitamins

When we think of nutrient requirements, energy requirement first comes to mind because, energy supplies the driving force necessary for the maintenance of life, growth, lactation, and work. However, consideration must be made also for similar requirement for protein, vitamins, and minerals.

Energy Requirements for Maintenance

Maintenance can be defined as that state in which there is neither gain nor loss of a nutrient by the body. Maintenance requirements are estimates of the amounts of nutrients needed to achieve such equilibrium states. Here feed is needed to keep intact the tissues of an animal which is not growing, working, or yielding any product. If this need for feed is not met, tissue breakdown occurs, which is commonly revealed by a loss in weight. This destruction of body tissue is referred to as the fasting catabolism.

Livestock are fed for production, and generally not for maintenance. Maintenance of an animal is an important 'overhead' of the livestock business. A dairy cow weighing 500 kg and producing 20 kg of 4% fat milk daily uses 37% of its total ME requirement for maintenance, versus 23% at a yield of 40 kg. That is why high milk producing animals are preferred for a profitable dairy enterprise.

Fasting Catabolism

In the absence of feed, the nutrients required to support the activities essential to life (*viz.* respiration, circulation, maintenance of muscular tonus, manufacture of internal secretions, etc.) come from the breakdown of body tissue itself. This destruction of body tissue is referred to as the fasting catabolism, and it can be measured in terms of the waste products eliminated through the various paths of excretion. Most of the tissue breakdown occurs to meet the demand of the fasting organism for energy for its vital processes.

Energy Metabolism of Fasting

The energy expended in the fasting animal is represented by the fasting heat production and this can be measured in the respiration calorimeter (Direct calorimetry), or can be obtained by one of the methods of indirect calorimetry. Its measurement provides a useful basis of reference for other phases of energy metabolism. Fasting catabolism of a given species provides a basis for studying the factors which affect it and for comparing the metabolism in different species.

Basal Metabolism

Fasting catabolism has to be measured at its minimum value just required for the maintenance of life. Such a minimum value is called basal metabolism, or basal metabolic rate (BMR). It has its most exact meaning in the case of humans, because it is with this species that the conditions which are essential for a true minimum value can most nearly be attained. The conditions for its measurement in man are 1. Good nutritive condition 2. Environmental temperature of approximately 25°C (thermoneutral environment) 3. Relaxation on bed prior to and during measurement 4. Postabsorptive state.

A good nutritive condition implies that the previous diet of the animal has been adequate. A poor state of nutrition tends to decrease the heat production during fasting. The temperature of 25°C is specified as it provides thermoneutral environment. Both these conditions are entirely realizable in the case of animals. The minimum muscular activity assured by the third condition is obviously much less subject to control in farm animals. The animal may be standing, lying down in addition to various miscellaneous movements. It has been reported that basal metabolism is 10 to 15% greater when animals are standing than while they are lying down, the horse being an exception. The fourth condition, postabsorptive state, implies a state of fasting in which a long enough time has elapsed since the ingestion of food to make sure that the heat increment due to its digestion and assimilation has been dissipated. Such a condition is readily obtainable in animals with simple stomachs in overnight fast, while in ruminants it cannot be obtained except after a prolonged period of fasting.

To determine if an animal has been reached a postabsorptive state, measurement of heat production to the point of a constant minimum level can be made. Measurement of the respiratory quotient (RQ) to the point that the nonprotein RQ of fat (0.7) is reached also indicates that a postabsorptive state has been attained. In ruminants a decline in methane excretion to a minimum level indicates a postabsorptive state. By third day of fasting it declines to 0.5 litre from 30 L in sheep and in cattle to 2 litres from 200 L per day. So the measurement of basal metabolism in the ruminant cannot have the exact significance as it has in humans.

Fasting Metabolism

In ruminants the value determined is referred as fasting metabolism rather than of the basal metabolism. Fasting metabolism refers to heat production at specified times after the last feeding. This should not be confused with the term fasting catabolism, which also includes energy voided in the urine of fasting animals. To avoid some of the problems associated with a four-day fast in ruminants, some workers have determined heat production over a specific time period after the last feeding and have referred this value as standard metabolism. The term resting metabolism has been used to denote the heat eliminated when an animal is lying at rest, though not strictly in a thermoneutral environment or in the postabsorptive state.

Units of Expressing Fasting Metabolism/Basal Metabolism

Heat production is obviously related to body size. Rubner developed the surface-area law, which states that the heat given off by all warm-blooded animals is directly proportional to their body surface. Lusk suggested that basal metabolism is approximately 1000 Kcal per square meter of body surface per 24 hours regardless of the size of the animal.

The surface area is not constant but varies with the position of the body. The fact that the skin is elastic causes its measurement to vary with conditions. Hence formulas were devised for computing surface area from body weight since surface area was proportional to some fractional power of weight. Brody and coworkers in the early 1930s found 0.734 to be the power of body weight best related to basal metabolism based on analysis of a very large number of basal metabolism data of mature animals of different species, ranging in weight from 0.02 to 4000 kg (mice to elephants). Later Kleiber in 1947 found the power 0.756 to provide the best fit for his data. Later, the NRC committee on Animal Nutrition had adopted, finally, the 0.75 power of weight as defining the metabolic body size of an animal.

Brody's original formula for basal metabolism (BM)

$$BM = 70.5 \ W^{0.734}$$

Kleiber's original formula

$$BM = 67.6 \ W^{0.756}$$

Both authorities agreed that the basal metabolism per day for adult homeotherms may be represented by the general formula: BM (Kcal) = $70 \ W^{0.75}$. The coefficient 70 represents an average value for the kilo calories of basal heat produced per unit of metabolic size in experiments with groups of adult mammals.

Basal metabolism is highest in the newborn and gradually drops during the growth period to the figure for the adult animal, and even during adult life. BMR declined about 8% per year of age. Basal metabolism is lowered by undernutrition but increased by emotional stimuli. Thyroid secretions augment heat production by increasing the heart rate, the respiration, etc. BMR declines with castration. It is quite variable among species, with sheep and swine being notably lower than cattle and poultry.

Methods Adopted to Estimate Energy Requirements for Maintenance

The energy requirement for maintenance is the minimum amount needed to keep the animal in energy equilibrium. Energy requirements are best determined by measurement of energy expenditure. Energy expended for maintenance of an animal is converted into heat and leaves the body. Thus an intake sufficient to offset the loss represented by the fasting metabolism would be the requirement if the animal is maintained under basal conditions.

Data on maintenance requirements of energy have mainly been obtained in four ways.

1. *Fasting metabolism as a basis for estimating maintenance requirements:* Dry non-producing, mature animals were fasted, kept in a thermoneutral environment and their heat production was determined (fasting

metabolism). This gives an estimate about the minimum quantity of net energy which must be supplied to the animal to keep it in energy equilibrium. This can be estimated by both direct and indirect calorimetry.

Direct calorimetry: A non-producing, adult, healthy animal in a postabsorptive state (3-5 days after the last feeding) is kept at 25°C in the animal calorimeter where there is an arrangement for the collection of faeces, urine, gases and the determination of sensible heat loss as well as heat loss by evaporation of water from lungs and skin surface.

Indirect calorimetry: Most of the work on energy requirement in India was conducted using the indirect calorimetry method. Open circuit respiration chamber is available at IVRI, Izatnagar. The fasting metabolism is only a portion of the energy required for maintenance, since it is only the energy required in a fasting animal, in a comfortable temperature, without voluntary activity.

Energy required for consumption and digestion of food, energy required for the increased respiration and heart rate due to walking and other movements, and that due to low or high environmental temperatures are not accounted for in the determination of basal heat production. The amount needed for activity is referred to as activity increment and obviously depends upon the activity. Birds kept in cages have different requirement compared to those in deep litter system. Cattle under feedlot require less than those under grazing or range conditions. Mitchell (1931) proposed that the net energy requirement for maintenance of poultry could be obtained by increasing basal metabolism by 50%. In case of cattle, sheep and swine the activity increments may be of the order of 20 to 30%. Adding factors such as activity increment to the fasting metabolism to obtain the maintenance energy requirement is called the factorial method of estimating requirements. Values obtained in this way often are not as reliable as those determined under practical conditions in feeding trials.

2. *Both short and long-term trials were performed with mature, non-producing animals fed at the maintenance level (if the energy content of their food is known).* In the short-term trials energy or nitrogen and carbon balances were determined to assess whether the animals were in energy equilibrium. In the long-term trials energy equilibrium was assumed to be the case if the body weight changes were absent or negligible (animals are not kept in calorimeters).

The use of feeding experiments to estimate the maintenance energy requirements under practical conditions has a greater problem of determining energy equilibrium than is true of measurements in a calorimeter. Some of

TABLE 1. Some Data[a] Obtained from a Comparative Slaughter Feeding Trial with Beef Steers.

S. No.	Item	Ad libitum	Near maintenance	How determined
1.	No. of steers	12	12	-
2.	Days fed	119	119	-
3.	Initial energy, Mcal	646	646	Calculated from the fat and protein content of an initial slaughter group
4.	Final energy, Mcal	1517	777	Calculated from the fat and protein content of the fed steers.
5.	Daily energy gain, Mcal	7.3	1.1	$\dfrac{(4) - (3)}{(2)}$
6.	Daily feed intake, kg	8.1	3.7	Measured during trial
7.	Fasting heat production, Mcal	5.8	5.8	Mathematical extrapolation of the data to zero feed intake.
8.	Feed for maintenance, kg	2.9	2.9	Mathematical extropolation of the data to zero energy gain.
9.	Net energy for gain, Mcal/kg	1.4	1.4	$\dfrac{(5)}{(6) - (8)}$
10.	Net energy for maintenance, Mcal/kg	2.0	2.0	$\dfrac{(7)}{(8)}$

(Feeding level spans the *Ad libitum* and *Near maintenance* columns.)

[a] Adjusted to equivalent body weights for the two feeding levels. Data source: Animal Science Department, University of California, Davis.

the studies referred to have been based on the energy intake necessary to maintain a constant body weight. Constant body weight, however, does not necessarily mean constant body energy. In addition, there is an added difficulty of feeding so that body weight gain or loss does not occur. It is much easier to feed for some gain and then correct for changes in weight.

3. Data on maintenance requirements were obtained (by conducting feeding trials with different levels of feed intakes) by extrapolation of intake of feed towards zero level of production.

Recently most of the work on nutrient requirements has been reported by following "Regression methods" to estimate maintenance requirements. Much more accurate corrections, could result from actual measurements of changes in body energy. This can be done by comparative slaughter experiments. NRC has used the experimental data of Garrett, Lofgreen and coworkers for the maintenance requirements of beef cattle and sheep, and for maintenance of growing heifers and bulls in case of dairy cattle.

Lofgreen and Garrett (1968) at California conducted a series of comparative slaughter studies to measure the NE requirements of beef cattle. By determining body composition and empty body weights initially and after a feeding period over the range from maintenance to *ad libitum* feeding it was possible to calculate the NE required for maintenance and gain (Table 1). Plotting the data of daily heat produced per unit metabolic body size versus daily ME intake per unit metabolic body size and then extrapolation to zero energy intake it was estimated that fasting heat production of beef cattle lies between 72 and 82 Kcal per unit metabolic body size with a mean of 77.

Dairy cattle:

$$NE_m = 80\ W^{0.75}\ (Kcal/day)$$

$$ME_m = 133\ W^{0.75}\ (Kcal/day)$$

$$DE_m = 155\ W^{0.75}\ (Kcal/day)$$

$$TDN_m = 35.2\ W^{0.75}\ (g\ TDN/day)$$

The energy values are expressed as kilocalories per day and W is expressed in kilograms.

4. *Change in live weight*

If it is not fed, an animal will get the energy it needs by breaking its own tissues. Obviously, this will cause a loss of body weight (Figure 1). Animal will gain or lose body mass according to whether its energy intake is greater or less than its maintenance energy requirement (MER). Hence the animal can be given varying amounts of dietary energy and the response data can be measured. Regressed data helps to find out at which energy intake energy balance (i.e. weight change) is zero. Data for yearling rusa (*Cervus timorensis*) stags are illustrated in Fig. 1. These studies generally last for several weeks as it is difficult to get a good estimate of live weight change in only a few days. Values for the MER of animals confined in stalls or small yards are (MJ ME/kg$^{0.75}$/day) 0.46 for cattle (NRC, 2001), 0.5 for rusa stags (Dryden et al., 2002), 0.44 for pigs (NRC, 1998) and 0.52 for horses (Vermorel et al., 1997).

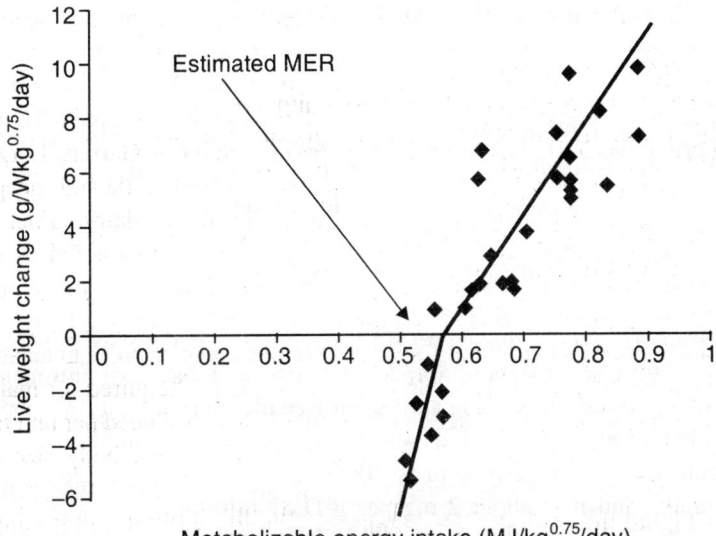

Figure 1 Change in body mass in rusa (*Cervus timorensis*) stags fed above- and below-maintenance energy intakes. (From M.C.Hmeidan and G.McL. Drde, 2000, Gatton, Australia.)

Protein Requirements for Maintenance

The amount of protein (N × 6.25) lost in the urine and faeces of animals, and additional losses, such as hair, skin, and hooves represent the amount of protein required for maintenance.

Endogenous-nitrogen metabolism: There is a minimum essential nitrogen catabolism incident to the maintenance of the vital processes of the body, even as is the case for energy. This catabolism is measured as the minimum urinary nitrogen excretion on a nitrogen-free, energy adequate diet and is called endogenous urinary nitrogen (EUN or UNe) Endogenous urinary nitrogen studies were initiated by Folin (1905). The greater part of the N in the urine of mammals not receiving food N is in the form of urea, the typical byproduct of amino acid catabolism, which arises from the turnover of body proteins.

Like basal metabolism, endogenous-nitrogen metabolism is a function of body size. Both represent the minimum catabolism essential to life, one would expect a relationship between them. Terroine and Sorg-Matter in 1927 reported that a relationship exists, for the first time, 2.3. to 2.9 mg nitrogen per kilocalorie BMR. Later in 1934, Brody and coworkers confirmed that relationship and is indicated by the following formula.

$$EUN \text{ mg/d} = 146 \text{ W}^{0.72} \text{ kg}$$

This interspecies equation was arrived at by the analysis of a body of data on minimum EUN excreted by mature animals of different species, ranging in weight from 0.02 to 500 kg. It was suggested that mammals excrete 2 mg of EUN per kilocalorie of basal metabolism, or 140 mg $N/kg^{0.75}$/day. EUN is highest in young animals and lowest during hibernation since EUN tends to reflect energy metabolism. EUN of Indian cattle was 0.02 g/kg BW while that of *Bos taurus* was 0.0289 g/kg BW.

Metabolic faecal nitrogen (MFN or FN_m): It consists principally of 'spent' digestive enzymes, abraded mucosa and bacterial nitrogen. It is difficult to obtain MFN using a nitrogen-free diet in ruminants. Mitchell used a well balanced protein such as 4% of defatted egg protein in rats instead of nitrogen-free diet. Egg protein is 100% absorbed. MFN is proportional to feed intake and it is about 2 mg per g DMI in rats.

In 1927 Titus introduced a technique with steers, which involved plotting of the total N intake as a function of the total faecal N excretion, using rations of varying protein content but of constant feed intake. He extrapolated the straightline thus obtained back to the point of zero protein intake and arrived at the estimated metabolic faecal N excretion for the feed in question. It is about 5 mg/g of DM intake. This is over twice the value for rats and would appear logical since both microbial residues and tissue desquamation would be expected to be higher in ruminants. The MFN values determined in Indian cattle were 0.35 g/100 g DMI and in buffaloes 0.34 g/100 g DM intake. These values are lower than the values determined in *Bos taurus*.

Endogenous urinary nitrogen and metabolic faecal nitrogen put together has come to 350 mg N/kg metabolic body size per day in ruminants. It is two to three times as great as in nonruminants.

Methods Adopted to Estimate Protein Requirements for Maintenance

The estimation of maintenance requirements for protein as compared with that of energy is more complicated because of the below mentioned reasons. Protein may also be used as a source of energy in case of energy shortage. An excessive supply of protein results in deamination of protein and utilization of the resulting N-free-substances as a source of energy, since deposition of protein in reserve tissue of mature animals is limited. The protein requirements can be estimated for maintenance based on calculations of the factors causing nitrogen losses from the body during maintenance. These factors include endogenous urinary nitrogen and metabolic faecal nitrogen. Losses of hair, feathers, and scurf are other factors that are involved. Although not strictly required for maintenance, factors such as growth of wool, feathers, or hooves do occur in animals otherwise being maintained. The term 'adult growth' is used to refer the growth and renewal of these epidermal tissues.

Protein requirements have been calculated by conducting nitrogen balance trials, feeding trials and factorial method where endogenous urinary nitrogen, metabolic faecal nitrogen, nitrogen loss through skin and biological values (BV) of proteins are estimated to assess the protein requirements.

1. *Nitrogen balance method:* Various rations containing different levels of protein are fed to the various groups of non-producing, adult, healthy animals. The rations are otherwise adequate in energy, minerals and vitamins required by the animals. Nitrogen balance is determined in the experimental animals. The minimum protein intake at which nitrogen equilibrium is achieved is the maintenance requirement. The experimental animals chosen for the studies must be in adequate protein nutrition at the start of the experiment.

   Disadvantage: It is a short-term measurement carried out under closely controlled conditions, and thus the question always arises as to how accurately the results apply to the long-term feeding.

2. *Feeding trial method:* Long-term feeding trials are conducted with non-producing, adult, healthy animals which are kept on different levels of protein with adequate intake of energy, minerals and vitamins. The level of protein at which the animal maintains its body weight without loss or gain over an extended period is considered the maintenance requirement of protein.

3. *Factorial method:* Protein requirements can be determined accurately by factorial method. Mostly this method has been followed throughout the world. In India many workers have followed factorial method where EUN and MFN are estimated to assess protein requirement (Kehar, 1944). Dermal losses of hair and scurf (2.2 g N/day) are also included. The net requirement, however, only covered replacing these losses, and the efficiency with which the absorbed protein is utilized (i.e., its BV) also must be considered. ARC assumed BV values of 70% for cattle and 65% for sheep. Since animals are being fed for productive purposes, the biological values for the combined function of maintenance and production are the ones of practical importance.

For pigs and poultry, protein requirements are usually stated for maintenance and production together.

Requirements for Growth

With the exception of the humans, the growth curves of many animals are quite similar (Brody, 1945). Typical growth curves are sigmoid in shape, showing that gains are faster in young animals than in older animals. Composition of the gains of growing animals change as they become older and larger. The water, protein, and ash content of the gain declines steadily, while the fat increases from 20% to in excess of 50% of the gain. Because of these variables, the assessment of requirements for growth is complicated.

In feeding standards for growing animals, requirements of both protein and energy for maintenance and growth are combined to give a single figure against the body weight. Strictly speaking this is not very accurate as calves of different breeds grow at different rates. Though the maintenance requirement of the different animals is practically the same for identical body weight, their extra requirement for growth will vary due to different rates of growth. The correct way is to calculate the maintenance requirement of a calf of a specified body weight plus to make provision for extra protein for its growth rate at that stage of its life.

Methods of Calculation of Protein Requirement

1. *A factorial method:* In the factorial method, the daily net requirement for protein is estimated as the sum of the requirement for maintenance and for the net accretion of body proteins. Maintenance requirement is the amount of protein required to replace the endogenous nitrogen losses from the body. The amount of protein needed for the tissue growth is determined by the rate of growth of fat-free tissue and its protein content.

For a calf weighing 70 kg with a DM intake of 2 kg per day, its EUN is 3.5 g and MFN is 7.0 g. The MFN value is lower than in adult animals because the young calf is kept on a diet having much less fibre. If the animal is gaining body weight at the rate of 0.6 kg per day, the amount of nitrogen stored in this gain will be 16 g per day. The total amount of N thus to be supplied in the diet will be 3.5 + 7.0 + 16 = 26.5 g per day. In terms of protein it will be (26.5 × 6.25) 166 g per day. Dermal losses may also be added. The BV of proteins for body building purposes is much less and is taken as 65% in the growing animals. Therefore the amount of digestible protein required will be 100/65 × 166 = 255 g. This value is for truely digested protein. Apparently digestible protein is $255 - (7 \times 6.25) = 211$ g. The requirement of protein generally taken in feeding standards is 0.22 kg for a calf weighing 70 kg and growing at the rate of 0.5 kg per day. This figure increases or decreases correspondingly with the increase or decrease of growth rate.

2. *Nitrogen balance studies:* Diets containing various levels of protein are fed to animals. The minimum amount of protein which ensures maximum nitrogen balance is taken as the estimate of the requirement.

3. *Based on feeding trials:* In this method diets containing various levels of protein are fed to animals and the lowest protein level which gives the maximum growth is taken as the protein requirement of growth.

Energy for growth and fattening: Energy requirements can be obtained by using 1. feeding trials and 2. factorial calculations.

Based on factorial calculations: The factors involved in the total net energy needs for growth and fattening include the needs for maintenance (basal metabolism, plus that for activity) and that deposited in the tissue gained. The NRC standards on energy requirements for growing and fattening beef cattle were established from NE values. They include a multiple net energy system whereby the daily requirements for maintenance were based on $NE_m = 77$ Kcal per W $kg^{0.75}$. Based on growth studies with steers and heifers, the NE requirements for gain of steers and heifers were calculated as NE_{gain}.

The NRC established the NE requirements for growth of dairy cattle on the same basis as was done for beef cattle. Requirements were also expressed in terms of DE, ME and TDN. The values for TDN had been previously established from feeding trials, but DE was calculated from TDN on the basis that 1.0 kg of TDN equals 4.409 Mcal of DE. The ME requirements of growing animals were computed from the requirements of NE_m and NE_g. ME is also calculated from DE by multiplying by 82%.

The ARC of Britain derived estimated requirements of energy for growth of ruminants on a factorial basis from a ME system proposed by Blaxter.

The basis for the energy requirements in NRC standards for growing sheep was the factorial estimates of Garrett and coworkers. But the recommendations were modified in view of results of feeding trials and for economic considerations.

Based on feeding trials: Estimating energy requirements from feeding trials is based merely on feeding different groups of animals with different levels of energy and determining the energy level that promotes the growth or fattening desired. Much of the earlier recommendations for beef and dairy cattle, swine, and sheep were on this basis. The energy requirements of growing and fattening swine in current NRC standards (1998) were based on feeding trials. Although these were expressed in terms of DE and ME, some of the values were converted from TDN. The ME was approximated as 96% of the DE values.

The energy requirements of growing poultry in both NRC and ARC standards were based on feeding trials.

Requirement for Milk Production

Energy Requirement

Energy requirement for milk production are based on the composition of the milk and milk yield and the efficiency of conversion of dietary energy into milk energy. Generally, the energy requirement increases with fat content of milk. Usually the milks are adjusted to a 4% fat equivalent by the formula to compare them on an equal-energy basis. Gaines Formula (W.L. Gaines and O.R. Overman 1938)

$$\text{Fat corrected milk (FCM) kg} = 0.4 \text{ (kg milk)} + 15 \text{ (kg fat)}$$

The following calculation illustrate how the energy requirement for the production of one kg of FCM can be estimated. The net energy content of 1 kg of FCM is 750 kcal; thus 750 kcal of NE is required for one kg of FCM. Efficiency of conversion of ME to NE of milk = 62%; Efficiency of conversion of DE to ME = 82%. Hence the DE required to produce one kg of FCM = 100 × 750/62 = 1210/0.82 = 1476 kcal DE. The amount of TDN required per kg of FCM = 1476/4400 = 0.335 kg.

Protein Requirement

Milk secretion represents a direct loss of protein to the animal body which needs to be replaced. Estimates of the efficiency of utilization of digestible protein for milk production vary from 60 to 70%; hence one kg FCM with 35 g of protein need 50 to 55 g digestible protein in the diet.

Requirements of Reproduction

The nutrient requirements of the breeding male per unit size above maintenance may be nearly comparable to those of the breeding female at the initiation of pregnancy. Thereafter, however, the nutritional needs of the pregnant female enhances. Two major criteria used in determining the requirements for reproduction are that the levels suggested must result in normal offspring and must prevent the maternal tissues from becoming depleted due to the demands of the foetus.

The requirements are for what has been called "the products of conception", that is, for the growth of the foetus and its membranes and for the growth of tissues related to reproduction, such as the uterus and the mammary tissues, plus the laying down of increased body reserves and for the increasing metabolism during pregnancy.

Energy: It has been reported that the deposition of energy is moderate during the first two-thirds of gestation and materially increases during the last one-third of the gestation. Further the heat increment of pregnancy, which is primarily due to the increase in the metabolism of the maternal tissue, accounts for more than three-quarters of the energy used throughout gestation; hence the additional requirement for energy above maintenance increases materially during the last trimester of gestation.

Protein: The requirement for protein during gestation closely parallels that of energy.

Avain Egg Production: Estimates of energy and protein requirements:

The nutritional requirements for egg production are affected by the size and breed of hen, the percentage production, and the composition of the egg. Scott and coworkers estimated the energy and protein requirements in 1969.

Energy: Estimates of the energy requirements for the average hen in production can be made by adding the costs of maintenance to those of producing one egg. For example, let us assume that a 1.8 kg hen lays seven eggs each weighing 54 g during ten days (70% production).[N] The requirements are calculated as follows.

Basal metabolic rate, kcal NE/day = 68 W kg$^{0.75}$; Activity increment is estimated at 50%.

Maintenance requirement = $68 \times 1.8^{0.75} \times 1.5 = 68 \times 1.55 \times 1.5$
$$= 159 \text{ kcal NE}$$
Energy content of one egg = 77 kcal NE; Daily energy requirement at 70% egg production = 77 × 0.70 = 54 kcal NE
Total requirement = 159 + 54 = 213 kcal NE
Average efficiency of utilization of ME for maintenance and egg production = 68%.

So Daily ME requirement = 213/0.68 = 314 kcal.

Protein: In considering the protein requirement for egg production, one must consider the quantity of protein deposited in the egg as well as that required for the maintenance of the hen.

Calculation of protein requirement per day

Maintenance of one hen	=	3.0 g of protein required
Production of one egg	=	6.0 g of protein required
Growth is nil and feather growth	=	0.1 g of protein required
Total requirement at 100% production		9.1 g

Daily requirement determined by feeding trial = 16.0 g

That is efficiency of protein utilization for maintenance and egg production is 57%. If egg production falls to 70%, then the daily requirement for egg production is 4.2 g and the efficiency of protein utilization falls to 46%. Also see P. 218.

Requirement for Vitamins and Minerals

The requirements for vitamins can logically be divided into two categories: the fat soluble vitamins and water soluble vitamins. The fat soluble vitamins are required for the maintenance of tissue and bone, whereas the B vitamins play roles in metabolism as enzyme cofactors and their requirement increase in parallel with of energy and protein.

Requirements for calcium and phosphorus are fairly well established because of their greater occurrence in the body and greater role of play in the body. Calcium and phosphorus make up the bulk of milk ash and hence the two minerals have received the most attention in relation to lactation. The minerals of major concern in the reproduction are calcium, phosphorus and iron.

The requirements for calcium and phosphorus for milk production can be calculated from the following: one kg of FCM contain about 1.3 g of Ca and 1.0 g of P. If the dietary Ca and P are used with an efficiency of approximately 60%, about 2.2 g of Ca and 1.6 g of P are required per kg of FCM.

For egg production as well, the minerals required in the greatest quantity are calcium and phosphorus. The requirement for calcium is especially high because it, as calcium carbonate, make up approximately 98% of the shell. Since the shell contains 2.2 g of calcium and only 50 to 60% of the dietary calcium is absorbed, then approximately 4 g of dietary calcium is required for each egg.

Factors that can alter nutrient requirements

1. *Individual animal variation:* Individual animals vary in their requirements of nutrients. Hence some margin of safety is desirable in formulating diets and especially with nutrients that are not very stable and may be slowly and gradually destroyed by long storage.

2. *Chemical composition of feeds:* Many factors affect the level of nutrients in feeds and these include soil type and level of fertilization; stage of maturity at harvesting; handling and storage methods; processing methods; exposure to varying temperature, humidity and other environmental factors; moisture level; rancidity level; variety of feed; time interval between harvesting, processing, storage and its use, etc.

3. *Variation in availability of nutrients in feeds:* There are differences in the availability of nutrients. For example, zinc in soybean meal (SBM) is less available than that in casein. This is due to the phytic acid in SBM forming a complex which makes zinc less available.

4. *Effect of higher level of performance:* The level of nutrient that may be satisfactory for the average producer is usually not adequate for the higher level of production. The higher producing animals have increased body metabolic heat from the products they produce. Hence they tend to be more susceptible to heat stress.

5. *Stress conditions:* Higher levels of nutrients are recommended for moderate or severe stress conditions. However, higher levels of nutrients should be used with caution because some can cause harmful effects if used at too high a level. Hence one should be careful when increasing nutrient levels are used to counteract stress. Well-balanced, nutritious diets should be the first line of defense against stress and infectious diseases.

6. *Intestinal flora:* The intestinal flora is affected by the type of diet and nutrients fed, antibiotic feed supplements and antibiotics used to treat diseases. Therefore, the intestinal synthesis of nutrients (vitamin K, biotin) or the requirements of nutrients by the intestinal microflora can change. This in turn will affect the requirement for certain nutrients in the diet.

7. *Antinutrients/antimetabolites in feeds:* There are certain compounds in feeds that can increase the need for certain nutrients. These include phytates that bind zinc; oxalates that bind calcium; avidin, streptavidin and stravidin (isolated from Streptomyces) that bind biotin; thiaminase destroys thiamin, goitrogens increase iodine needs, gossypol increases iron needs. Certain antimicrobial drugs may also increase the need for certain nutrients. Rancidity in feeds may destroy vitamins A, D, E, C, biotin, and possibly other nutrients. Similarly trypsin inhibitor, tannins, saponins, isothiocyanate, moulds, etc present in feed also influence the nutrients in feeds.

8. *Nutrient interrelationships:* Examples of these interrelationships are:

Choline and methionine

Methionine and cysteine

Phenylalanine and tyrosine

Niacin and tryptophan

Calcium, manganese and copper

Zinc, copper and protein

Copper, zinc and iron

Vitamin D, Ca, P, and Mg

Iron and phosphorus

Molybdenum, copper and sulphur

Sodium and potassium

Biotin and pantothenic acid

Vitamin B_{12} and methionine

Vitamin E, selenium and sulphur amino acids

Because of these interrelationships, the requirement of many nutrients will be modified by the level of other nutrients. Excess calcium may increase the need for phosphorus, Mg, Zn, Cu, Fe and total sulphur amino acids.

9. *Quality of water:* Water is a source of minerals and other compounds. Nitrates, sulfites, and other chemicals in the water can destroy certain nutrients. High levels of sulfates and other compounds in water may cause diarrhoea and other digestive disturbances.

10. *Energy content of diet:* The energy content of the diet will definitely affect nutrient needs. For example, amino acid requirements increase as the caloric density increases. The need for other nutrients in the diet may be either increased or decreased depending on the level and kind of fat in the diet.

11. *Variation in deficiency symptoms:* Single nutrient deficiencies are seldom encountered under farm conditions. Conditions such as reduced appetite and growth or unthriftiness are common to malnutrition in general. Nutritional deficiencies may exist without the appearance of definite deficiency symptoms. These may be called borderline deficiencies. Many deficiency symptoms do not appear in an average- or low-producing group of animals.

12. *Nutrient requirements for immunity:* Nutrient levels that are adequate for growth, feed efficiency, gestation, and lactation may not be adequate for normal immunity and for maximizing the animal's resistance to disease.

13. *Moulds in feeds:* Moulds in feeds may affect the availability of biotin. Streptomyces moulds are found in soil, mouldy feeds, manure and litter.

14. Environmental temperature and humidity affects the nutrient needs. Destruction of nutrients by rancidity, light or irradiation; feed additives, enzymes, hormones; toxins in feeds; managemental practices affect nutrient needs of the animals.

15. Long term studies involving growth, reproduction, and haematological, histopathological and related data are needed to determine the nutrient requirements more accurately.

16. Some nutrient requirements are worked out using purified diets. This is to be kept in mind while applying this information to the farm animals fed on natural diets because of some difference in the availability of nutrients in the natural diets. For example, zinc in soybean protein is less available than that in purified casein for pigs; similarly vitamin D needs were higher with a soybean protein diet than with a purified casein protein diet.

After perusal of so many factors that affect the nutrient requirements of animals, it is concluded that there are no exact nutritional requirements but only approximate requirements.

4

Feeding Standards — History — their uses and Significance

Definition and Expression of Feeding Standards

Feeding standards are statements of the amounts of nutrients required by animals. Feeding standards may be expressed in quantities of nutrients or in dietary proportions. Various units are used for feeding standards. It is obviously desirable that the units used in standards should be the same as those used in the evaluation of feeds.

Feeding standards may be given separately for each function of the animal (e.g. for maintenance, for pregnancy) or as overall figures for the combined functions (e.g. for maintenance and pregnancy).

Variations exist between animals, and also between feeds and these variations in the requirement of nutrients by the animals and the variations in the amount of nutrients present in the feeds are to be borne in mind when applying feeding standards to formulate rations. It is for this reason feeding standards should be considered as guides and flexible rules in computation of rations to individual animals and groups of animals in a farm.

History of Feeding Standards

German workers were responsible for early development of feeding standards for farm animals.

Albrecht Thaer (1752-1828) (a German) in 1810 published 'hay equivalents' as measures of relative value based on determining the materials in feeds extractable with water (and other solvents). He used meadow hay as a unit to compare other feeds. Einhoff, Thaer's associate, isolated fibre from straw, barley, lentils and beans by macerating them and washing with water.

Boussingault (1830-1845), Henneberg and Stohmann (1860; German scientists), Henry (1904), and Armsby (1917) all credited Thaer with this concept and with originating hay equivalents.

William Prout, in 1827, recognised protein, fat and carbohydrate as essential organic nutrients. Liebig in 1830s developed simple analytical methods. Grouven (a German) formulated the first feeding standard with protein, carbohydrate and fat contained in the feed for farm animals in 1859. Henneberg and Stohmann found that the total nutrients contained in the feed are not the correct guide and only the digestible nutrients are available.

Wolff's standard: Emilvon Wolff (a German Scientist) in 1864 devised a feeding standard based on digestible protein, digestible fat and digestible carbohydrates derived from results obtained in feeding trials. This standard has not considered the quantity and quality of milk produced. The maintenance and production requirements were not separately considered. Keeping these shortcomings in mind Professor Kuhan published feeding standard in 1867 based upon the maintenance and production requirements along with quantity of milk production. Wolff's standards were published annually without fundamental change until 1897, when they were modified by G. Lehmann (a German Scientist) to become Wolff-Lehmann standards for various classes of animals.

These standards took into account the quantity of milk produced only but not of its quality. Atwater brought the Wolff's standards to the attention of American workers in 1874 in the annual report of the Connecticut Board of Agriculture. In 1880 these standards were also published by Armsby in his book "Manual of Cattle Feeding". As a result, the Wolff standards commenced to be used in the United States.

In 1884, Professor Fjord formulated Scandinavian Feed Unit Standard. This standard is of comparative type similar to 'hay equivalent'. He considered one pound of common grain such as maize, barley or wheat as one unit for comparing different feedstuffs.

In 1890 Atwater proposed a feeding standard based on the "available fuel values" of the feeds. Available fuel values were obtained by the use of Rubner's factors applied to digestible nutrients.

Rubner's factors:

Protien	4.1 Kcal/g
Fat	9.3 Kcal/g
Carbohydrates	4.1 Kcal/g

Since the Rubner factor for protein contained a deduction for urine losses of 1.25 Kcal per gram of protein, Atwater's value took account both faecal and urine losses.

In 1898 W.A. Henry published the first edition of his book 'Feeds and Feeding' containing composition of American feeds. He calculated nutritive ratios as follows

DCP: Dig. carbohydrates + Dig. EE × 2.4

Later the factor 2.4 has been replaced by 2.25.

During 1903-1914, T.L. Haecker (1907; an American) published feeding standard for dairy cows showing that the nutritive requirements varied not only with the quantity of milk produced but also with its quality, especially its fat content. He was also the first to separate the requirements for maintenance from the requirements of production. Savage (an American) published his feeding standard in 1912 by increasing the protein requirement 20% above the standard of Haecker since it was too low especially in protein. He expressed requirements in terms of DCP and TDN for protein and energy, respectively. He further stated that about 2/3 requirement of the DM should be met by feeding roughages and the remaining 1/3 from concentrates. Fat content of milk was also considered.

Frap's Feeding Standard: Frap formulated his feeding standard which was based on DM, DCP and productive values.

Kellner's S.E. System: Kellner (a German scientist) published 'Starch equivalent system' in 1907. It was based upon the net energy and digestible true protein. See p. 250 of Principles of Animal Nutrition and Feed Technology for calculation of SE of feedstuffs.

Morrison's Feeding Standard: Morrison, F.B. published his own feeding standard in 1915 in the 15th edition of "Feeds and Feeding" under the authorship of Henry and Morrison. They were then called "Modified Wolff- Lehmann standard' which were later called as "Morrison's Feeding standard". These standards were expressed in terms of DM, DCP and TDN. Morrison indicated the nutrient requirement of animals in a range rather than in one figure. Later they were revised in 1936, 1948 and in the year 1956. Morrison included the allowances for Ca, P and carotene, DCP, TDN and Net energy. The average of Morrison's standards have been accepted for Indian Livestock.

Armsby Feeding Standard: Armsby (an American scientist) published feeding standard based on true protein and net energy values in 1917. By means of the respiration calorimeter, he determined the net energy available for productive purposes. The NE values of some feeds have actually been determined, and most of the values have been computed from the Table of Morrison's digestible nutrients. Armsby standard is not as widely used as are the standards based on digestible nutrients. Kellner feeding standard and Armsby feeding standard are based on production value (net energy).

ARC Standard: In UK a techincal committee was set up to develop the standards in 1959, by the Agricultural Research Council (ARC) which later came to known as Agricultural and Food Research Council (AFRC). Between 1960 and the mid-1980s, feeding standards in the UK were drawn up by research scientists and then translated into practical manuals by extension workers of the Ministry of Agriculture, Food and Fisheries (MAFF) and associated Governmental and commercial organizations. In 1983 AFRC set up a single organization for the UK, Technical Committee on Responses to Nutrients (TCORN) and this became responsible for both revising the standards and producing practical manuals. Requirements are given for ruminants, pigs and poultry in three separate reports, each of these reports furnished extensive summaries of the literature upon which the requirements are based.

NRC Standard: In USA the committee on Animal Nutrition under the auspices of the National Academy of Sciences-National Research Council (NRC) and US Department of Agriculture (USDA) has been publishing the Nutrient Requirements for all types of farm animals since 1945.

Broadly feeding standards may be divided into 3 main groups

Comparative type feeding standards such as Thaer's hay equivalents and Fjord's Scandinavian feed unit standard.

Production type feeding standards such as Kellner's feeding standard and Armsby feeding standard.

Digestible nutrient type standards such as Wolff's, Wolff-Lehmann's, Haecker's, Savage's, Frap's, Kellner's, Morrison's, etc.

Usefulness and Limitations of Feeding Standards

1. Feeding standards serve as guides in feeding animals and in estimating the adequacy of feed intakes and of feed supplies for groups of animals or people.

    In practical feeding operations it is frequently desirable to take economic factors into account. Thus, modifications (in feeding standards) may be called for in the interest of obtaining the rate of gain or level of milk production that seems the most economical in terms of current feed costs and the market price of the product.

2. No standard can be a complete guide to feeding because other factors such as palatability and the physical nature of the ration must also be taken into account.
3. Further, environment may change nutrient requirements.

Merits and Demerits of Various Feeding Standards

As mentioned earlier, it is obviously desirable that the units used in feed-ing standards should be the same as those used in the evelution of feeds.

Energy Evaluation: It is not tenable to consider one nutrient more important than another, since all must be available to the animal in adequate amounts if efficient production is to be maintained. However, an animal's requirement for energy is the primary consideration from a quantitative and economic position. Energy is most often the factor which limits livestock production, and meeting the energy requirements for maintenance and production is the major cost associated with feeding animals. The best unit for expressing the energy value is the one which takes into account all the losses incurred by the animal in utilising the energy present in feeds.

TDN and DE Systems

The TDN and DE system of feed evaluation have been and continue to be used because these measures are useful as first approximations of a feed's value as a source of energy, and a considerable and valuable volume of knowledge exists concerning the proximate composition and the TDN or DE value of feedstuffs.

Merits

1. TDN is a measure of apparent DE but is expressed in units of weight or per cent rather than energy *per se.*
2. TDN value provides a relative measure of the DE content of feed; 1 kg TDN = 4.409 Mcal DE.
3. It is easy to determine the TDN content of feedstuffs; proximate composition of feeds and faeces and digestion trial are to be done.
4. Digestible energy can readily be determined by using a bomb calorimeter to measure the GE of feed and faeces. No chemical analyses are required.

Demerits

1. TDN system takes into account only the losses of nutrients in the faeces but not the other losses from the body.

2. TDN system overevaluates the energy value of poor quality roughages in relation to concentrates specially so in hot environment because (i) TDN does not consider large amounts of energy wasted in the digestion of fibrous feeds in the form of gases and heat increment and (ii) ether extract of forages largely comprise other than true fat. So a kg of TDN in roughage has less value for productive purpose than a kg of TDN in concentrate.

3. Certain species of forage were found to have high gross energy and high TDN values due to essential oils but low ME values.

4. The measurement of DE takes into account the losses only through faeces.

SE and ME Systems

The total digestible nutrients system in the United States, Canada and India and Starch equivalent (SE) system in Europe have been widely used since early 1900s. The SE system was replaced by the ME system devised by Blaxter in the UK. The ARC has adopted the ME system since 1980. ME goes a step beyond DE or TDN (since energy losses in urine and GPD are corrected), and provides a more accurate measure of the value of a feedstuff.

It has been common to use ME as a measure of feed value for poultry because their faeces and urine are excreted through a common orifice; it is actually easier to determine ME than DE for them.

Merits of ME System

1. ME represents a more accurate measure since losses in urinary and gaseous products of digestion are also accounted for.

2. ME provides a more satisfactory measure of nutritive value than do TDN or DE.

3. ME is cheaper and easier to obtain than NE values.

4. The efficiency of utilization of ME takes into consideration the purpose for which it is fed, level of feeding and caloric density of the diet.

Demerits

1. The requirement of the animal and feed value are given in terms of NE and ME, respectively.
2. The large differences in the efficiency of utilization of ME are primarily due to wide variation in the energy losses as heat increment.

Net Energy Systems of Feed Evaluation for Ruminants: Net energy is more scientifically sound for expressing energy requirements and energy value of feeds. The British (ARC, 1965) have adopted a procedure proposed by Blaxter (1962) which adjusts the ME value of a feedstuff or diet according to the efficiency with which it is used for a particular purpose.

In Rostock, East Germany, many years of energy balance experiments originating with the classical work of Kellner (1905) have resulted in a proposal by Nehring *et al.* (1969, 1970) that net energy values be expressed in terms of net energy for fattening (NE_f).

In the US there has been a slightly different approach to the development of net energy systems for feed evaluation, though the theoretical basis is identical to that used by the British and German scientists.

Garret, Lofgreen and coworkers in 1968 from California University have proposed a net energy system for beef cattle which assigns two net energy values to each feedstuff, NE_m and NE_g. Since the partial efficiency of energy utilization for maintenance is higher than the partial efficiency of energy used for production and storage of fat and protein, the NE_m value for a ration or a feedstuff is always higher than the NE_g value. Equations have been derived which give an animal's requirement for maintenance and growth in terms of NE_m and NE_g.

A research team (Moe, Flatt, Tyrrell and coworkers) working in the USDA laboratory at Beltsville, Maryland, have conducted a large number of energy balance trials with lactating dairy cows. The efficiency of energy use for maintenance (NE_m) and lactation (NE_l) is generally similar and it is different from the efficiency of energy use for fattening. This finding has resulted in the suggestion that the energy requirements and feed values for the lactating cow could be expressed in terms of NE_l.

The NE value of a feed depends on whether it is used for maintenance, fattening, growth or milk production. Metabolizable energy is used with different degrees of efficiency for maintenance and body gain in non-lactating animals but is used with similar degrees of efficiency for maintenance and milk production in lactating animals. For this reason NRC tables (1988) gave three NE values for feeds: NE_m, NE gain and NE lactation.

NE_m is the value of feeds for the maintenance of non-lactating animals (dry animals).

NE_g is the NE value of feeds for the deposition of body tissue in growing males and females and mature bulls.

$NE_m + NE_g$ = Total energy needs of growing cattle. In lactating animals, the NE value of feeds as well as requirements for all physiological functions is described in terms of single value as NE milk (NE_l), since energy is used with similar degrees of efficiency for maintenance and milk production.

Protein Evaluation: The present system of expressing the protein requirement for ruminants and the nutrient content of feedstuffs to satisfy these requirements in terms of DCP, available protein or CP is inadequate and unsatisfactory. The DCP system regards the ruminant as a monogastric and takes no account of the ability of the ruminant to utilize NPN.

Available protein system of ARC (1965) did not consider protein and energy interrelationships and the large contribution made by undigested microbial protein to faecal N loss. Further, biological values were used to describe dietary proteins which are not relevant to the ruminant. Expression of protein requirements in terms of CP, in the USA, is based on the assumption that all the nitrogen is present as protein and that all the proteins contain 16% N. Also refer Chapter 15 of *Principles of Animal Nutrition and Feed Technology.*

New Protein Systems

Metabolizable protein system proposed by NRC in the USA, Rumen degradable and undegradable protein system proposed by ARC (1980) for the UK (The UK Metabolizable protein system), True protein digested in the small intestine (PDI) system of France and a similar system proposed by Germany are the new protein systems. Important features of these systems are consideration of two protein synthesizing systems, rumen microbes and ruminant tissues and linking of protein needs to available energy.

ARC (1980) recognizes that dietary protein should be considered in terms of RDP and UDP. The system is fully described in the report of the Agricultural and Food Reserch Council (AFRC 1992) Technical Committee on Responses to Nutrients, No. 9. The microbial demand for protein is stated in terms of Effective Rumen Degradable Protein (ERDP). The demand for amino acids at tissue level is quantified in terms of truly digestible protein required to be absorbed from the small intestine and designated as 'Metabolizable Protein' (MP). Also see figure 2 in Chapter 5 (Page no. 90)

The NRC (1989) gave the protein requirements as rumen Degradable Intake Protein (DIP) and Undegradable Intake Protein (UIP).

Recommended Dietary Allowances Versus Nutrient Requirements

An individual's requirement for nutrients is influenced by numerous interdependent physical, environmental, social and dietary characteristics. Thus people vary widely in their needs. Since it is not practical to determine each individuals exact needs, the allowances have been set high enough to take care of almost all healthy people. 'Recommended Dietary Allowances' were given for humans by the NRC Food and Nutrition Board in the first place. Later NRC started publishing the Recommended Nutrient Allowances for Farm Animals from 1944 and were used up to 1964. These allowances were set higher than average determined requirements to provide a margin of safety. In 1953, the Committee on Animal Nutrition of NRC decided not to include such margins in future recommendations and thus NRC 'Nutrient Requi-rements' of Domestic Animal series have been issued from time to time.

The term 'requirement' implies that it is the minimum amount of a given nutrient needed to promote a given body function to the optimum in a perfectly balanced ration. After 1964 the committee considered nutrient requirements to represent values sufficient to promote maintenance, optimum production and prevention of all symptoms of deficiency.

The NRC 1989 for Dairy Cattle are designed to meet the needs of those individual animals that have higher than average requirements for essential nutrients and not those that have merely average requirements. Thus, the requirement values are higher than average and in this respect, provide a margin of safety for animals whose requirements are average or below average.

Publications on Nutrient Requirements

* Nutrient Requirements of Livestock and Poultry by S.K. Ranjhan, 2nd Rev. Ed. ICAR, 1998.
* Nutrient Requirement of Animals–Cattle and Buffalo (ICAR-NIANP), 2013
* Nutrient Requirement of Animals–Sheep, Goat and Rabbit (ICAR-NIANP), 2013
* Nutrient Requirement of Animals–Poultry (ICAR-NIANP), 2013
* Nutrient Requirement of Animals–Pigs (ICAR-NIANP), 2013
* Nutrient Requirement of Animals–Equines (ICAR-NIANP), 2013
* Nutrient Requirements of Ruminants in developing countries by L.C. Kearl, 1982.
* Nutrient Requirements of ruminant livestock, ARC 1980, 1984.

* Nutrient Requirements of domestic animals series by
  National Research Council of National Academy of Sciences,
  USA.

1. Nutrient Requirements of Dairy cattle, sixth Rev. Ed., Update 1989; 7th edition 2001
2. Nutrient Requirements of Beef cattle, sixth Rev. Ed., 1984, 2001
3. Nutrient Requirements of Sheep, sixth Rev. Ed. 1985
4. Nutrient Requirements of Goats, 1981
5. Nutrient Requirements of Small Ruminants, 2007
6. Nutrient Requirements of Horses, fifth Rev, Ed., 1989; sixth Rev. 2007
7. Nutrient Requirements of Swine, ninth Rev. Ed., 1988; 10th ed., 1998
8. NRC, 2012. Nutrient requirements of swine 11th Ed. National Academy Press, Washington, DC.
9. Nutrient Requirements of Poultry, ninth Rev. Ed., 1994
10. Nutrient Requirements of Dogs, Rev. Ed., 1985
11. Nutrient Requirements of Cats, Rev. Ed., 1986
12. Nutrient Requirements of Dogs and Cats, 2006
13. Nutrient Requirements of Mink and Foxes, Rev. 1982
14. Nutrient Requirements of Rabbits, second Rev. Ed., 1977
15. Nutrient Requirements of Laboratory Animals, fourth Rev. Ed., 1995; 1998
16. Nutrient Requirements of Nonhuman Primates 2003
17. Nutrient Requirements of Fish 1993

While the nutritional requirements of all animals are broadly similar, the sources from which nutrients are obtained differ widely from species to species. Animals are carnivores, herbivores or omnivores.

Because the nutrients in plant leaves are held within cellulose walls and animals lack an enzyme (cellulase) to break them down, many herbivores have a symbiotic relationship with gut microorganisms capable of transforming cellulose and other structural polymers into a useful energy source. This microbial action simultaneously release the protein-rich cell contents. In ruminants, hamsters, the stomach has evolved a special fermentation chamber, while in others, such as rabbits, rodents and horses, the caecum, a large diverticulum of the hind gut, fulfils a similar function. The contribution of this microbial action to nutrition varies from species to species. Refer Chapter 6 of *Principles of Animal Nutrition and Feed Technology* for greater details.

5

Nutritional Requirements of Indian Cattle and Buffaloes

Evolution of Indian Requirements for Cattle and Buffaloes

The first published reference document on scientific feeding of animals in India appeared as ICAR bulletin No. 25 entitled "Nutritive Value of Indian cattle feeds and the feeding of animals by Sen (1957).

Sen and Ray (1964) came up with the first Indian standards for dairy cattle based on mid-Morrison values of 1954. Thereafter, these were revised by Ray and Ranjhan (1978). Kearl (1982) independently compiled data on the nutritional requirements of different livestock species and nutritive values of different feedstuffs from several developing countries in a systematic manner. The ICAR published the first report on the nutrient requirements of livestock and poultry in 1985. The second revised edition has been brought out in 1998 under the authorship of Dr. S.K. Ranjhan.

The Western data, on which the Morrison standard is based, pertains to the animals which are larger in body size and body weight and are superior in their productive performance. The Indian cattle are smaller in size, lower in body weight, low in production and are adapted to the adverse climatic and poor feeding conditions. So lot of work has been done in India in ICAR Institutes and the State Agricultural Universities to determine the energy and protein requirements for Indian cattle and buffaloes.

Energy and Protein Requirements for Maintenance

Energy requirement in dry animals for maintenance is low (61 to 104 kcal/ $W kg^{0.75}$) whereas in lactating animals it is high (113 to 160 kcal/ $W kg^{0.75}$). Since in the case of milch cows BMR is higher than the dry animals (Brody,

1945), the maintenance requirements are higher (5-10%) in the milch animals.

NPN compounds such as urea can be used to replace about 30% of the protein requirements of the dairy cattle and buffaloes after the rumen functions are established. Easily available carbohydrates should be incorporated in diets whenever urea is fed.

Taking 122 kcal of ME (33.74 g TDN) and 2.84 g of DCP per unit metabolic body size, the maintenance requirements were calculated for Zebu cattle, buffaloes and crossbred animals (ICAR, 1998; Table 1). The DCP and TDN system is more popular in India because these values are available for a large number of animal feeds.

In view of changes achieved in the productivity of Indian livestock and in the nutritive value of available (including newer byproducts) feedstuffs since 1998, further revision regarding the nutritional requirements of Indian cattle and buffaloes was considered essential. ICAR (2013) provided an up to date and comprehensive review of published research data in India and abroad in its publication on "Nutrient Requirements of Cattle and Buffalo". Buffaloes manage to digest fibre more efficiently than the cattle, largely

TABLE 1 Daily Nutrient Requirements for Maintenance for Cattle and Buffaloes (Ranjhan, 1998).

Body weight kg	Dry feed kg	DCP g	ME Mcal	TDN kg	Ca g	P g	Carotene mg	Vitamin A 1000 IU
1	2	3	4	5	6	7	8	9
Maintenance of Mature Cows/Buffaloes**								
200	3.5	150	6.0	1.7	8	7	21	9
250	4.0	170	7.2	2.0	10	9	26	11
300	4.5	200	8.4	2.4	12	10	32	13
350	5.0	230	9.4	2.7	14	11	37	15
400	5.5	250	10.8	3.0	17	13	42	17
450	6.0	280	12.4	3.4	18	14	48	19
500	6.5	300	13.2	3.7	20	15	53	21
550	7.0	330	14.4	4.0	21	16	58	23
600	7.5	350	15.5	4.2	22	17	64	26
650	8.0	370	16.2	4.5	23	18	69	28
700	8.5	390	17.3	4.8	25	19	74	30
750	9.0	410	18.0	5.0	26	20	79	32
800	9.5	430	19.1	5.3	27	21	85	34

**During the first and second lactation, in order to allow the growth of the lactating cows/buffaloes, add about 20 and 10 per cent of the maintenance allowance.

because of higher rumen volume, efficient rumination, nitrogen recycling capacity and increased retention time in the rumen (ICAR, 2013).

For estimating the nutrient requirements of cattle and buffaloes for maintenance, Kearl (1982) adopted 118 kcal and 125 kcal, respectively, per kg metabolic body size, while Paul and Lal (2010) adopted 128 kcal in buffaloes per kg metabolic body size. No targeted nutrient requirements were published during the last decade in India and hence, available data are not enough to assign different maintenance energy requirements for Indian cattle and buffaloes. Thus, a common value of ME requirement has been adopted by ICAR (2013) to propose maintenance energy requirements for cattle and buffaloes (Table 2).

TABLE 2 Maintenance requirements for DM, energy and protein of lactating cattle, buffalo/day*

BW (kg)	DM (kg)	TDN (kg)	ME (Meal)	MP (g)	RDP (g)	CP (g)
200	4.32	1.92	6.94	141	220	259
250	5.4	2.28	8.24	167	260	306
300	6.48	2.62	9.47	191	298	351
350	7.56	2.95	10.67	214	335	394
400	8.64	3.27	11.82	237	370	436
450	9.72	3.58	12.94	259	405	476
500	10.8	3.88	14.04	280	438	515
550	11.88	4.18	15.10	301	470	553
600	12.96	4.47	16.15	321	502	591
650	14.04	4.75	17.18	341	533	627
700	15.12	5.03	18.19	361	563	663
750	16.2	5.31	19.19	380	593	698
800	17.28	5.58	20.17	399	623	733

*ICAR (2013)

It is well understood now that protein digestibility is influenced significantly by the source of protein and energy and also their dietary levels. Hence a single value of DCP requirement cannot be assigned with reasonable accuracy (ARC, 1980 and 1982). All the more, the data generated during the last two decades reveal that the DCP system itself is erroneous. Therefore, an alternative approach **'the metabolizable protein (MP) system'** has been followed in the revised ICAR (2013) nutrient requirements in order to be in tune with the times. The equation MPm (g/d) = 2.65 g/kg $W^{0.75}$ has been used to arrive at the protein requirement (Table 2). The digestible microbial true protein (DMTP) along with digestible undegraded dietary protein (DUP) or digestible rumen undegraded protein (RUP) constitute the metabolizable protein (MP) of the feed (please see page no. 112 for detailed description).

Nutrient requirements of cattle and buffalo for production

The requirements for TDN and DCP have been calculated per kg of milk production taking 1188 kcal of ME per kg of 4% fat corrected milk (FCM) and 132 g digestible nitrogen for 100 g of milk nitrogen (ICAR, 1998; Table 3).

TABLE 3 Nutrient Requirements per kg of Milk Production[*].

Fat (%)	DCP g	ME Mcal	TDN kg	Ca g	P g
3.0	40	0.97	0.270	2.5	1.8
4.0	45	1.13	0.315	2.7	2.0
5.0	51	1.28	0.370	2.9	2.2
6.0	57	1.36	0.410	3.1	2.4
7.0	63	1.54	0.460	3.3	2.6
8.0	69	1.80	0.510	3.5	2.8
9.0	75	2.06	0.500	3.7	3.0
10.0	81	2.16	0.600	3.9	3.2
11.0	85	2.34	0.650	4.1	3.4

[*]Ranjhan, S.K. 1998. Nutrient Requirement of Livestock and Poultry, ICAR, New Delhi.

In ICAR (2013) the ME and MP values of cow and buffalo milk were computed as per fat % and CP concentrations (CP value in milk was taken as 3.5% and 4.5% for cattle and buffaloes, respectively). The 132 g digestible nitrogen / 100 g milk N (ICAR, 1998) is on lower side, considering the data of nitrogen utilization efficiency in cattle and buffaloes. It was opined (ICAR, 2013) that DCP values given in ICAR (1998; Table 3) milk production requirements were significantly lower considering the utilization efficiency of MP as 68%, and felt more studies warranted. However, because of the limitations of DCP, metabolizable protein values are calculated. The requirements for milk production per kg milk in cattle (Table 4) and in buffaloes (Table 5) are presented.

TABLE 4 DM, energy and protein requirements for milk production / kg milk in cattle.

Fat %	DM* (kg)	TDN (kg)	ME (Meal)	MP (g)	RDP (g)	RUP (g)	CP (g)
3	0.450	0.290	1.05	51	44	44	96
4	0.510	0.330	1.20	51	50	37	96
5	0.570	0.370	1.34	51	56	30	96
6	0.640	0.410	1.50	51	62	23	96
7	0.700	0.400	1.64	51	69	15	96

* Digestibility of feed; ICAR (2013)

TABLE 5 DM, energy and protein requirements for milk production / kg milk in buffaloes

Fat %	DM* (kg)	TDN (kg)	ME (Meal)	MP (g)	RDP (g)	RUP (g)	CP (g)
4	0.550	0.360	1.29	66	54	60	124
5	0.610	0.400	1.43	66	60	53	124
6	0.670	0.440	1.58	66	66	46	124
7	0.740	0.480	1.73	66	72	39	124
8	0.800	0.520	1.88	66	78	31	124
9	0.860	0.560	2.02	66	85	24	124
10	0.930	0.600	2.17	66	91	17	124

* Digestibility 65%; ICAR (2013)

Major mineral and trace mineral requirement for maintenance and milk production are provided (ICAR, 2013; tables 6, 7, 8 and 9) in the appendix I. A table of data (Table 5) on levels of NDF and non-fibrous carbohydrate to be maintained in the TMR for dairy animals to ensure their optimum rumen health is also provided in appendix I.

In case of feeding heavy yielders with high planes of nutrition there is depression in the digestibility of the feed. To compensate for depression, 3% extra feed may be given for each 10 litres of milk produced above 20 kg.

During the last trimester of gestation an additional amount of 90 to 130 g of DCP and 1.0 to 1.1 kg TDN have to be provided to cattle and buffaloes of 350 kg to 500 kg body weight (ICAR, 1998). During the pregnancy nutrients are required for the development of foetus and membranes.

After six months of pregnancy, the growth of fetus increases significantly. The nutrient requirements for pregnancy of cattle and buffaloes are presented in Tables 6 and 7. Ready reckoner for calculation of animal's body weight (BW) from body measurements in the farmers' house is provided in the appendix I.

TABLE 6 Pregnancy requirements of energy and protein for Cattle/ day**

Month of gestation	DM* (kg)	TDN (kg)	ME (Meal)	MP (g)	RDP (g)	RUP (g)	CP (g)
6-7	0.85	0.64	2.30	109	96	56	169
7-8	0.99	0.74	2.67	143	112	85	216
8-9	1.13	0.84	3.05	178	128	113	263

* Concentrate having 75% TDN or 2.71 Mcal/kg DM; ** Average birth weight of calf 25 kg; ICAR (2013)

TABLE 7 Pregnancy requirements of energy and protein for buffalo/day**

Month of gestation	DM* (kg)	TDN (kg)	ME (Meal)	MP (g)	RDP (g)	RUP (g)	CP (g)
6-7	1.0	0.8	2.76	131	115.4	67	203
7-8	1.2	0.9	3.21	172	134.2	101	259
8-9	1.4	1.0	3.66	214	153.0	136	316
9-10	1.5	1.1	4.11	255	171.8	171	373

* Concentrate having 75% TDN or 2.71 Mcal/kg DM; ** Average birth weight of calf 30 kg; ICAR (2013)

TABLE 8. Daily Nutrient Requirements of Cattle and Buffaloes (Kearl, 1982).

				CATTLE								BUFFALOES					
				Protein				Vit			Protein				Vit
BW kg	Gain kg	DMI %BW	TDN kg	To-tal g	Di-ges-tible g	Ca g	P g	A 1000 IU	DMI %BW	TDN kg	To-tal g	Di-ges-tible g	Ca g	P g	A 1000 IU
Maintenance and Growth															
100	0	2.2	1.0	167	90	5	5	5	2.4	1.09	163	80	4	4	5
	0.5	3.0	1.6	379	254	15	9	6	2.8	2.47	373	254	14	11	6
150	0	2.0	1.4	231	123	6	6	6	2.2	1.48	223	109	5	5	6
	0.5	2.8	2.2	474	305	16	10	9	2.7	2.86	486	319	14	12	9
200	0	1.9	1.8	285	152	6	6	8	2.0	1.84	288	135	6	6	8
	0.5	2.6	2.8	554	348	16	12	12	2.6	3.22	543	341	14	13	12
250	0	1.8	2.0	337	180	9	9	9	1.9	2.17	327	160	8	8	9
	0.5	2.5	3.2	623	383	16	14	13	2.4	3.55	604	374	15	12	12
300	0	1.7	2.4	385	206	10	10	10	1.9	2.49	377	183	9	9	10
	0.5	2.3	3.7	679	411	19	14	13	2.3	4.01	663	402	17	16	13
350	0	1.6	2.6	432	231	12	12	12	1.8	2.79	426	205	10	10	12
	0.5	2.3	4.1	731	433	20	16	18	2.2	4.45	703	416	17	15	15
400	0	1.6	2.9	478	256	13	13	13	1.8	3.09	469	227	11	11	13
	0.5	2.2	4.6	772	447	21	18	17	2.1	4.88	740	428	17	16	16
450	0	1.5	3.2	528	279	14	14	14	1.7	3.37	515	248	12	12	14
	0.5	2.1	5.0	805	456	22	20	17	2.0	5.31	758	424	16	16	17
500	0	1.5	3.4	567	302	15	15	15	1.7	3.65	556	268	13	13	14
	0.5	2.1	5.4	831	457	23	21	19	1.9	5.27	786	433	16	16	18

Requirements for zero gain indicate for maintenance; Requirements for 0.5 kg gain indicate for maintenance and growth; Gain of 0.5 kg was chosen to compare them with those of Indian requirements.

During the last 60 days, live weight of pregnant animal increases by about 25 to 35 kg depending upon the breed and their condition. Besides the requirement for foetal growth and uterus, nutrients are also deposited in reserve that may be utilized for milk production in early lactation. The calcium, phosphorus, carotene and vitamin A requirements are 7-9 g, 4-7 g, 30-42 mg and 12-17 thousand IU vitamin A respectively (ICAR, 1998).

Additional quantity of concentrate mixture (75%-TDN) is recommended for pregnant cows (0.9 to 1.1 kg/d) and buffaloes (1.0 to 1.5 kg/d) to support the growth of fetus during the last 3 months of gestation (ICAR, 2013).

Growth: At birth, calf is as good as a non-ruminant animal, being in its pre-ruminant stage, which may last up to three months. The most critical period in the calf life is the initial 2-3 weeks, during which the digestive system develops rapidly with regard to digestive secretions and enzymatic activities. Accordingly, the feeding system of calf has been divided into three phases (Davis and Clark, 1981), depending on their age to get good overall performance (Table 9A). These are liquid feeding phase (requirements are met from colostrum and milk/milk replacer), transitional phase (liquid diet plus calf starter and hay) and ruminant phase (calf derives nutrients from solid feed through microbial fermentation in the reticulo-rumen).

TABLE 9A   Nutrient requirements for pre-ruminant calves*

Age (day)	BW (kg)	ADG (g)	CP (g)	DCP (g)	TDN (g)	ME (Mcal)	Ca .(g)	P (g)	Vit A (g)	Vit D (g)
0-15	25	200	114	80	400	1.5	2.5	1.5	1.5	200
16-30	30	300	129	90	500	1.7	3.0	2.0	1.5	250
30-60	40	300	180	125	800	2.4	3.5	2.5	1.7	250
60-90	50	350	215	150	1000	3.6	4.0	3.8	2.0	300

*Source: ICAR (1998)

A good number of growth trials have been conducted on cattle and buffalo calves in India. However, comprehensive studies that work out the nutrient requirements for growing calves are limited and hence, data on MP, RDP and RUP requirements is lacking. Hence, NRC and ARC data have been used. Requirements in terms of DM, energy and protein for growing heifer calves and bull calves are presented in Table 9B (ICAR, 2013) only for 0.5 kg gain per day and only from 70 kg to 300 kg weight range. The reader may view the complete data in 'ICAR (2013) requirements'. The literature on growing calves reveals that their maintenance requirements are higher than that of dry animals.

TABLE 9B DM, energy and protein requirements of male & female cattle and buffalo calves (ICAR, 2013)

BW (kg)	Weight gain (kg/d)	DM (kg)	TDN (kg)	ME (Meal)	Total MP (g)	RDP (g)	RUP* (g)	CP (g)
Female cattle and buffalo calves								
70	0.4	1.8	1.28	4.63	178	278	127(78)	406
100	0.5	3.1	1.75	6.32	221	345	142(81)	487
200	0.5	5.6	2.74	9.90	267	418	108(34)	525
300	0.5	7.2	3.61	13.04	310	484	85	569
Male cattle and buffalo calves								
70	0.4	1.8	1.36	4.91	201	314	153(97)	467
100	0.5	3.0	1.83	6.60	248	388	174(105)	562
200	0.5	5.2	2.87	10.38	293	457	131(50)	588
300	0.5	6.9	3.79	13.69	333	521	96(4)	617

*Values in the parenthesis are indispensible requirements of RUP, otherwise growth rate will decrease.

Use of Maintenance Requirement Values in Practice

Although there are situations under which farm animals are fed for maintenance only, for the most part they are fed primarily for productive purposes. Here maintenance values serve as basic figures to which additions are made in accordance with number of calvings, milk production, gestation, etc. to calculate the total requirments of nutrients and to formulate a ration.

BIS Specifications for Bone Meal (Steamed)

According to the BIS not less than 90% of material should pass through 1.18 mm IS sieve and should have the following specifications (Table 10).

TABLE 10. BIS Specifications for Bone Meal

Moisture,	Max	7.0%
Ca,	Min	32.0%
P,	Min	15.0%
C. fat,	Max	1.0%
Fluorine,	Max	0.06%
AIA,	Max	1.0%

The meal should be free from Salmonella and Anthrax spores. Specifications for mineral mixture are presented in Table 11.

TABLE 11. BIS Specifications for Mineral Mixtures Containing Salt (Type I) and without Salt (Type II) for Supplementing Cattle Feeds. (IS 1664 : 1992)

S. No.	Characteristic	Type I	Type II
i)	Moisture, per cent by mass, Max	5	5
ii)	Calcium, per cent by mass, Min	18	23
iii)	Phosphorus, per cent by mass, Min	9	12
iv)	Magnesium, per cent by mass, Min	5	6.5
v)	Salt (chlorine as Sodium chloride), per cent by mass, Min	22	-
vi)	Iron, per cent by mass, Min	0.4	0.5
vii)	Iodine (as KI), per cent by mass, Min	0.02	0.026
viii)	Copper, per cent by mass, Min	0.06	0.077
ix)	Manganese, per cent by mass, Min	0.1	0.12
x)	Cobalt, per cent by mass, Min	0.009	0.012
xi)	Fluorine, per cent by mass, Max	0.05	0.07
xii)	Zinc, per cent by mass, Min	0.3	0.38
xiii)	Sulphur, per cent by mass, Max	0.4	0.5
xiv)	Acid insoluble ash, per cent by mass, Max	3	2.5
xv)	Spores of Bacillus anthracis, Clostridium spp	Nil	Nil

Note: The values specified for requirements (ii) to (xiv) are on moisture free basis.

Specifications for Bypass Protein Feed

The National Dairy Development Board, Anand, has initiated massive project on the production of bypass protein feed with the following specifications.

S. No.	Characteristics	Requirement
1.	Moisture, per cent by mass, Max	10
2.	CP (N × 6.25), per cent by mass, Min	30
3.	EE, per cent by mass, Min	3.5
4.	CF, per cent by mass, Max	8
5.	AIA, per cent by mass, Max	2.5
6.	UDP, per cent by mass, Min	20
7.	RDP, per cent by mass, Max	9

Note: The values for characteristics 2 to 7 are on moisture free basis.

Specifications for Urea Molasses Mineral Block

The NDDB, Anand has developed Urea molasses mineral blocks which contain molasses 45%, urea 15%, mineral mixture 15%, salt 8%, calcite powder 4%, bentonite 3% and cotton seed meal 10% with the following specifications.

S. No.	Characteristic	Requirement
1.	Moisture, per cent by mass, Max	3.5
2.	CP (N × 6.5), per cent by mass, Min	58.0
3.	CF, per cent by mass, Max	2.0
4.	Total ash, per cent by mass, Max	34.0
5.	AIA, per cent by mass, Max	3.0
6.	Calcium per cent by mass, Max	4.0
7.	Phosphorus, per cent by mass, Min	1.5
8.	Sulphur, per cent by mass, Min	1.0
9.	Urea, per cent by mass, Max	15.0

Note: The values for characteristics 2 to 9 are on moisture free basis.

Concentrate Mixtures for Cattle and Buffaloes

Two categories of cattle feed *viz.*, Type I and Type II (Table 12) have been prescribed by the Bureau of Indian Standards (BIS). These are suitable to be fed to cows and buffaloes yielding more than 10 litres of milk if it has to

TABLE 12. BIS Specifications for Cattle Feeds[*].

Item	Type I IS: 2052, 1979 Reaffirmed 1990	Type II IS: 2052, 1979 Reaffirmed 1990
Moisture, % max	11	11
Crude protein, % min	22	20
Ether Extract, % min	3	2.5
Crude fibre, % max	7	12
Acid insoluble ash, % max	3	4

[*]All are on moisture free basis, except moisture
[**]Requirements for the following characteristics shall be complied with and declared by the manufacturer after periodical testing:

Characteristic	Requirement
Common salt (as Na Cl), % by mass, Max	2.0
Calcium (as Ca), % by mass, Min	0.5
Phosphorus (as p), % by mass, Min	0.5
Vitamin A, IU/kg, Min	5000

These compound feeds should be in the form of a meal, cubes or pellets. The feed shall be free from harmful constituents, metallic pieces and adulterants. The feed shall also be free from fungal growth and insect infestation and from fermented, musty, rancid or any other objectionable odour. The proportion of urea when incorparated shall not exceed 1% by mass. When urea has been added to cattle feed, it shall contain not less than 10% by mass of easily digestible carbohydrates like molasses, cereal grains, etc.

be cost-effective. A majority of dairy farmers in India possess two or three cows/buffaloes yielding about 2 to 4 litres of milk. They cannot afford to pay the high cost of cattle feeds conforming to Types I and II of BIS specifications. The nutritional parameters prescribed for the Type I and Type II do not allow the incorporation of abundantly available NCFR and AIBP.

In order to encourage majority of the farmers to use compound feed, CLFMA felt necessity to introduce additional categories (Table 13) to feed animals of different production capacities. Based on milk yield and body weight, the dairy cattle were classified as follows.

TABLE 13. CLFMA Specifications for Compound Feeds for Dairy Cattle and Buffaloes.

Item	Dairy Special	I	II	III
		Types of Feed		
Moisture, % Max	12	12	12	12
CP, % Min	22	20	18	16
UDP, % Min	8	-	-	-
EE, % Min	3	2.5	2.5	2
CF, % Max	7	7	12	14
AIA, % Max	3.5	4	4.5	5
Recommended levels of feeding, kg/day cows/buffaloes				
Low yielders[c]				
Maintenance				1.0 (1.0)[a]
Production (kg/kg milk)				0.5 (0.5)
Medium yielders				
Maintenance			1.0 (1.5)	
Production (kg/kg milk)			0.5 (0.5)	
High yielders[b]				
Maintenance		1.0 (1.5)		
Production (kg/kg milk)		0.4 (0.5)		

[a] Values in the parentheses are for buffaloes;
[b] For cows yielding 20 kg milk-maintenance 1.5 kg and for every kg of milk yield 0.4 kg of Dairy special.
[c] Fifty g extra per kg milk for every additional 0.5% milk fat over 4%

Cows

(i) **Low yielders** (BW 350 kg, Milk yield 1-7 kg, Average 4 kg/day)
(ii) **Medium yielders** (BW 400 kg, Milk yield 8-14 kg, Average 11 kg/day)

(iii) High yielders (BW 450 kg, Milk yield 15-21 kg, Average 17 kg/day)

Buffaloes

(i) Low yielders (BW 400 kg, Average milk yield 4 kg/day)
(ii) Medium yielders (BW 450 kg, Average milk yield 8 kg/day)
(iii) High yielders (BW 500 kg, Average milk yield 12 kg/day)

Formulating Concentrate Mixture/Complete Feed by Using the Pearson Square Method and Algebraic Method: I Pearson Square Method

Example 1: When only two feeds are involved: A farmer has home-grown maize (8.8% CP) and he purchases a protein supplement (40% CP) containing minerals, vitamins. Formulate a concentrate mixture with 16% CP.

Procedure

1. Draw a square at the left side of the page.
2. Insert the % crude protein desired in the final mixture (16%) in the middle of the square.
3. Place maize with its crude protein (8.8%) on the upper left corner and protein supplement with its crude protein (40.0%) on the lower left corner (for this method to work one feed must be above the desired level of protein and the other below).
4. Subtract the % crude protein in maize (8.8) from the % crude protein desired in the mixture (16.0) and place the difference (7.2) on the corner of the square diagonally opposite from the maize. This amount is supplement.
5. Subtract the % crude protein desired in the mixture (16.0) from the % crude protein in the supplement (40.0) and place the difference (24.0) on the corner of the square diagonally opposite from the supplement. This amount is maize.

Maize   8.8   24

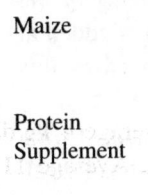

16

Protein
Supplement   40   7.2

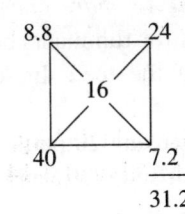

———
31.2
———

Ration

Maize :   24/31.2 × 100 = 76.92%
Supplement : 7.2/31.2 × 100 = 23.08%

        100.00%

Examples 2: *When two or more feeds are involved:* In formulating a pig feed, grains like maize and oats are used in a 2:1 ratio to circumvent the higher crude fibre level of oats. Formulate the pig feed using maize, oats and a protein supplement.

Procedure:

1. Draw a square
2. Place the % crude protein desired (14.0) in the middle of the square.
3. Separate the feeds into two groups, specify the proportion of each feed in each group and calculate the weighted average, % protein in each group. Maize and oats were grouped together in the proportion of 2:1 with the supplement being used alone. The average % of protein in the maize and oats must then be calculated as follows.

$$\begin{array}{rcl} 2 \times 8.8 & = & 17.6 \\ 1 \times 11.7 & = & \dfrac{11.7}{29.3/3} = 9.77\% \end{array}$$

4. Place 2 maize + 1 oats with its calculated % of crude protein (9.77) on the upper left corner of the square and 40% supplement (40.00) on the lower left corner.
5. Subtract diagonally and proceed with the calculation as in the previous example.
6. Divide the final figure for maize + oats into 2/3 maize and 1/3 oats.

Figure

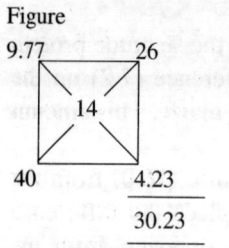

9.77   26

14

40   4.23
_____
30.23

Ration on % basis
Maize + oats = 26.0/30.23 × 100 = 86.01%
Supplement = 4.23/30.23 × 100 = 13.99%

Maize = 86.01 × 2/3 = 57.34% or parts
Oats = 86.01 × 1/3 = 28.67% or parts
Supplement   = 13.99% or parts
_____
Total   = 100.00

Example 3: *With a fixed percentage of one or more components of the ration:* In formulating concentrating mixtures for ruminants urea is added at 1%, molasses at 10% to reduce the cost of the feed. In such cases this example is useful.

Formulate a 14% CP concentrate mixture using 20 parts of oats (11.7% CP), 3 parts of mineral and vitamin supplement and maize and soybean meal.

Procedure:

1. Calculate the CP contributed by 20 kg oats in a 100 kg mixture and this the CP contributed by 23 kg since the mineral and vitamin supplement do not contribute any protein.

   $20 \times 0.117 = 2.34$ kg CP

   $100 - 23 = 77$ kg of maize and soybean meal should supplement the remaining, i.e. $14.00 - 2.34 = 11.66$ kg.

2. Calculate what % of protein will be needed in the maize (8.8%) and soybean meal (45.8%) combination to provide 11.66 kg of protein per 100 kg.

   $11.66 / 77 \times 100 = 15.14\%$

3. Figure

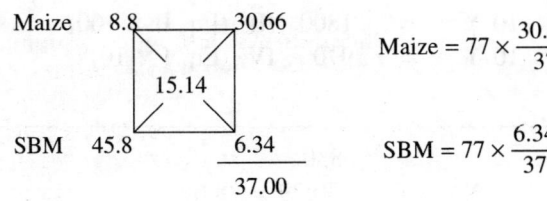

$$\text{Maize} = 77 \times \frac{30.66}{37} = 63.81$$

$$\text{SBM} = 77 \times \frac{6.34}{37} = 13.19$$

4. Final ration

Oats	=	20.00
Minerals and vitamins	=	3.00
Maize	=	63.81
Soybean meal	=	13.19
		100.00

II Algebraic Method

Example 1: A farmer has the following ingredients

	CP	TDN
	%	
Groundnut cake	44	71
Gingilly cake	34	78
Sorghum grain	9	75
Maize grain	10	75
Rice bran	11	60

Compute a concentrate mixture with 18% CP and 70% TDN. Incorporate mineral mixture and salt at 2 and 1%, respectively.

Procedure:

1. Divide the ingredients into two groups based on their CP content and calculate the average CP.

$$\text{Oil seed cakes} = \frac{44 + 34}{2} = \frac{78}{2} = 39$$

$$\text{Grains and bran} = \frac{9 + 10 + 11}{3} = \frac{30}{3} = 10.0$$

2. Restrictions: Mineral mixture and salt = 3%
   Let X be kg of oil seed cakes for 97 kg mixture
   Let Y be kg of grains and bran for 97 kg mixture

X	+	Y	=	97	I	
0.39 X	+	0.1 Y	=	18	II	(minerals and salt do not contribute crude protein)
39 X	+	10 Y	=	1800	III	(Eq. II × 100)
10 X	+	10 Y	=	970	IV	(Eq. I × 10)
-		-		-		

$$29 X = 830$$
$$X = 830/29 = 28.6$$
$$Y = 97 - 28.6 = 68.4$$

$$\text{Groundnut cake} = 28.6 \times \frac{44}{78} = 16.1$$

$$\text{Gingilly cake} = 28.6 \times \frac{34}{78} = 12.5$$

Sorghum	=	68.4 × 9/30 = 20.5
Maize	=	68.4 × 10/30 = 22.8
Rice bran	=	68.4 × 11/30 = 25.1

Final Ration		CP	TDN			
Sorghum grain	20.5	1.845	15.375			
Maize grain	22.8	2.28	17.1			
Rice bran	25.1	2.761		15.06	CP	= 18.22%
Groundnut cake	16.1	7.084	11.43		TDN	= 68.72%
Gingilly cake	12.5	4.25	9.75			
Mineral mixture	2.0	-	-			
Salt	1.0	-	-			
Total	100.0	18.22	68.72			

Feeding of Dairy Cattle and Buffaloes: Formulation of Rations — Balanced Ration and its Characteristics

Ration: A ration is the feed offered for a given animal during a day of 24 hours. The feed may be given at a time or in proportions at intervals.

Balanced ration: A balanced ration is one that furnishes nutrients in such proportions and amounts that it will properly nourish a given animal for 24 hours (Morrison, 1956). In addition, the required nutrients must be contained in the amount of dry matter (DM) the animal is able to consume in the 24 - hr period; otherwise the ration can not be considered balanced.

Desirable Characteristics of a Ration

1. The ration should have highly digestible feed ingredients. For example, feather meal contains 87% CP but its digestibility is as low as 15-20%. Therefore it is not the amount which is present in the feed is important but how much is digested by the animal, i.e., DCP and TDN. The ration should be balanced.

2. The feed must be palatable. Evil smelling, musty, mouldy feed should not be given. If unpalatable, improve the palatability by the addition of salt and molasses.

3. Variety of feeds in the ration makes it more palatable. A balanced combination of proteins, vitamins and other nutrients are furnished by incorporating many feeds in a ration.

4. The ration should contain enough of mineral matter. This is especially important in case of milch animals since each litre of milk had more than 0.7% ash.

5. The ration should be fairly laxative; otherwise the animal may suffer from constipation. Hence succulent green fodders should be included in the ration.

6. Green succulent fodders have cooling effect. They aid the appetite and keep the animal in good condition. They are bulky, easily digestible, rich source of carotene, other vitamins and minerals. Leguminous green fodders are rich in proteins and calcium.

7. The ration should be fairly bulky to satisfy the hunger. If it is too bulky the animal will fail to get all its nutrient requirements.

8. Avoid sudden change in the diet; it may cause tympanitis, impaction, etc. All changes of food must be gradual and slow.

9. Maintain regularity in feeding. The time of feeding should be evenly distributed so that the animals are not kept too long without feed.

10. Feed should be properly prepared to render it more digestible and palatable. e.g. grinding of grains, chaffing of coarse fodders, moistening of dry fodders, soaking of cotton seed and other cakes before feeding.
11. Economy in labour and cost: The cost of feed and labour charges should be minimized to make rearing of livestock profitable.

Computation of Ration for Cattle and Buffaloes

Computation of rations involve translating the recommendations contained in feeding standards into actual formulation of feed mixtures and feeding practices. In computing rations for ruminants the dry matter, digestible protein (DCP), energy (TDN), minerals and vitamin A are given consideration.

Dry matter: The DM requirement of an animal depends on its body weight and its status of productivity. Cattle generally eat daily 2.0 to 2.5 kg DM for every 100 kg of body weight. Buffaloes and crossbred animals are slightly heavy eaters and their DM consumption varies from 2.5 to 3.0 kg per 100 kg body weight. In ruminants bulk is essential and the DM allowance is divided as follows.

Total DM
┌─ 2/3 as roughage ──── ┌─ 2/3 dry roughage
│   └─ 1/3 green roughage*
└─ 1/3 as concentrates

*If the green fodder is a legume, the proportion of green fodder may be reduced to 1/4 DM of the total roughage component and the remaining 3/4 is dry roughage.

Requirement of other nutrients for maintenance, growth, milk production, gestation and work are given separately. Refer the 'Nutritional Requirements of Indian cattle and buffaloes'.

Partitioning of DM between Roughages and Concentrates: An Example
A 400 kg crossbred cow require 10 kg dry matter per day.

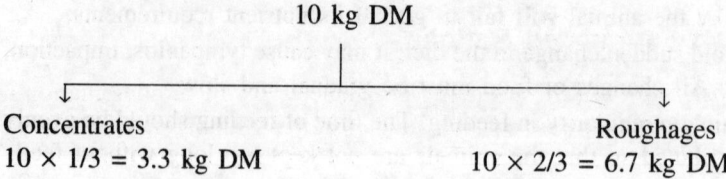

10 kg DM

Concentrates
10 × 1/3 = 3.3 kg DM

Roughages
10 × 2/3 = 6.7 kg DM

If green legume is available

DM as green roughage $6.7 \times 1/4$ = 1.7 kg;
(e.g. subabul green fodder (34% DM) = 1.7/0.34 = 5 kg)
DM as dry roughage $6.7 \times 3/4$ = 5 kg

It nonlegume green fodder is available

DM as green fodder $6.7 \times 1/3$ = 2.2 kg; [e.g. Hybrid
napier/Para grass (25% DM]   = 2.2/0.25 = 8.8 = say 9.0 kg)
DM as dry roughage $6.7 \times 2/3$ = 4.5 kg

Methods Employed in Formulating a Ration

Pearson's square method: Pearson's square method has been used for ration formulation for many years. However, it cannot handle inequalities and ranges, and rations are independent of price of the feed ingredients. Further, this method can balance only one nutrient at a time and so has limited application in diet formulations as situations demand balancing many nutrients at a time.

Trial-and-error method: The trial-and-error method is very popular to formulate rations. As the name implies, the formulation is manipulated until the nutrient requirements are attained and thus ration is balanced. Ration formulation by trial-and-error method can be done manually on paper or with the aid of computer spreadsheet programmes like Excel. It is laborious and takes more time to arrive at a fairly satisfactory solution.

Linear programming: The use of linear programming (LP; page 82) in ration formulation came into being in late 60's in feed mixing plants and animal farms. The experience of LP applications over the years proved that this programme alone is not sufficient to solve the complicated demands for precision animal nutrition (PAN).

Linear and stochastic programming method: Current trend is to integrate the advantage of LP and different other optimization programmes for solving the varying nutritional problems. One such method is called Stochastic programming (stochastic is a Greek word meaning 'skillful at aiming'). This method came into being for effective incorporation of nutrient variability into the formulation process so that the requirement of the animal is met with a measured level of certainty.

Computer-Formulated Rations

'Least cost' ration: If a ration is balanced using a combination of ingredients with the lowest possible total cost, the resulting mixture is called a "least cost" ration.

Formulating a ration to fulfill the nutrient needs of the animal at the lowest possible cost is difficult by hand. The 'simplex method' (Heady and Candler, 1966) can be used for such calculations, but it requires a tremendous amount of time when large numbers of feeds and nutrient requirements are considered.

Linear Programming: The technique employed to calculate least-cost and profit maximizing rations is called linear programming. A simple definition of linear programming is the "maximizing or minimizing of some function subject to constraints". In the case of livestock rations, it is the minimizing of the cost of a ration or maximizing the income above feed cost.

Computer programmes have been developed that allowed the calculation of optimum and least-cost rations in a matter of seconds. Some of the programmes are available from mainframe computers over telephone lines to remote computer terminals (Bath and Bennett, 1980); also some programmes have been developed to run on microcomputers, thus making both the computer hardware and software available at a reasonable cost to many dairymen.

With the use of computerized linear programming models, the prices of available feed ingredients as well as their nutrient contents can be considered when formulating rations. With computer formulations many more specifications and/or restrictions are feasible as compared to hand calculations. Accuracy and speed of calculation are the major advantages of computer formulation.

Nutrient requirements in terms of the nutrients, the minimum or maximum amounts of each nutrient is entered. Then for each feed to be considered, the current price, nutrient composition and percentage limitations are considered. Using this information, the computer picks the mixture of feed ingredients which will satisfy the nutrient levels specified with the least cost. Limits may also be included on individual feed ingredients. For example, salt and urea can be locked at the fixed amount. Level of molasses may be restricted for either mechanical or nutritional reasons.

Limitations

1. Nutrient density within the mix: If nutrient levels specified for the mix are low, the computer will add a low cost ingredient as a filler to reduce the cost of the ration. While the ration price may be very low, the filler may be of no benefit to the animal. In this manner, a least cost mixture may not produce least cost production.

    Conversely, if the nutrient density of the mix is specified too high, the computer is forced to use feeds with concentrated nutrients which will rise the cost of production even though the mix is least cost at the specifications set.

2. The 'Associative effects' of feeds are not considered.

Steps in Formulating a Ration

1. Calculate the probable DM intake (DMI) of the animal in question.
2. Calculate the nutrient requirements of the animal.
3. Determine the amounts of available ingredients that must be fed to fulfill the animal's nutrient requirements within its expected DMI limits.

Feeding of pregnant animals

Pregnant animals are to be offered extra nutrients during (Table 6 and 7) the last two months of gestation. The aim is that by the end of gestation period the cows and buffaloes should not only gain their initial body weight but also put on an extra 25 to 30 kg of body weight. This is necessary to enable the animal to withstand the stress of parturition and to maintain the persistency of milk production during the subsequent lactation period. The provision of extra nutrients should be given in the form of concentrate mixture and not as forage because roughages are not as efficient as concentrates in increasing the body weight. The rest of the ration must contain sufficient green feeds so that the colostrum secreted after parturition should be rich in vitamin A.

Feed intake decreases around 15% during the last week before calving. During the last 3 days prior to calving, the amount of concentrate mixture should be reduced and a little warm bran is fed to keep the animal in laxative condition before calving.

Feeding of milch animals

After parturition, the cow/buffalo should be given fresh warm water and a mash consisting of 1 kg wheat bran, 1-1.5 kg ground/cooked grain, 0.5 kg jaggery and 25 g each of common salt and mineral mixture. This mash may be continued for 3 to 4 days after calving; the regular feed is gradually introduced to the cow. The nutrient requirements of a lactating cow/buffalo can be conveniently divided into two parts, *viz.* maintenance requirement and milk production requirement. If the lactating animal is in first and second lactation, extra allowance, needed to take care of growth production, has also to be added (Table 1).

The maintenance requirement of lactating animals for energy is higher by 10% than in dry animals. During early lactation dry matter intake falls around 15-20% after parturition, while the requirements for milk synthesis continue to increase up to 6-7 weeks post-parturition, which often results in negative energy balance in lactating animals.

In feeding high-milk yielder, quality feed i.e., nutrient dense feed need to be given. Ration should contain a minimum 25% DM from forages. Forage should be of superior quality and 30 to 50% of this should be from leguminous crops. Concentrate mixture supplementation should be given ideally in installments and not more than 1 kg at a time, in order to control the drop in the rumen pH. Hence the ration may be in the form of complete feed or total mixed ration (TMR). Frequency of feeding is four times a day. To ensure proper nutrient intake, optimum roughage concentrate ratio need to be maintained.

Lactation curve

Following calving, the milk production starts rising and reaches a peak by about 7 weeks and then gradually falls by the end of lactation (305 days). Increments in feed intakes occur more slowly than the increases in milk yield. Cow/buffalo is able to consume less energy than she is expending. Hence milch animals use their own body tissues for about 12 weeks after calving to provide energy in addition to that consumed.

Lactation curve has a characteristic shape. It consists of four phases.

First phase '10–12 weeks': During the 10-12 weeks of lactation, milk production increases rapidly while milk fat percentage inversely follows the lactation curve. Dry matter intake rises after calving but lags behind the needs of the rapidly increasing milk production. The cow is able to consume less energy than she is expending. This is a most difficult phase for feeding and the cow / buffalo loses body weight over this period. Higher weight loss may lead to metabolic disease and impaired fertility.

Second phase '12–24 weeks': During phase two, DMI is at its maximum. The cow / buffalo should no longer be in negative balance.

Third phase 'week 24– till end of lactation': Phase three is the period when yield begins to fall. During this period the cow / buffalo should be able to restore weight lost in early lactation as well as supporting the increasing demands of the developing fetus. It is generally more profitable to improve the condition of the cow / buffalo in late lactation rather than in the dry period, since lactating cows use energy more efficiently for weight gain (75% efficient) compared to dry cows (59% efficient).

Fourth phase 'dry period': Phase four is the dry period of 60 days. The dry period is between the 'end of one lactation and the beginning of the next'. The purpose of a dry period is to allow the cow's udder an opportunity to regenerate secretory tissue and to allow the digestive system to recover from the stress of high levels of feed intake. Rations are predominantly based on good quality forage and should be supplemented with vitamins and minerals.

Steaming Up: During the latter weeks of the dry period (14 days prior to calving) the rumen of the cow / buffalo should be prepared for the diet it is going to be fed in early lactation. Rumen microflora and fauna take 10-14 days to adjust to a new substrate i.e., post-calving diet. Feeding large amounts of concentrates before calving is necessary so that the cow / buffalo can store sufficient resources to be drawn on in early lactation. This proactive feeding is known as 'steaming up'. Feeding concentrates is helpful to stimulate the restoration of the rumen papillae which in turn increases post-calving absorption from the rumen.

Lead feeding / challenge feeding

Calving to peak milk production: Once the pregnant animal calves the milk letdown is initiated and the milk production in dairy animals increases for 80-90 days. As the animal increases production during the first 3 months, it is beneficial to calculate her production needs and continue to add little extra nutrients to take care of the increasing production. Feeding a bit more then, is what is called lead feeding. This is also called challenge feeding. High milk producing animals are fed increasing quantity of feed challenging them to produce at their maximum potential. Best grades of hay, high grain level, undegradable intake protein (UIP) to meet as much as one-third of the total protein requirements, sodium bicarbonate as a rumen buffer to avoid acidosis are offered.

Rations for Cattle and Buffaloes: Some Examples

All these examples are calculated based on ICAR (1998) nutrient requirements.

Example 1: Computation of a ration for a dry cow weighing 400 kg.

Computation of a ration includes noting down the requirements of the animal and formulation of a ration using the available feedstuffs. In this example, three rations have been suggested utilizing the home-grown fodders. Common salt and mineral mixture are to be supplemented.

	RM* kg	DM kg	DCP kg	TDN kg	Ca kg	P kg	Carotene mg
Requirement of the animal	-	5.5	0.25	3.0	0.017	0.013	42
Ration I							
Green grass (25, 1, 12, 0.07, 0.04)**							
(Hybrid napier/Para/Guinea)	25	6.25	0.25	3.0	0.0175	0.01	–
Ration II							
Green grass (25, 1, 12)	10	2.5	0.1	1.2	0.007	0.004	–
Leguminous green fodder (15, 2.5, 10, 0.3, 0.05) (Berseem/Lucerne/cowpea)	6	0.9	0.15	0.6	0.018	0.003	–
Rice straw/ Wheat straw (90, 0, 44, 0.5, 0.12)	3	2.7	0	1.32	0.015	0.0036	–
Total	–	6.1	0.25	3.12	0.033	0.0066	–
Ration III							
Green grass (25, 1, 12)	10	2.5	0.1	1.2	0.007	0.004	–
Rice straw/wheat straw (90, 0, 44)	3.5	3.15	0	1.54	0.0175	0.0042	–
Groundnut cake (90, 42, 71, 0.2, 0.7)	0.35	0.315	0.147	0.249	0.0007	0.0025	–
Total	–	6.0	0.247	3.0	0.025	0.011	–

*Raw Material.

**% Composition of the feed in the order of DM, DCP, TDN, Ca and P.

The rations formulated supplied more TDN than required and it is good to furnish a little extra. This holds good in case of other nutrients also. In formulating rations, concentrate mixtures, with specific DCP and TDN, may also be formulated (see example 4 for details) to supply the balance of nutrients of the ration.

Example 2: A farmer has a 350 kg cow giving 4 to 6 kg of milk. Formulate a ration using rice straw, perennial green grass (from field bunds), rice bran, wheat bran, groundnut cake.

1. The dry matter requirement is 8.75 kg at the rate of 2.5 kg per 100 kg BW.

2. Nutrient requirement:

Function	DCP kg	TDN kg	Ca g	P g	Carotene mg	Vit. A 1000 IU
Maintenance	0.230	2.7	14	11	37	15
Production per kg milk 4% fat	0.045	0.315	2.7	2.0		
4 kg of milk	0.180	1.260	10.8	8.0		
6 kg of milk	0.270	1.890	16.2	12.0		
Total requirement for 4 kg milk yield	0.410	3.96	24.8	19.0	37	15
Total requirement for 6 kg milk yield	0.500	4.59	30.2	23.0	37	15

3. Formulating the ration for cow yielding 4 kg milk

Feedstuff	RM kg	DM kg	DCP kg	TDN kg	Ca kg	P kg
Ration I						
Rice Straw (90, 0, 44)	5	4.5	0	2.2	0.025	0.006
Green grass (25, 1.5, 15)	6	1.5	0.09	0.9	0.0042	0.0024
Wheat bran (90, 10, 68, 0.1, 0.8)	1.0	0.9	0.10	0.68	0.001	0.008
Deoiled Rice bran (90, 6, 60, 0.08, 1.5)	0.6	0.54	0.036	0.36	0.005	0.009
Groundnut Cake (90, 42, 71)	0.5	0.45	0.21	0.355	0.001	0.0035
	-	7.89	0.436	4.495	0.0317	0.0289

Feedstuff	RM kg	DM kg	DCP kg	TDN kg
Ration II				
Rice straw	5	4.5	0	2.2
Green grass	6	1.5	0.09	0.9
Deoiled rice bran	2	1.8	0.12	1.2
Groundnut cake	0.5	0.45	0.21	0.36
	-	8.25	0.42	4.66

Ration III

Rice straw 5	4.5	0	2.2	
Green grass	10	2.5	0.15	1.5
Deoiled rice bran	1	0.9	0.06	0.6
Groundnut cake	0.5	0.45	0.21	0.36
	-	8.35	0.42	4.66

Formulating the ration for cow yielding 6 kg milk

Ration I

Rice straw 5	4.5	0	2.2	
Green grass	6	1.5	0.09	0.9
Wheat bran	1.5	1.35	0.15	1.02
Deoiled Rice bran	1.0	0.9	0.06	0.6
Groundnut cake	0.5	0.45	0.21	0.36
	-	8.70	0.51	5.08

Ration formulation may also be done as explained here.

	4 kg yield		6 kg yield	
	DCP kg	TDN kg	DCP kg	TDN kg
Total requirement of the cow	0.410	3.96	0.500	4.59
Nutrients met from the roughages (5 kg rice straw and 6 kg green grass)	0.09	3.10	0.09	3.10
Nutrients to be supplied from concentrate mixture	0.32	0.86	0.41	1.49

A 2 kg concentrate mixture meets the requirement of the cow yielding 4 kg milk while the other one needs 2.5 kg mixture. The composition of the concentrate mixture: Groundnut cake (extr) 14, Sunflowerseed cake (extr) 15, Tapioca thippi 11, Wheat bran 10, Deoiled rice bran 30, Molasses 16, Urea 1, Mineral mixture 2 and Salt 1%. DCP 15.94%; TDN 62.7%.

Example 3: A farmer has been given a crossbred Jersey cow giving 10 kg of milk with 5% butter fat. Weight of the cow is 400 kg. Formulate a ration for the cow using locally available feedstuffs (Rice straw, hybrid napier green grass, groundnut cake and deoiled rice bran).

i. DM requirement @ 2.5 to 3 kg/100 kg BW is 10 to 12 kg
ii. Nutrient requirement:

Function	DCP kg	TDN kg	Ca g	P g	Carotene mg	Vitamin A 1000 IU
A. Maintenance	0.250	3.0	17	13	42	17
B. Milk production	0.510	3.7	29	22	-	-
Total	0.760	6.7	46	35	42	17

iii. Ration formulation

Feedstuffs	RM kg	DM kg	DCP kg	TDN kg	Ca kg	P kg
Rice straw (90, 0, 44)	5	4.5	0	2.2	0.025	0.006
Hybrid napier (25, 1, 15)	15	3.75	0.15	2.25	0.0105	0.006
Groundnut cake	1	0.9	0.42	0.71	0.002	0.007
Deoiled rice bran	3	2.7	0.18	1.80	0.0024	0.045
Calcite	30 g	-	-	-	0.0102	-
Salt	30 g	-	-	-	-	-
	-	11.85	0.75	6.96	0.0501	0.064

Example 4: Compute a ration for a 350 kg BW cow yielding 11 kg of FCM in its second lactation.

i. DM requirement = 8.75 to 10.75
ii. Nutrient requirement:

Function	DCP kg	TDN kg	Ca g	P g	Carotene mg	Vitamin A 1000 IU
A. Maintenance	0.230	2.7	14	11	37	15
B. Growth allowance during 2nd lactation (10% of maintenance)	0.023	0.27	1.4	1.1	3.7	1.5
C. Milk production	0.495	3.465	29.7	22	-	-
Total	0.748	6.435	45.1	34.1	40.7	16.5

iii. Ration formulation

Feedstuff	RM kg	DM kg	DCP kg	TDN kg
Rice straw	5	4.5	0	2.0
Green grass	6	1.5	0.06	0.72
	-	6.0	0.06	2.72

Difference of nutrients to   2.75 to
be met from concentrates   4.5 kg DM, 0.688   3.715

If TDN of the concentrate mixture is 75%;

Quantity of concentrate mixture required $= \dfrac{3.715}{0.75} = 4.95$ or say 5 kg

Therefore, % DCP of the

concentrate mixture $= \dfrac{0.688}{5} = 0.1376 = 13.76\%$

Ration for the cow:		**Composition of the concentrate mixture %**	
Rice straw	5 kg	Maize	32.0
Green grass	6 kg	Wheat	15.0
Concentrate mixture 5 kg		Deoiled rice bran	10.0
with 13.8% DCP		Wheat bran	10.0
75.0% TDN		Groundnut cake (extr)	5.0
0.5-0.7% Ca		Coconut cake	10.0
0.3-0.4% P		Soybean meal	10.0
		Molasses	5.0
		Mineral mixture	2.0
		Salt	1.0
			100.0

Example 5: Compute rations using a sole leguminous green fodder or rice straw and a proprietary concentrate mixture for a cow (400 kg BW) yielding 10 kg milk with 5% BF per day.

Nutrient requirement

Function	RM kg	DM kg	DCP kg	TDN kg
Maintenance			0.250	3.0
Milk production 10 kg with 5% BF			0.51	3.7
Total requirement			0.76	6.7

Ration I:

Leguminous green fodder Berseem /Lucerne/Cowpea (15, 2.5, 10)	70	10.5	1.75	7.0

Experiments conducted at NDRI, Karnal and IVRI, Izatnagar have shown that *ad libitum* feeding on berseem green fodder (70 kg berseem) supported milk production up to 10 kg per day. Minerals are to be given to balance the ration. The problem of bloat, which has been reported occasionally, can be avoided by introducing greens gradually, offering 1 kg in the form of hay or wilted forage.

Ration II:

Rice straw (90, 0, 44)	6	5.4	0	2.64
Concentrate mixture (90, 15, 75)	5.5	4.95	0.825	4.125
Total	–	10.35	0.825	6.765

The composition of the concentrate mixture: Maize 32, Wheat 15, Deoiled rice bran 10, Wheat bran 10, Groundnut cake (extr) 5, Soybean meal 10, Coconut cake 10, Molasses 4, Urea 1, Min. mixture 2 and Salt 1 per cent.

Feeding Cattle and Buffaloes by Thumb Rule Method

Although the conventional method of ration formulation is based on scientific experimentation, the common farmer finds difficult to follow the computation on bodyweight basis. The following thumb rule may guide them to feed their livestock satisfactorily. This is based on practical experiences rather than scientific basis as discussed in the conventional method.

1. Maintenance Ration

Feedstuff	For zebu cattle	For crossbred cows and buffaloes
a. Straw	4 kg	4-6 kg
b. Concentrate mixture		
14-16% DCP 68-72% TDN	1-1.25 kg	2.0 kg

2. Extra Allowance during Pregnancy

During the last trimester of pregnancy, a further quantity of 1.25 and 1.75 kg concentrate is recommended for Zebu and Crossbred cow/buffalo, respectively.

3. Extra Allowance for Milk Production

Additional amount of 1 kg concentrate mixture is required for every 2.5 kg of milk over and above the maintenance requirement in case of Zebu cattle and 2.0 kg of milk in case of buffaloes. Cow milk is assumed to contain 4% BF while buffalo milk 6%. The concentrate mixture contains 20% CP, 65% TDN, 0.5-0.7% Ca and 0.3-0.4% P.

Computation of Ration for a Herd

When a large number of animals in a farm are to be fed a balanced ration, it is impracticable to compute rations on individual animal basis. Usually, the herd is divided into several groups like dry cows, dry and pregnant cows, cows in milk, infant calves (up to 6 months of age), young stock (6 months to one year of age), young males (1 year to 2 years), young heifers (1 year to 2 years), bulls, bullocks, etc. By doing so, the individuals present, in any particular group (based further on live weight) may not vary widely from each other, so that liberal feeding standard for each group will provide a sufficient margin of safety in the provision of nutrients to meet the requirements of all the individuals in that group.

It is customary to provide the maintenance ration primarily through roughage if good quality roughage is available, or some concentrate mixture is supplemented to the roughages like straw and concentrate mixture is provided to meet the production requirements.

The average body weight of the animals in a herd is taken to compute the ration for the maintenance purpose and depending upon the amount of milk produced, (in case of milch animals) the concentrate mixture is fed at the rate of 1 kg for every 2.5 kg of milk produced if it is a cow and 1 kg for every 2 kg of milk produced if it is a buffalo.

Example: Herd average body weight = 400 kg; Furnish a feeding programme.

Maintenance requirement = 0.254 kg DCP, 3.03 kg TDN

Maintenance Rations

Three alternate rations are furnished hereunder.

Ration A. 25 kg green grass (hybrid napier/para/guinea grass)

Ration B. 10 kg green grass, 3.5 kg paddy straw and 350 g of groundnut cake

Ration C. 10 kg green grass, 6 kg leguminous green fodder and 3 kg paddy straw

Concentrate mixture is formulated by using either Pearson square method or algebraic method. Such a mixture is offered to meet the production requirement of animals in the herd.

Examples of Concentrate Mixtures

1.
Groundnut cake (exp)	15		
Gingilly cake	14		
Jowar	20	DCP	= 16.4%
Maize	22	TDN	= 72.4%
Deoiled rice bran	26		
Mineral mixture	2		
Salt	1		
	100		

2.
Groundnut cake	15		
Jowar	20		
Maize	22	DCP	= 11.37%
Tapioca thippi	14	TDN	= 70.45%
Deoiled rice bran	26		
Mineral mixture	2		
Salt	1		
	100		

3. | | |
    | --- | --- |
    | Groundnut cake | 12 |
    | Maize | 21 |
    | Wheat bran | 30 |
    | Deoiled rice bran | 25 |
    | Molasses | 9 |
    | Mineral mixture | 2 |
    | Salt | 1 |
    | | 100 |

    DCP = 11.18%
    TDN = 68.11%

4. | | |
    | --- | --- |
    | Groundnut cake | 10 |
    | Wheat bran | 30 |
    | Deoiled rice bran | 25 |
    | Tapioca thippi | 15 |
    | Molasses | 16 |
    | Urea | 1 |
    | Mineral mixture | 2 |
    | Salt | 1 |
    | | 100 |

    DCP = 11.96%
    TDN = 62.24%

5. | | |
    | --- | --- |
    | Sunflower cake | 10 |
    | Deoiled rice bran | 30 |
    | Wheat bran | 25 |
    | Tapioca tippi | 15 |
    | Molasses | 16 |
    | Urea | 1 |
    | Mineral mixutre | 2 |
    | Salt | 1 |
    | | 100 |

    DCP = 9.86%
    TDN = 62.14%

6. | | |
    | --- | --- |
    | Groundnut cake (extr) | 14 |
    | Sunflower seed cake (extr) | 15 |
    | Tapioca thippi | 11 |
    | Wheat bran | 10 |
    | Deoiled rice bran | 30 |
    | Molasses | 16 |
    | Urea | 1 |
    | Mineral mixture | 2 |
    | Salt | 1 |
    | | 100 |

    CP = 21.34%
    DCP = 15.94%
    TDN = 62.73%

Exercise on ration formulation

Exercise 1: Compute a ration for a crossbred cow of 500 kg BW yielding 20 kg milk with 4% BF in its third lactation.

Requirements:

Function	DM kg	DCP kg	TDN kg	Ca g	P g
Maintenance		0.296	3.69	20	15
Production		0.900	6.32	54	40
Total	15	1.196	10.01	74	55

Ration

Feedstuff	RM	DM	DCP	TDN Ca	P
	←		kg		→
Hybrid napier/para green fodder					
Rice straw					
Maize grain					
Groundnut cake					
DORB					
Minerals					

Exercise 2: Compute a ration for a crossbred cow weighing 400 kg yielding 10 kg milk with 4% BF in its 2nd lactation.

Requirements:

Function	DM kg	DCP kg	TDN kg	Ca g	P g
Maintenance		0.254	3.03	17	13
Production		0.450	3.16	27	20
Growth		0.025	0.30	2	1
Total	10	0.729	6.49	46	34

Ration

Feedstuff	RM	DM	DCP	TDN	Ca	P
		←		kg		→
Para grass (green)						
Groundnut straw						
Rice straw						
Maize grain						
Groundnut cake						
DORB						
Minerals						

Feeding of Calves — Importance of Colostrum; Milk Replacers and Calf Starters

Requirements for growth: The nutrient requirements of growing calves may be divided into two phases, namely preruminant growth period, that is before the rumen is anatomically and physiologically developed and postruminant growth, that is after the rumen has been developed. Daily nutrient requirements are presented in Table 8 and 9A.

Preruminant Growth (from Birth to 3 Months of Age)

The nourishment of the calf should be taken care of much before it is born. That is why extra nutrients should be provided during the last two months of gestation. The expectant dam should also be provided with 15 to 20 kg of green fodder daily so that the colostrum secreted will be rich in vitamin A. Vitamin A content of colostrum is normally dependent on the type of ration given to the cow prior to parturition. If green fodder was not offered, the calf should be given at least 10,000 IU of vitamin A in its first feed within a few hours after its birth. For the next 7 days, the dosage may be reduced to 5000 IU per day. Carotene cannot replace vitamin A in feeding infant calves, as they are unable to convert carotene into vitamin A. Thereafter, the dosage may be 1000-2000 IU daily, in case the cow is not receiving any green fodder. If the cow is fed liberally with green fodder, vitamin A supplementation can be stopped.

Practical Calf—Feeding Schedule

Under the natural system of rearing, the calf sucks milk from its mother's udder as long as the latter is in milk. Usually the calf is allowed to suck for a few seconds only to induce letdown of milk, and later a little quantity of milk is left in the udder after milking. The allowance of milk to the calf is mostly insufficient and the calves fail to grow at a proper rate.

The calves, in all well-organized farms, are separated (weaned) from their mothers soon after parturition and then hand fed with measured quantities of milk (at 1/10 of the body weight) in a bucket or pail. The calf can be trained to drink colostrum and later milk from a pail with due care. It must be remembered that calf's natural instinct is to suck milk from its mother with its mouth turned upwards so that the ingested milk flows directly into omasum and abomasum through the esophageal groove.

Colostrum: The first feed or the colostrum should be given fresh as milked from the mother within 2 hours. Colostrum should not be warmed, as due to the presence of large quantities of protein, it will clot during heating.

During the first 3 days of its life the calf should receive colostrum. The feeding of colostrum is important because of the following.

(i) The protein content of colostrum is 17% as against only 3.5% in ordinary milk. A major portion of the protein is globulin in nature. Globulins are found in blood but are present only in traces in ordinary milk. The globulins of colostrum contain antibodies which help the body system in fighting diseases and are called immunoglobulins (IgM, IgG, IgA). The newborn calf has little or no reserve of antibodies (antibodies cannot pass through the placental membranes) and its intestinal wall permits the passage of whole globulin at least during the first 12 hours of its life. Later in life, intact proteins are not absorbed.

(ii) The high content of vitamins (A, D and E) and minerals (Ca, Mg, Fe, and P) help the calf to resist infections.

(iii) The laxative action of the colostrum helps the calf in evacuating the accumulated faecal matter from its intestines. The faecal matter if not excreted may undergo fermentation and release toxins, causing ill-health or even death.

Refrigeration of colostrum–Need for instant cooling of the colostrum container

The bacteria will not yet have had time to replicate, if colostrum is fed to a newborn roughly within one hour after it is collected from the mother. When colostrum availability is more than the requirement, it may be kept in a refrigerator to avoid the bacterial growth. However, about 77% of refrigerated colostrum contains such a high bacterial count (more than 100,000 colony forming units/ml), that it can make the calves sick (Emmy Koeleman of All About Feed, 6 Aug 2014). It was concluded that the bacteria are grown during the storage of the colostrum. Hence there is a need to cool the colostrum container instantly to inactivate the bacteria.

When bacteria are introduced into colostrum they do not begin to grow immediately and need lag phase. Bacteria in freshly milked colostrum (temperature of colostrum equals to the animal body temperature) double in 20 minutes. At 15°C this doubling (or generation) time is about 2.5 hours. At refrigerator temperature of 4.5°C generation time is over 24 hours. Hence, when the colostrum is to be stored put the container in an ice water bath first, which reduces the temperature to 15°C within half an hour, before storing the container in the fridge.

Artificial colostrum: If colostrum is not available, **artificial colostrum** can be made as follows. Take 275 ml of warm water, add the contents of one raw egg (55 g), 3 ml of castor oil, 10,000 IU of vitamin A, 525 ml of warm whole milk and 80 mg of aureomycin; Mix well and feed at 40°C. This is sufficient for one meal. The calf should be fed thus three times a day. Whole milk is given from the fourth day onwards till it attains three months of age. The milk is given after warming it to a temperature of 40°C.

From the 15th day of its age a small quantity of good hay, preferably a legume hay, and a little calf starter may be offered (Table 14). Early introduction of solid feed helps in the rapid development of rumen; drenching of rumen fluid collected from adult animals also helps to achieve this.

TABLE 14 Feeding Schedule of Calves up to 3 Months of Age*.

Age of calf	Whole milk	Calf starter	Good quality hay
1-3 days	Colostrum @ 1/10th BW in 3 feeds	-	-
4-7 days **	Whole milk @ 1/10th BW in 3 feeds	-	-
8-14 days	Whole milk @ 1/10th BW	-	-
15-21 days	Whole milk @ 1/10th BW	A little	A little
22-35 days	Whole milk @ 1/15th BW	100 g	Ad lib
Up to 2 months	Whole milk @ 1/20th BW	250 g	Ad lib
2-3 months	Milk is gradually reduced and tapered	500 g	Ad lib

*This schedule is satisfactory to produce a daily growth rate of 0.5 kg in crossbred calves.
**Milk replacer can be given directly after colostrum feeding or after one week of age.

Milk replacers: Milk replacer is usually fed in the gruel form. The amount is gradually increased with a simultaneous decrease in the amount of whole milk. It should have good quality ingredients. The saved milk is available for human consumption.

Example 1.

Dried skim milk	50.00
Dried whey	30.00
Dextrose	8.00
Oat flour	5.00
Brewer's yeast	5.00
Irradiated yeast	0.26
Trace minerals	0.04
Stabilized Vit. A supplement	1.70
	100.00

Example 2.

Wheat flour	10.00
Fish meal	12.00
Linseed meal	40.00
Coconut oil	7.00
Linseed oil	3.00
Butyric acid	0.30
Citric acid	1.40
Molasses	10.00
Mineral mixture	3.00
Aurofac	0.30
Milk	13.00
	100.00
Rovimix	15 g

This has been developed at NDRI, Karnal.

Calf starter: It is a solid feed consisting of ground grains, oil cakes, animal protein supplements and brans fortified with vitamins, minerals and antibiotic feed supplements. It should contain 23-26% CP, DCP 18.8–19.5% and 75% TDN. Use of antibiotics helps in checking the occurrence of scour. The daily allowance of antibiotic preparation is generally 3 to 6 g.

A calf needs a relatively large proportion of protein in its ration so as to furnish the basic building blocks (amino acids) for the rapid growth of its tissues. The proportion of protein in the ration should be less as the animal grows older. The quality of protein given to the calf depends on the age of the calf. Since the rumen is not developed, the protein in the calf ration should be of high BV. Milk replacers and calf starters should contain some animal proteins. If calves receive sufficient milk up to the age of 2 months, the supply of good quality protein is ensured. Once the rumen is developed, the microflora present in the rumen can convert inferior type of protein into better quality microbial protein, which can be utilized by the animal by digestion in the abomasum and further.

Growth rate of calves up to 3 months of age is similar in bull and heifer calves and thereafter heifer calves grow at a slower rate.

Calf starter is a crucial link for proper rumen development and successful weaning. As per NRC (2001), a good quality calf starter should contain 18 % CP. Studies conducted at Veterinary College, Mannuthy, Kerala (Jini et al., 2015) revealed that phase feeding can be practiced in pre-ruminant crossbred calves with calf starter containing 15% CP in milk feeding phase (1 to 6 weeks) and 18% CP in weaned phase (6 weeks to 20 weeks), without any adverse effect on their growth performance, compared to those fed on calf starter with 24% CP both in milk feeding and weaned phase.

Feeding Schedule of Calves from 3 Months to 1 Year

From the third month onward cultivated green forages (Hybrid napier, Para, Guinea, Maize, etc.) can be given at the rate of 2 kg per day, raising the quantity to 5 to 10 kg at 6 months of age. Simultaneously the quantity of hay can be reduced. Green leguminous forages like berseem or lucerne should be wilted in the sun for 3-4 hours before feeding to minimize bloat. Type I concentrate mixture may be offered at the rate of 0.75 kg, 1 kg and 1.5 kg per calf during 4th, 5th and 6th month of its age. The quantity of concentrate mixture is adjusted depending upon the quality and quantity of the forage offered.

After 6 months of age (Murrah buffalo calf-54 kg; crossbred calf-45 kg), individual feeding of calves may be discontinued. The males and females should be kept in separate paddocks. The calves can be maintained on a high quality roughage ration plus a minimum amount of concentrate so as to effect economy in maintenance.

Assuming a daily body weight gain of 0.45 kg from the 7th to 24th month of age, 2 kg concentrate mixture with 16% DCP and 70% TDN and 15 to 20 kg of green fodder should be provided to each calf. If leguminous fodders are available in plenty and fed to appetite, the amount of concentrate mixture can be reduced to 1 kg a day. When the main roughage is a straw or stover, 2.5 kg of concentrate mixture should be given daily to calves of 6 months to 1 year of age and 3 kg mixture for older growing stock. These feeding schedules do provide higher DCP than suggested and it is not harmful.

The research works carried out by K.T.Sampath & coworkers and T.K.Walli & coworkers since 1990s revealed that animals up to the age of 12 to 18 months may be benefitted by supplementing bypass protein (RUP) in their diet (Table 9B) to achieve higher growth rate, productivity and efficiency. Formaldehyde treated oil cakes are proven to be effective as sources of bypass protein (RUP). Further, it has been recommended that a level of 50% of the CP as bypass protein that is required for improving the growth and milk production under straw based feeding system.

Normal Rate of Growth of Indian Cattle and Buffaloes

A growth rate of 0.4 kg per day is quite satisfactory for calves of Sahiwal and Tharparker breeds. The crossbred calves grow at the rate of 0.5 kg/day. Buffalo calves are generally heavier than cow calves of the same age. So this fact has to be kept in mind while formulating ration, and the feeding schedule should be adjusted according to their body weight and not according to the age.

Feeding of Growing Animals

Feeding of bull calves: Animals which are earmarked to be raised as future breeding sires should generally be kept on a liberal amount of milk for the first 6 months or more of their life. Milk is also supplemented with calf starter from 2 weeks of age onwards along with good quality hay.

After 6 months of age, a bull calf should have a somewhat larger amount of concentrates. Bull calves from 6 to 12 months and those from 1 to 2 years of age should be given 2.5 and 3.0 kg, respectively, of Type I concentrate mixture. Cost of feeding can be reduced through introduction of nutritious forages. But the quantity of concentrate mixture should not be cut down below 1 kg per head per day. Care should be taken that the bull calves do not become unduly fat and lethargic.

Young males to be used for draft purpose should only be castrated at 12 to 15 months of age and their feeding schedule should be identical to that of heifers. To economise the cost of feeding, these animals can be fed solely on green fodders and hay from 1 year of age. Leguminous fodders (green) like lucerne/cowpea can be fed at 20-25 kg per head per day together with rice straw or stovers.

Male buffalo calves are reared for meat production and these are generally fattened before slaughter. They are usually sent for slaughter at about 1 year of age. As the feed efficiency for fat laying is less, such animals are generally given extra feed in order to induce more rapid gain in weight. The supply of CP and TDN should be increased by at least 50% over the figures for growing calves (Table 9B) from the time the calves attain a body weight of about 200 kg until they are marketed.

Feeding of Bulls in Service

The nutrient requirements of breeding bulls as proposed initially by Sen and Ray (1964) and retained by Ranjhan (1978) (Table 15A) and ICAR (2013) (Table.15 B) are presented. In view of non-availability of comprehensive Indian data on breeding bulls, ICAR (2013) requirements are derived by adding 10% of maintenance energy needed per hour to corroborate the findings of NRC(1989).

TABLE 15A Nutrient Requirements of Breeding Bulls (Sen, Ray and Ranjhan, 1978).

Live weight kg	DCP g	TDN kg	ME Mcal	Ca g	P g	Carotene mg	Vit. A 1000 IU
400	380	3.6	13.0	18	13	40	16
500	450	4.5	16.2	20	15	53	21
600	530	5.4	19.4	22	17	64	26

TABLE 15B Daily energy and protein requirements of cattle/buffalo breeding bull*

BW (kg)	DM (kg)	TDN (kg)	ME (Meal)	MP (g)	RDP (g)	RUP (g)	CP (g)
350	6.5	3.46	12.5	214	335	59	394
400	7.6	3.82	13.8	237	370	65	436
450	8.6	4.18	15.1	259	405	71	476
500	9.7	4.52	16.3	280	438	77	515
550	10.8	4.86	17.5	301	470	83	553
600	11.9	5.18	18.7	321	502	89	591
650	13.0	5.50	19.9	341	533	94	627
700	14.0	5.82	21.0	361	563	99	663
750	15.1	6.13	22.1	380	593	105	698
800	16.5	6.43	23.2	399	623	110	733

*ICAR (2013)

Breeding bulls are to be fed good quality fodders (green as well as dry) together with concentrates to keep them in thrifty condition as per the requirements. The bull should be regularly exercised to keep it in prime condition. Overfeeding should be avoided as it leads to excessive fattening which lowers the libido. Bulls should get high energy ration, preferably bypass fat supplements, during hot and humid summer months.

Feeding of heifer calves

Example: Formulate a ration for a growing heifer weighing 150 kg. The dry matter requirement will be about 4 kg per day. Nutrient requirements of the animal at a daily growth rate of 0.5 kg and the ration are presented hereunder:

	RM kg	DM kg	DCP kg	TDN kg	Ca g	P g	Carotene mg	Vit. A 1000 IU
Requirement		4.0	0.35	2.6	13	12	16.25	6.5
Ration		←		kg		→		
Green grass (Hybrid napier) (25, 1, 12)	10	2.5	0.1	1.2	0.007	0.004		
Concentrate mixture (90, 12.5, 70)	2	1.8	0.25	1.4	0.0096	0.0184		
	–	4.3	0.35	2.6	0.0166	0.0224		

The composition of the concentrate mixture: Groundnut cake 15, Jowar 20, Maize 22, Tapioca thippi 14, Deoiled rice bran 26, Mineral mixture, 2 and Salt, 1%. (Ca 0.48%; P 0.92%.)

Feeding of Working Bullocks

Increased muscular work results in an oxidation of large amounts of nutrients in the body. In the contraction of muscle, the immediate energy requirement is met by break-down of creatine phosphate and adenosine triose phosphate. In the muscle, the amount of these high energy phosphate compounds is very limited. During the subsequent relaxed state of the muscle, these compounds are resynthesized through the energy furnished by the oxidation of glycogen in the muscle and also glucose is brought to the muscles in the blood.

The source of all potential energy in skeletal muscle is the absorbed products of digestion from the diet. Theoretically, therefore, only carbohydrates need to be supplied to meet the extra energy required for work. However, fats also can be utilized as their catabolism can be used by the system to furnish energy through the carbohydrate aerobic oxidation cycle.

When food supply is adequate, a working animal first draws upon the carbohydrates and fats in the feed. If the supply is inadequate, the body fat is used for the purpose and as a last resort muscles and other protein tissues are used. Thus, as long as there is a sufficient supply of carbohydrates in the feed, an ox at work needs no more protein than required for maintenance except probably when the work done is very hard.

In formulating a ration for working bullocks, it is nevertheless necessary to give some supplemental protein for two reasons.

1. When the feed intake of an animal is higher than what is required for maintenance, the digestibility of the ration as a whole is diminished.
2. For the proper utilization of feed carbohydrates in the rumen, there should be a proper ratio between energy and protein, otherwise the digestibility of crude fibre will be greatly diminished, leading to a shortage in energy supply.

Additional protein may also be desirable for working animals to compensate for the losses through sweating.

As systematic work has not been carried out on working bullocks, research work done on horses has been used to derive the nutrient requirements. Horses at slow walk require 4 kcal ME/kg BW/h (NRC, 1978). Since bovines move at a slower pace than the horses, energy required, by cattle and buffaloes is often assumed to be 75% of the horses. These values for energy along with 10 and 20% increase in CP have been used for computing the respective requirements (ICAR, 2013).

The nutrient requirements of the working animals (Table 16 and Table 17A and 17B) depend upon the labour performed. The heavier the work the greater should be the proportion of easily digestible carbohydrates in the ration. For bullocks the work has been categorized into two types, normal and heavy work. Normal work consists of 6 hrs of carting or 4 hrs of ploughing, and heavy work consists of 8 hrs of carting or 6 hrs of ploughing (ICAR, 1998).

TABLE 16 Nutrient Requirements for Working Bullocks and Buffaloes (Sen, Ray and Ranjhan, 1978).

Live Weight kg	Normal Work*				Heavy Work**			
	DM kg	DCP kg	TDN kg	ME Mcal	DM kg	DCP kg	TDN kg	ME Mcal
200	4.00	0.24	2.0	7.2	5.0	0.25	2.7	9.5
300	5.80	0.33	3.1	11.4	7.0	0.42	4.0	14.4
400	7.60	0.45	4.0	14.4	9.8	0.57	4.8	17.3
500	9.40	0.56	4.9	18.0	11.2	0.71	6.4	23.0
600	11.2	0.66	5.8	20.8	13.40	0.82	8.0	28.8

*6 hrs of carting or 4 hrs of ploughing.
**8 hrs of carting or 6 hrs of ploughing.

TABLE 17A Daily energy and protein requirements of cattle/buffalo working bullocks (light work 4 hr)*

BW (kg)	DM (kg)	TDN (kg)	ME (Meal)	MP (g)	RDP (g)	RUP (g)	CP (g)
300	6.5	3.70	13.3	210	323	58	380
350	7.6	4.15	15.0	236	363	65	427
400	8.6	4.59	16.6	261	401	72	472
450	9.7	5.01	18.1	285	438	79	515
500	10.8	5.42	19.6	308	474	85	558
550	11.9	5.83	21.0	331	509	91	599
600	13.0	6.22	22.5	353	544	97	640
650	14.0	6.60	23.8	375	577	103	679
700	15.1	6.98	25.2	397	610	109	718

*ICAR (2013)

TABLE 17B Daily energy and protein requirements of working cattle and buffalo (heavy work 8 hr)*

BW (kg)	DM (kg)	TDN (kg)	ME (Meal)	MP (g)	RDP (g)	RUP (g)	CP (g)
300	6.5	4.93	17.8	229	353	63	415
350	7.6	5.53	20.0	257	396	71	466
400	8.6	6.12	22.1	284	438	78	515
450	9.7	6.68	24.1	311	478	86	562
500	10.8	7.23	26.1	336	517	93	609
550	11.9	7.77	28.0	361	556	100	654
600	13.0	8.29	29.9	386	593	106	698
650	14.0	8.81	31.8	409	630	113	741
700	15.1	9.31	33.6	433	666	119	783

*ICAR (2013)

Example: Compute a ration for a working bullock weighing 400 kg and doing 6 hrs of ploughing each day (heavy work). The available feeds are rice straw, guinea grass (green), gingilly cake, ground maize and wheat bran.

(i) Dry matter requirement is 8-10 kg per day
(ii) The DCP and TDN requirements are 0.57 kg and 4.8 kg, respectively.
(iii) Ration formulation

Feedstuff	RM kg	DM kg	DCP kg	TDN kg
Rice straw (90, 0,44)	3	2.7	0	1.32
Guinea grass (green) (25, 1.5, 15)	15	3.75	0.225	2.25
Ground maize (90, 7.4, 84.9)	0.5	0.45	0.037	0.425
Wheat bran (90, 10, 68)	1.2	1.08	0.12	0.816
Gingilly oil cake (90, 38, 78)	0.5	0.45	0.19	0.39
Total	–	8.43	0.572	5.2

The green fodder meets the requirement of vitamin A. Gingilly cake and wheat bran are good sources of calcium and phosphorus, respectively. With incorporation of mineral mixture (30 g), salt (30 g) and contributions from all feedstuffs ensure the supply of macro and micro minerals. Maize along with bran and cake promote higher production of propionic acid in the rumen to keep the blood glucose content at an optimum level.

Alternative Method

	DM kg	DCP kg	TDN kg
Nutrients provided through roughages	6.45	0.225	3.57
Nutrients to be provided through concentrates		0.347	1.23

A suitable concentrate mixture may be offered to meet the nutrient requirements. 0.347/0.16 = 2.17 or say 2.2 kg concentrate mixture meet the digestible protein requirement. This concentrate mixture should contain 16% DCP and 63% TDN.

Exercise

Compute a ration for a breeding bull of 500 kg BW (ICAR, 1998).

Use the given feedstuffs.

	RM kg	DM kg	DCP kg	TDN kg	Ca g	P g
Requirement		12.5	0.450	4.5	20	15

Guinea grass (green)
Cowpea green fodder
Rice straw
Maize grain
Sesame cake

Feeding of Protein to Ruminants

Introduction

The protein requirement of ruminants is considered in terms of nitrogen requirement of the rumen microorganisms and amino acid requirements of the host animal. The nitrogen requirement of the rumen microbes is met from non-protein nitrogen (NPN) compounds present in the diet and saliva and from dietary protein degraded in the rumen i.e., rumen degraded protein (RDP). The amino acid requirement of the host animal is met from the microbial protein and the rumen undegraded dietary protein (UDP). The amino acid and peptide requirement of the rumen microbes are obtained through the RDP fraction.

Requirement of Rumen Microbes

Rumen microorganisms require protein, carbohydrates, phosphorus, sulphur, cobalt, etc. Protein provides ammonia, amino acids, peptides while carbohydrates provide fermentable energy. Phosphate is needed for the synthesis of nucleic acids which contain 10-20% of the nitrogen present in the microbes. Sulphur is needed for the synthesis of methionine and cysteine.

Protein Degradation in the Rumen

Dietary protein is degraded, at different rates but often rapidly, by the microbial action in the rumen (Figure 1). Protozoa may make some contribution but it is likely that bacteria are mainly responsible and a number of bacterial species have been shown to possess proteolytic activity. The

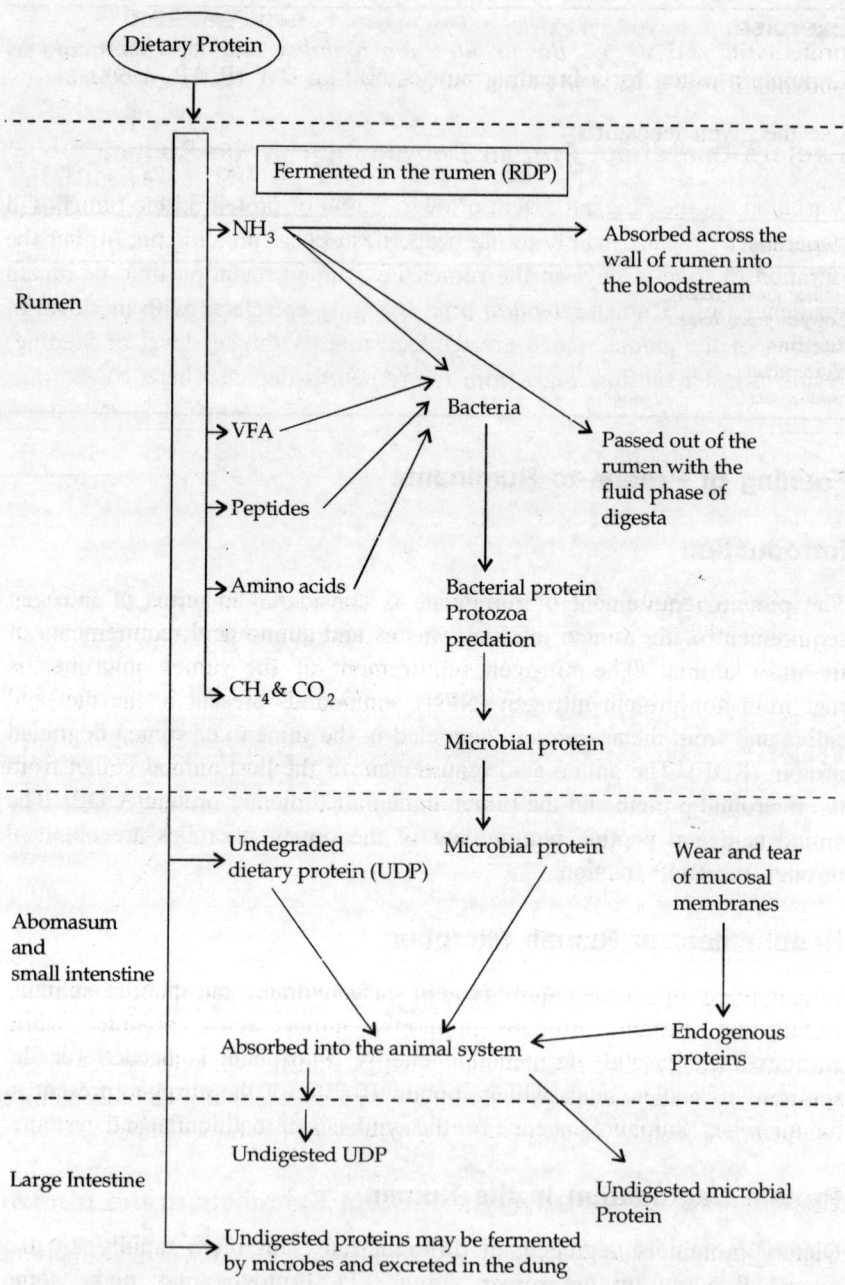

Figure 1. Fate of Dietary Protein in Ruminants.

proteolytic activity of *Bacteroides amylophilus* and *B. ruminicola* is maximum over a wide pH range of 6 to 8.

Factors that affect Protein Degradation in the Rumen

Variations in the rate and extent of degradation of protein in the rumen will generally be related mainly to the properties of that protein and, further the duration of time it stays in the rumen i.e., rumen retention time or rumen residence time. Rumen retention time is highly correlated with the level of feeding of the animal, since greater feed intakes (higher level of feeding) result in faster outflow rates from the rumen as depicted here:

	Level of feeding	Outflow rate
a)	Animals fed at a low level of feeding, about 1 X maintenance	0.02/h
b)	Calves, low yielding dairy cows (<15 kg milk/d), beef cattle and sheep on higher levels of feeding but less than 2 X maintenance	0.05/h
c)	High yielding dairy cows, greater than 2 X maintenance	0.08/h

Contrary to the earlier assumption that higher the protein soluble greater the rumen degradability, it has been reported that the molecular structure (sulphur-sulphur cross linkages) of some soluble proteins renders them resistant to degradation. The rate of rumen fluid turnover can affect actual rumen degradation of protein next to its molecular structure. If flow rate from the rumen is rapid, some of the normally degradable protein may be flushed from the rumen before it can be degraded. Similarly, when the rate of rumen turnover is slower, some of the normally bypass protein may be broken down in the rumen due to excessive long exposure to the rumen fluid.

Factors that affect Microbial Protein Synthesis in the Rumen

The factors that affect microbial cell synthesis in the rumen are supply of nutrients to meet the needs of rumen microbes for their maintenance and growth, rumen fluid turnover or dilution rate, microbial cell turnover in the rumen and frequency of feeding. Type and amount of nutrients available from the diet and synchronisation of their release matters much importance in their effective utilisation for growth of rumen microbes who form microbial protein after death.

Where is the Need for Bypass Protein?

The earlier concept of "Feed the rumen microbes which in turn feed the ruminant animal" is not valid and the need to provide UDP or bypass protein to ruminants arises under the following situations:

(a) In early lactation period of high yielding (more than 15 kg/day) milch animals.
(b) In case of rapidly growing (1 kg/day) calves.
(c) Further, in case of animals thriving only on poor quality roughages sufficient quantities of microbial protein is not synthesized as this process is an energy dependent process.

In all these situations protein requirements are met from microbial protein synthesized in the rumen and the rumen bypass protein (UDP), which are absorbed at duodenal level. Protein quality is important and bypass protein is required for high growth and milk production.

Protein Protection from Rumen Degradation

Protein that is fermented in the rumen is largely wasted because essential amino acids are deaminated and fermentation of 1 g of protein generates only half the ATP that would be produced from 1 g of carbohydrate. The main objective of protecting proteins from ruminal degradation is to provide greater amounts of essential amino acids to the productive ruminant. It has long been recognised that it is possible to increase the amino acid supply to the ruminant animal by treating dietary protein in such a way as to reduce its susceptibility to microbial attack in the rumen which eventually increases its UDP or bypass protein content.

Methods such as heat treatment, formaldehyde and tannic acid treatments have been developed to protect the protein from rumen degradation without affecting its digestibility at the intestinal level. Heating causes denaturation of protein and this may be beneficial because of reduced ruminal degradation partly by blocking reactive sites for microbial proteolytic enzymes and partly by reducing protein solubility. Heat developed during expeller process of oil seed extraction and extrusion cooking are beneficial to ruminants. That is modest amount of 'heat damage' is beneficial. Formaldehyde treatment is also effective. The optimum level appears to be 0.5-1.5% of the crude protein for concentrate diets and 1.3-2% for hay.

Protection of amino acids: Protected amino acids are, nowadays, added to diets, as feed additives. Several laboratories have devised encapsulation procedures to protect amino acids from ruminal degradation without impairing their intestinal release and absorption. Protection is given by coating or mixing methionine, for example, with a combination of fats or fatty acids and sometimes by addition of carbonates, kaolin, lecithin, glucose or other products. Another method of protection is structural manipulation of amino acids, e.g. glycosylation which make them resistant to ruminal degradation.

DL-2-Hydroxy-4-(methylthio) butanoic acid (HMB, methionine hydroxy analog) coated with Ca-soaps of palm fatty acids was found to be inert in the rumen and was used as a source of methionine for high producing cows.

Relation between Bypass Protein and Voluntary Feed Intake

As early as in 1965, Egan and Moir showed an interesting appetite-stimulating effect from bypass protein. Single infusions of casein administered to sheep into the duodenum produced substantial and rapid increases in the voluntary intake of a diet low in nitrogen content. Later several studies reported increased feed intake when formaldehyde treated feed protein or feedstuffs naturally rich in UDP such as fish meal was supplemented to straw diets at catalytic level. Such supplemental protein can influence physical control (by its effect on digestion and rate of movement of digesta) as well as metabolic control (by providing amino acids at duodenal level to the animal which influences the metabolic response to the diet) of feed intake.

Protein Requirement of Ruminants

The ruminant animal derives its requirement of amino acids from microbial proteins synthesized in the rumen and the dietary proteins which escape degradation in the rumen. Hence the use of the term "CP" when referring to ruminant needs for nitrogen is imprecise. Further, it becomes obvious that one cannot state the protein requirements for ruminants as digestible crude protein (DCP) in the diet because:

1. dietary proteins are largely degraded in the rumen,
2. the extent to which degraded N is utilized by rumen microbes is related to the amount of energy fermented, and
3. the faecal excretion could be altered by manipulating the site of fermentation between the rumen and the caecum.

Several new systems have been proposed such as metabolizable protein system in the USA, rumen degradable and undegradable protein system of the UK and true protein digested in the small intestine (PDI) of the France. The fundamental principle underlying these new systems is that nitrogen requirements of a ruminant animal is most logically considered as a requirement for nitrogen by rumen microorganisms and a requirement for protein by host ruminant animal. Metabolizable protein is that part of the dietary protein undegraded in the rumen and the microbial protein, which are absorbed by the host animal and is available for use at tissue level. Metabolizable protein is defined as the total digestible true protein (amino acids) available to the animal for metabolism after digestion and absorption of the feed in the animal's digestive tract (Figure 2). Protein requirement of the animal is calculated in terms of RDP required plus UDP required for its metabolizable energy requirement and tissue protein requirement.

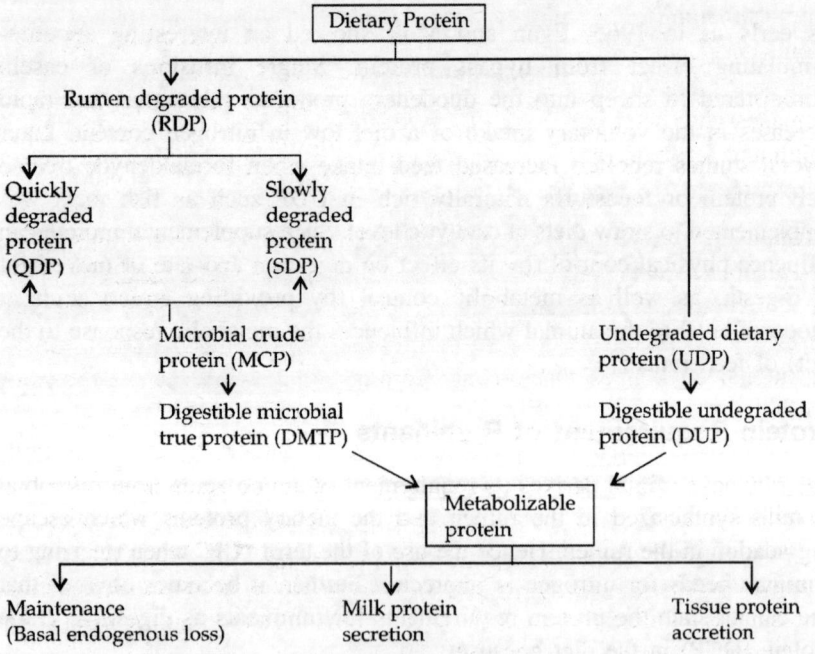

Figure 2. Use of Dietary Protein in Ruminants.

Feeding of Fat to Ruminants

Fat is a high energy dense nutrient. Fat in the diet of ruminants varies from negligible amounts to levels in excess of 10% of the dry matter in leafy forages or where animals are able to select leaf tip materials. Most of the lipid in pasture plant materials are in the form of phospholipids and glycolipids. The major long chain fatty acid components are linolenic (50%), linoleic (10%) and palmitic (15%) which make up 60% of the total.

The complex lipids of plants are rapidly hydrolysed in the rumen by bacterial lipases to fatty acids, galactose and glycerol. Galactose and glycerol are fermented to volatile fatty acids (VFAs). The fatty acids are largely unsaturated and as soon as they are released they are adsorbed onto particles in the rumen where they are hydrogenated by microbes. These long chain fatty acids–now largely stearic, palmitic and oleic acids are absorbed only from the intestines. Rumen bacteria incorporate some of the long chain fatty acids into their cellular components.

Milk Fat Synthesis: Long chain fatty acids (LCFAs) are used for the milk fat synthesis. The higher the availability of LCFAs, the better the ruminants can cope with high milk production. Often milk fat is synthesized from short chain fatty acids particularly acetic acid which is a fermentation end product. It is known that the conversion of acetic acid into milk fat demands glucose which could otherwise be used for lactose production. A minimum fat level of 3% is required in order to spare glucose for lactose synthesis, etc.

Rumen bypass/Rumen inert Fats: Profitable commercial dairy production requires dairy cows with very high average milk production level i.e. "high-output" dairy cows. Such cows now can produce more than 9000 litres per lactation. However, high-output cows present characteristic nutritional challenges that are not common in feeding lower production cows.

Just after calving, the cow must generate an increasing amount of milk, but with a diminished capacity to consume feed to support that much output of milk, inevitably mobilising the nutrients from body stores provoking a loss of weight. The requirement of protein and most other nutrients, except energy, can be met. The first three months of lactation is a critical period. The diminished ingestion capacity make it obvious to add fat to the diet. But the rumen is very sensitive to the high level of fat in the diet, which can negatively affect fermentation in the rumen - physical coating of the fibre and that of the microorganisms reducing the digestibility, reduction in the absorption of cations and toxic effects on the cellulolytic flora. This suggests the need for a source of fat that does not affect ruminal fermentation and is readily assimilated by the cow in the later part of the digestive system. This is the rationale for "rumen bypass"/rumen inert fats.

Manufacture of Rumen Protected Fats: Rumen protected fats have been developed based upon two types of mechanisms:

1. One is based upon the melting point of fatty acids. Rumen protected fat products containing saturated fats are manufactured with saturated or hydrogenated fatty acids. These fatty acids remain in a solid state at environmental temperatures but melt at temperatures above 50-55°C. So, these fats remain in a solid state at the rumen temperature of 38-39°C and are insoluble in the ruminal liquid. They remain inert in the rumen and are digested in the small intestine. But this type of bypass fat is relatively less digestible due to the high proportion of saturated fatty acids.

2. Fatty acid calcium salts

In order to maximise fat digestibility in the ruminant's small intestine while protecting the fat in the rumen, bypass fat products composed of calcium salts of fatty acids were developed based on saponification of fatty acids. These are also known as calcium soaps. These compounds are formed of saturated and unsaturated fatty acids joined to calcium ions to form salts. The rumen protection mechanism here is based upon the acidity level or pH of the rumen and small intestine. The calcium salts remain intact (little or no dissociation of calcium soaps would be expected, as the pKa is between 4 and 5) in the neutral acidity of rumen (6.2 - 6.8 pH) and remain insoluble in the ruminal liquid but dissociate in an acid environment (pH 2-3) of the abomasum and the fatty acids are "freed". The free fatty acids are soluble and are absorbed in the intestine more efficiently (upto 95%) [The composition of calcium salt products is almost equal parts of saturated fatty acids (Palmitic and stearic) and mono-unsaturated fatty acids (oleic). The total melting point is nearly 38°C]. However, it has been reported that calcium soaps of unsaturated oils can be extensively hydrogenated.

Apart from these two methods, a method first developed about 25 years ago involved the encapsulation of an emulsion of oil by formaldehyde - treated proteins. Refer Chapter 9 in *Principles of Animal Nutrition and Feed Technology.*

Rumen protected fats support the high energy demands of early lacta-tion in the high-output dairy cow (without affecting the rumen fermenta-tive digestion) with minimum loss of weight (Excessive loss of body weight causes fertility disorders, ketosis and lower milk production).

Common Sources of Rumen Inert Fats/Rumen Bypass Energy

1. *Megalac*[R] Concentrated protected energy (30 MJ ME/kg) from Volac International Ltd.; Feed it during the first 100-150 days of lactation.

2. *Ener GII*^{TM} Calcium salts of long chain fatty acids from Bioproducts.
3. *SoyPreme*^{R} Rumen bypass protein and rumen inert fat from Borregaard Lignotech UK Ltd.
4. Nutrijoule (84% bypass fat) 0.5-2.5% in feed; Vetcare.
5. Nutrisacc powerpack 100g/ animal/day as a top dress; Vetcare.

FEEDING OF HIGH YIELDING COWS/BUFFALOES

Feeding of Milch Animals during Early Lactation: Problems

The milk yield of crossbreds (above 15 kg per day) is many times more than the local animals. The rate of milk letdown in the first six weeks of lactation is so high that the secretion of nutrients into the milk exceeds the rate of uptake of nutrients from the digestive tract. The nutrient deficit is compensated by the diversion of nutrients from the body reserves (mobilisation of body protein and fat) resulting in weight loss. Too large a loss in body weight can prove harmful and uneconomical.

The appetite of the animal during the early lactation (up to 8 weeks) is reduced by 2 to 3 kg. So all the nutrient needs of the animals are to be provided within this appetite limit. It is difficult to meet the nutrient requirements, particularly the energy requirement of such high yielders (more than 15 kg per day in case of cows and 12 kg per day in case of buffaloes) through normal concentrate mixtures and fodder. High energy diets are to be formulated and challenge feeding has to be adopted. And adequate fibre (36% NDF in the total ration) is critical for maintenance of normal milk fat. Usually, all such cows and buffaloes will remain under negative energy balance during first 2-3 months of lactation.

Rumen filling effect

Fibre degradation rates of straws and stovers are lower due to their higher NDF (and higher lignin) concentration resulting in their longer retention time in the rumen and causing rumen fill, which then limits the intake of DM. To maximize the dry matter intake in case of high producing dairy animals, they need to be fed diets with lower rumen filling effect. These include non forage fibre sources like agro-industrial byproducts such as soy hulls, beet pulp, cottonseed hulls, corn gluten feed, distiller's grain etc. Fibre that is less lignified clears from the rumen faster, allowing more space for the next meal.

High yielding animals, therefore, receive more of their energy requirements from concentrates and non-forage sources such as byproducts (soy hulls, cottonseed hulls, etc) rather than from straws. Hence their diets may not contain the optimum NDF level. Maintaining efficient rumen fermentation is important for optimum rumen health and productivity. It is recommended that the dietary levels of minimum NDF and maximum non-fibrous carbohydrates (NFC) in the ration (see table No 5 in appendix I) should be followed to maintain the efficient fermentation in the rumen.

Dry matter intake

Cows should reach peak dry matter intake (DMI) between 10 to 13 weeks after calving. At this time the animal should be consuming approximately 4% of its body weight. For much (if not all) of this time the animal will be in negative energy balance leading to weight loss. Excessive body weight loss, especially in fresh cows, can lead to health and reproductive problems that can adversely affect the profitability of a dairy enterprise. Maximizing feed intake during this time can mitigate the extent of negative energy balance of the animal allowing for increased production, improved reproduction and better animal health.

Wallace et al. (1998) monitored and found that healthy cows ate nearly 6.8 kg more dry matter in the first 20 days after calving compared to the sick ones with an event such as a retained placenta, metritis, ketosis or a displaced abomasum. The same trend was observed in milk production as healthy cows produced about 9 kg more. One way to insure better DMI is with a more consistent total mixed ration (TMR), while quality and uniformity of feed are equally important.

Vitamin A and immune functions of dairy cows

Due to their high rates of metabolism, dairy cows experience considerable oxidative stress, resulting in susceptibility to disease pathogens. Vitamin A is an important factor in improving immune function and attenuating oxidative stress. The effect of supplementation of vitamin A at two levels has been studied in dairy cows (550kg body weight and 21kg milk yield/day) on antioxidant status and immune function (Jin et al., 2014). These results suggested that supplementation of the diet with 220 IU of vitamin A/kg of body weight may enhance the antioxidant and immune functions of dairy cows and implied that the vitamin A requirement necessary to ensure beneficial immune and antioxidant functions of dairy cows is higher than the current recommended dose that ensures optimum production performance.

Feeding of oilseeds

In the light of advances made in the field of protein metabolism, the protein requirements in ruminants are calculated based on rumen protein degradability. Mobilization of body reserves during early lactation can be prevented by feeding high fat, high protein oilseeds such as cottonseed which supply both protein and long chain fatty acids (LCFAs) for post-ruminal (Bypass protein and bypass fat) digestion.

Feeding Soybean to High Yielding Cows/Buffaloes

Soybean has to be fed as both whole oil seed and solvent extracted soybean meal to cows during lactation, more so during the first 3 to 5 months, to overcome the negative energy balance. A milch cow was fed 6 kg of concentrate mixture (Maize 40%, soybean meal 30%, groundnut meal 10%, rice polish 10%, molasses 7%, mineral mixture 3%), 1 kg of soybeans, 30 kg green fodder and *ad libitum* wheat straw throughout the 10 months of lactation. The cow yielded 4836 kg milk during the lactation period. It was inferred that better milk yield persistency seemed to be as a result of supplementing extra energy and additional protein from one kg whole soybean.

Twenty Murrah buffaloes yielding 9.2 kg milk per day were used to assess the usefulness of feeding full fat soybean on milk production traits. The study was conducted for 11 weeks. Milk Fat Booster (MFB) was prepared by mixing soybean 60%, soybean meal 30% and maize 10% (CP 36%, EE 10%). Each animal was offered fat booster 2 kg, cottonseed cake 1 kg, maize 2 kg and straw *ad libitum*. The results showed an improvement in fat per cent from 6.69 to 7.48 while there was not much difference in milk yield. Since most of (high yielding) cows and buffaloes are expected to be in negative energy balance during first trimester of lactation, the soybean feeding can be advantageous to boost milk or milk fat percentage. (Source: S.P. Arora and D. Bhosale "Future of feed industry in dairy sector in India" Technical Bulletin of American Soybean Association).

Level of Nutrition and Reproduction

Low levels of protein and energy in the diets of cows and buffaloes are liable to affect the reproductive system in a number of ways, such as disturbing the estrous cyclicity, prolonging postpartum anoestrous period, and increasing number of services per conception. The mechanism of inhibitory action is on the hypothalamus affecting the release of LH releasing factor from anterior pituitary.

In case, the energy requirement is met fully from time to time during lactation, there may be further increase in milk production as well as better persistency from such cows.

High protein diets are reported to be beneficial for higher milk production and superior growth rate. It has been estimated that two-third of increase in milk yield is due to adequate protein and one-third is a result of optimum energy in the rations.

Metabolic Disorders

The diseases associated with imbalance in 'input' of dietary nutrients and 'output' from animal products (like foetus production, milk, etc.) are clubbed under metabolic disorders. Metabolic disorders occur shortly after calving include milk fever and ketosis primarily. Following calving, the dairy cow/buffalo undergoes a transition from a relatively high roughage diet to a lactation diet that generally includes grains, brans, oilseed meals. During this period, the amount of energy required for maintenance of body tissues and milk production usually exceeds the amount of energy available from the diet. This nutrient deficit makes the dairy animal susceptible to metabolic diseases/disorders.

Milk Fever or Parturient Paresis

Milk fever is characterised by low blood calcium and paralysis. It is usually observed within 40 hours postcalving. Milk fever is a misnomer. The milch animals do not develop fever; on the contrary, body temperature may be depressed. There is a fall in serum calcium levels in all cows during calving. However, when the fall is high, cows develop this disease. This disease is more prevalent among high yielding cows. Mature cows are susceptible usually in 5-10 years age group, although rare cases have been observed in first and second calving. Blood calcium is low in milk fever, but a low dietary intake is not the cause. It seems probable that the parathyroid glands fail to mobilize blood calcium rapidly enough to meet the drain at parturition which results from the onset of active milk secretion. Thus the cows develop hypocalcaemia (see blood calcium dynamics, p. 119) and tetany. High dietary calcium prior to calving is not helpful, but rather harmful. It increases the incidence of milk fever because the parathyroid becomes less active during the prolonged period of high dietary supply.

Dietary Cation Anion Balance (DCAB) and Milk Fever

During feed production and ration formulation, DCAB calculations (see appendix, p. 449) help to predict how a feed will affect the acid-base balance of animals. Normally, rations fed to herbivores have a positive DCAB value, as evidenced by the alkaline urine (calcium loss in alkaline urine is low) commonly encountered in such animals. Various salts, like calcium chloride, magnesium sulphate or ammonium chloride, may be added in order to produce acidifying diets, which is a desirable feature of diets used before calving in dairy cows prone to develop hypocalcaemia.

Why do you Acidify Diets of Pregnant Cows Nearing Parturition?

Increasing calcium absorption and enhancing bone resorption before parturition can prevent milk fever. Both processes are stimulated when a diet that leads to a negative calcium balance is fed during the last part of pregnancy.

An acidifying diet fed before calving will greatly increase the calcium loss through urine. This calcium loss enhances calcium turnover in bone and increases calcium absorption. The cow will therefore be primed for the sudden increase in calcium demands at parturition, and for maintaining plasma calcium in the normal concentration range at parturition, when faced with the calcium losses through colostrum. Hence, feeding a diet containing anionic mineral mixture is effective (as it creates mild metabolic acidosis and initiate calcium resorption) for the prevention of hypocalcemia. Anionic mineral mixture consists of calcium chloride 33.4, magnesium chloride 33.3, sodium chloride 18.3, magnesium sulphate 8.3 and calcium hydrogen phosphate 6.7 percent. Approximately 90 g of anionic mixture/day is recommended for three weeks prepartum (ICAR, 2013).

Prepartum DCAD and transition animals

Transition period is the duration of 2-4 weeks prior to calving through 2-4 weeks after calving. This period is also called as periparturient period. A prepartum negative dietary cation-anion difference (DCAD) balancing has consistent impact on transition animal health and early lactation performance.

A prepartum negative DCAD diet significantly minimizes the occurrence of milk fever (below 5.8 mg/dl serum calcium) and subclinical hypocalcemia (SCH; below 8.5 mg/dl serum calcium). Calcium is not just required to milk production, but it is also needed for smooth muscle contraction. Therefore, it is a key player in expulsion of the fetus and contraction of the uterus post-calving, teat closure after milking and rumen contraction. In other words, most cows afflicted with milk fever are more likely to succumb to other transition disorders including retained placenta, metritis, mastitis, ketosis or displaced abomasum. Thus proper DCAD implementation improves transition animal health, early lactation milk yield and ultimately profitability from dairy enterprise.

Blood calcium dynamics

Dairy cattle derive the minerals from water, feed and fodder and the minerals are required for optimal productivity. The input of minerals through feed and water must balance their output through faeces, urine and milk to maintain the animals' health. If the output exceeds input, the animals obtain the required ones from its body resources (through mobilization process) for a shorter period. But continuous imbalance develops into productivity related problems.

Blood calcium levels in cows and buffaloes with milk fever

Normal lactating cow	8.4-10.2 mg/dl
Normal at calving	6.8-8.6 mg/dl
Slight milk fever	4.9-7.5 mg/dl
Moderate milk fever	4.2-6.8 mg/dl
Severe milk fever	3.5-5.7 mg/dl

The drop in blood calcium level is usually accompanied by a drop in blood phosphorus and increase in blood potassium and magnesium levels. Calcium is critically important to normal nerve and muscle function. Acetylcholine requires calcium to properly stimulate muscle movement.

Guidelines for managing Ca intake include restriction of high-calcium forages (legumes) during the dry period and supplementation of dry cow diets with anionic salts. Urine pH is affected by changes in the cow's acid-base status. Checking the urine pH can help the farmer monitor the effectiveness of a ration containing anionic salts. Urine pH of 8.0-7.0 indicates a positive DCAB status.

Hypogalactia in dairy animals

Cows at freshening are more susceptible because of the sudden spurt in turnover of fluids, minerals and organic constituents for milk biosynthesis in functional alveoli of the mammary gland. In functional hypogalactia, the lactating cow or buffalo, irrespective of breed/genotype, gives sub-optimal milk production because of imbalanced nutritional states, attributable to deficiency of minerals (Ca, P and Mg) often coupled with negative energy balance (NEB; hypoglycemia).

Ketosis

Ketosis or acetonemia often occurs during the first 6 weeks following calving which is caused due to inadequate supply of glucose precursors to maintain the adequate blood glucose level.

As has been studied earlier the entrance of acetyl CoA into the TCA cycle is contingent upon an adequate supply of oxaloacetate. Under conditions of nutritional and/or physiological stress, where energy demand exceeds the available tissue glucose, fat is mobilized to acetyl CoA. It can not be converted to energy via the TCA cycle and is thus converted to ketones.

Such conditions exist in cows and buffaloes just after parturition (heavy glucose demand for milk production; milk contains about 100 times the concentration of sugar as does blood), in sheep just before parturition (heavy glucose drain to the foetus) and in humans after a long siege of vomiting [limited food (CHOs) consumption]. Under these conditions the level of ketones in the blood increases (Acetonemia) and since two of them (acetoacetic acid and β hydroxy butyric acid) are highly acidic, an acidosis develops. The ketones appear in the urine, acetonuria. Acetone is exhaled via the lungs and in severe cases is readily detectable as a sweet odour. Other signs of ketosis include anorexia, hypoglycemia and in cows and buffaloes a spectacular drop in milk production.

Pathways of Ketone Bodies Production and Use

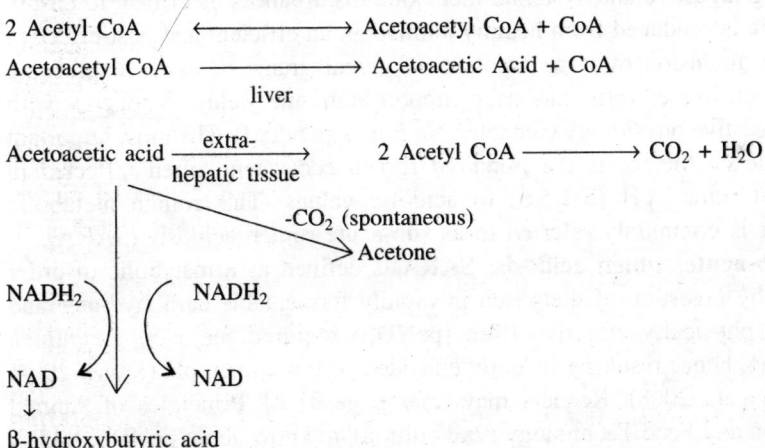

The carbon dioxide transporting power of the blood is lessened and cellular oxidation is decreased. This is a serious condition which in extreme conditions result in coma and death.

Treatment: Sodium propionate, propylene glycol and glycerol feeding. Injecting ACTH, adrenal glucocorticoids stimulate glucose production from body protein. Before inappetence occurs, increasing the dietary energy intake is effective.

How to ensure effective support for the dairy animal's energy metabolism at the start of lactation?

Glycerin and propylene glycol: The onset of lactation is associated with major challenges for high-yielding cows. As a rule, feed intake can barely keep pace with the soaring demand for energy. The result is a negative energy balance, which is even more pronounced in animals with excess condition at the time of calving. The animals mobilize body fat, leading to stress on the liver and consequently to an increased susceptibility to problems such as metritis and mastitis. Feeding glucoplastic substances such as glycerin and propylene glycol and a high dose of vitamin B_{12} can ensure effective support. This oral feed supplement has to be given on the day of calving and the following two to five days based on the need. Consequent to this administration, increased blood levels of vitamin B_{12} and reduced free fatty acid content with marked enhancement in appetite in the animals have been observed.

Ruminal acidosis

Meeting energy and nutrient requirements of dairy cattle/buffaloes, while avoiding digestive and systemic metabolic disturbances, is critical to ensure that milk is produced from healthy animals in an efficient and cost-effective manner. Inclusion of large amounts of cereal grains or easily degradable byproducts in feed formulations to support high milk yields do not cope with their digestive physiology (see table No 5 in appendix I). The most important consequence thereof is the impaired rumen ecosystem, often reflected in declined rumen pH (5.2-5.8) to acidotic values. This rumen metabolic disorder is commonly referred to as sub-acute rumen acidosis (SARA).

Sub-acute rumen acidosis: SARA is defined as a metabolic disorder caused by ingestion of diets rich in rapidly fermentable carbohydrates and lacking physically effective fibre (peNDF) required for adequate rumen buffering, hence resulting in 'daily episodes' of low rumen pH (Stone, 2004; Zebeli et al., 2008). Readers may refer page 31 of 'Principles of Animal Nutrition and Feed Technology (2nd edition)' to know about peNDF. SARA is an important digestive disorder of high-producing cattle that results in major changes in the rumen ecosystem, disrupting the symbiosis among rumen microbial communities and the epithelial tissues of the host's gastrointestinal tract.

Prolonged systemic inflammation can cause (1) significant changes in the energy and lipid metabolism in different body tissues, (2) immune suppression and increased susceptibility to various diseases and (3) artificially increase host's requirements in energy and nutrients, lowering the efficiency of energy and feed use by the animal. It is emphasized the need to formulate diets with adequate peNDF to enhance the metabolic health of dairy cow/buffalo.

Rumination-Eructation

The ruminant can be considered to be a superorganism because it has a symbiotic relationship of life between the cells of the animal's body and the rumen microbes (DePeters and George, 2014). Ruminant means to chew over again hence the designation of 'cud chewing'. Out of the four compartments of the ruminant stomach (Figure 3), rumen along with reticulum serves as site of anaerobic fermentation. There are coronary grooves in the rumen creating sacs. There is a cranial groove that separates the reticulum and rumen, and in cattle, buffalo, sheep and goat the two compartments are easily distinguished with the reticulum having a honey combed appearance. These compartments are lined with finger like projections called papillae that absorb nutrients (e.g.VFA). Reticulo-rumen functions together in the rumen cycle (coordinated contractions) to support the acts of eructation and rumination.

The contractions of the rumen cycle are important for mixing of new feed with microbes, distribute the end products of fermentative digestion for absorption by the mucosa papillae, and pass the digesta to the omasum. Eructation (release of gases produced during anaerobic fermentation) is a quiet process that involves eructated gas passing up the esophagus and into the trachea and the lungs to be respired.

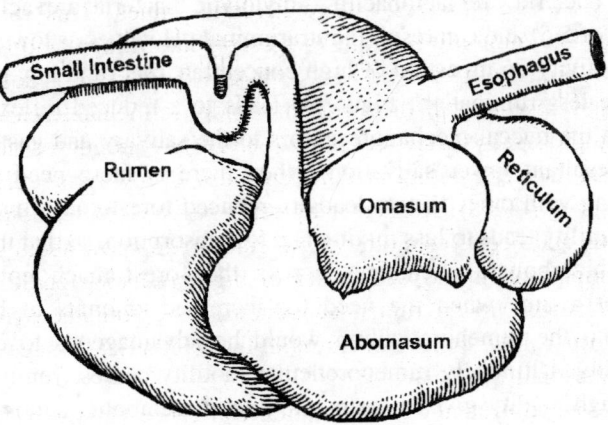

Figure 3 Ruminant stomach (http://biobook.nerinxhs.org/bb/systems/digestion/1000px-Abomasum-ia-omaso.svg.png)

Rumination involves regurgitating the bolus of digesta (cud) into the mouth where it is chewed eventually to be re-swallowed. Cud chewing (crushing and grinding of fibrous feed particles by the molars) enhances microbial digestion, stimulates saliva production, and the buffers present in saliva help to maintain rumen pH when the bolus is re-swallowed. Digesta leaves the reticulum via the reticulo-omasal orifice. The omasum, with its many leaves or laminae, controls flow of digesta to the abomasum.

Occurrences in the rumen: Roughage diet versus concentrate diet

Maintaining healthy animals is key component of animal welfare. Ensuring good rumen health in dairy cattle is key for the maintenance of efficiency and productivity, and thus herd profitability. In dairy cattle, the rumen environment is designed to function optimally within a pH range of 6.2-7.2, for which a certain amount of peNDF in the diet is a must.

With high-roughage diets (Figure 4), high rates of salivation are evoked by several reflex mechanisms. This gives adequate alkali to buffer the VFAs produced at low rates by the slow cellulolytic fermentation. With high-concentrate diets, much lower rates of saliva and hence lower alkali are produced, since the reflex stimuli for salivation are less compared to that with the high-roughage diet. The low alkali availability and high VFA production rates culminate in acidic environment.

Intraruminal conditions below 6.2 pH inactivate the propionate bacteria. Hence accumulation of lactic acid occurs and this leads to more acidity. The dominant bacteria are lactobacilli (amylolytic bacteria are active till the rumen pH of 5.5) and can result in intraruminal pH values as low as 4.6. Less chewing activity on ingestion of high concentrate diet (and low particle size also evoke less rumination; Figure 4) leads to a reduced reflex excitatory drive from the buccal mechanoreceptors to the salivary and gastric centres.

The resultant lower salivation (when there is more need of salivary alkali) along with other factors leads to reduced forestomach motility. This reduced motility leads to less mixing and less absorption, so that the potential for VFA-bicarbonate exchanges across the forestomach epithelium is lessened at a time when the need for increased amounts of bicarbonate moving into the rumenoreticulum would be advantageous to combat the rising acidity. Ultimately rumenoreticular motility ceases (ruminal stasis).

The high acidity gives rise to a systemic metabolic acidosis and also breaks down the integrity of the forestomach lining. This leads to multiple ulceration of the epithelium (rumenitis) and the entry of largely anaerobic bacteria into the portal venous system. The bacteria may cause liver

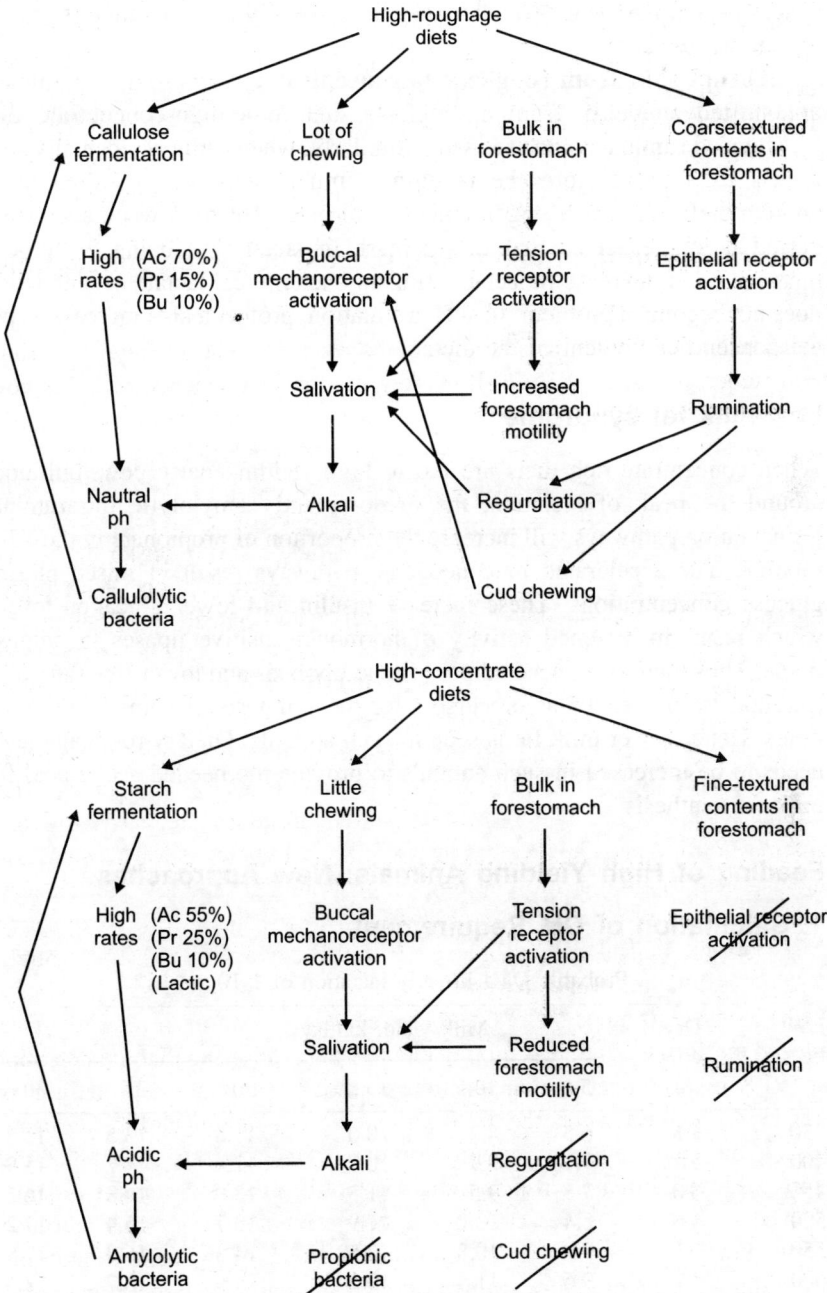

Figure 4 Occurrences in the rumen (Source: page 466 of Duke's Physiology of Domestic animals 12th ed (2004) by W.O. Reece]

abscesses and may lead to fatal toxaemia. Clinically this condition is known as ruminal acidosis.

Abrupt shift from roughage to concentrate: When ruminant animals are shifted suddenly from a roughage diet to a high-concentrate diet pronounced ruminal acidosis is seen. Similarly, when cattle accidentally gain access to a grain store the resulting ruminal acidosis is called more appropriately the 'grain engorgement syndrome'. Up to 4 week-adaptation period is suggested so that the increase in lactate-producing bacteria is matched by an increase in lactate-utilizing bacteria and lactate accumulation does not become a problem. In such a situation, protozoa also increase as per the concentrate content of the diet.

Low-milk fat syndrome

When concentrate-rich diets are fed to high-yielding dairy cows/buffaloes around the peak of lactation, the predominantly amylolytic intraruminal fermentation pathways will increase the proportion of propionate in the VFA mixture. The accelerated gluconeogenic pathways result in raised plasma glucose concentrations. These increase insulin and lower glucagon levels, which result in lessened activity of hormone-sensitive lipases in adipose tissue. Thus there is reduced adipose tissue lipolysis and lower free fatty acid (plasma) levels needed as precursors for the synthesis of some of the milk lipids. Hence lower milk fat is seen in such animals. Dietary roughage level needs to be increased in such animals to provide the needed acetic acid for milk fat synthesis.

Feeding of High Yielding Animals: New Approaches

1. Calculation of DM Requirement

Probable DMI in early lactation of 1-10 weeks*

LW kg	Dry cow	Milk yield, kg/day					
		5	10	15	20	25	30
350	4.8	6.5	8.3	10.0	11.8	13.5	15.3
400	5.4	7.1	8.9	10.7	12.4	14.2	15.9
450	6.0	7.8	9.5	11.3	13.0	14.8	16.5
500	6.6	8.4	10.2	11.9	13.7	15.4	17.2
550	7.3	9.0	10.8	12.5	14.3	16.0	17.8
600	7.9	9.6	11.4	13.2	14.9	16.7	18.4

* In mid lactation of 10-29 weeks, DM has to be increased by 1.7 kg/day; In late lactation of 30 weeks onwards, DM has to be increased by 4.1 kg/day.

A new system has been proposed in MAFF Technical Bulletin 33 to assess the DM appetite of the cow from both body weight and milk yield. The DM requirement calculation is based on 2.5% of body weight plus 10% of milk yield.

2. Calculation of Protein Requirement

If the ARC (1980), (1984) and NRC (1989) protein feeding recommendations are compared, there is considerable difference in the levels of protein recommended. The UDP recommended by NRC is much higher than the UDP recommended by the ARC. Comparison of NRC and ARC protein feeding in cows producing up to 30 kg of milk per day had revealed that the ARC-UDP is adequate. The difference between ARC-UDP and NRC-UDP for milk production in the range of 5 to 15 kg is about 300 g per day.

A. Protein requirement for maintenance is based on live weight.

B. Protein requirement for growth: The requirement of body tissue protein (TP) for live weight gain or loss is estimated by the ARC (1980) as 150 g per kg of gain and -112 g TP per kg of body weight loss.

C. Protein requirement for milk production: For milk production TP requirement is dependent on the protein content of the milk and this can be calculated from the SNF (Solids not fat) content which is closely correlated with the protein content.

Tissue protein for maintenance based on LW

LW (kg)	TP (g/day)
300	56
350	60
400	64
450	67
500	69
550	72
600	74

Tissue protein for milk production (based on SNF% of milk)

% SNF	TP (g/kg milk)
8.4	30.5
8.5	31.3
8.6	31.8
8.7	32.5
8.8	33.1
8.9	33.8
9.0	34.4
9.1	35.1
9.2	35.7
9.3	36.4
9.4	37.0
9.5	37.7

3. Calculation of Energy Requirement

The animal needs ME for maintenance (ME_m), lactation (ME_l) and gain in weight (ME_g). ME that is needed in the ration is the sum of ME_m, ME_l and ME_g. The animal obtains its ME from the daily ration which is fed. ME values vary from 5.5 to 7.0 for low energy feeds (e.g. cereal straws) to high values for the cereal grains and compounded feeds which normally have ME values of 10-14 MJ/kg DM.

ME for Maintenance		ME for Lactation (MJ/kg milk)	
Live Weight (kg)	ME (MJ/day)	% SNF	4.0% BF
350	40	8.4	5.13
400	45	8.5	5.17
450	49	8.6	5.20
500	54	8.7	5.24
550	59	8.8	5.27
600	63	8.9	5.31
		9.0	5.34
		9.1	5.37
		9.2	5.41
		9.3	5.44
		9.4	5.48
		9.5	5.51

(a) ME for maintenance (ME_m)

$$ME_m \ (MJ) = 0.578 \ W \ kg^{0.75} \qquad K_m = 0.72$$

(b) ME for lactation (ME_l)

ME_l (MJ) = yield (kg) $\times$ 1.694 (0.386 BF + 0.205 SNF – 0.236)

(K_l = 0.62 i.e. in order to produce 62 MJ of NE in the milk, the cow needs a dietary intake of about 100 MJ of ME)

(c) ME for gain or ME from loss in weight

In the case of suckler cows and high yielding dairy cows there is a cyclic process of accumulation and oxidation of body fat. These animals loose weight for the first 4 to 10 weeks after parturition when energy demand is high and put it back again in the latter part of lactation and in the dry period.

$$\text{Energy required for 1 kg gain} = \frac{20^*}{0.62^{**}} \times 5\% \text{ as safety factor}$$

$$= \frac{20}{0.62} \times 1.05 = 34 \text{ MJ}$$

* 1 kg of mature body tissue contains 20 MJ NE
** Efficiency of use of ME for live weight gain in lactation is the same as that for the production of milk.

ME available to the cow

When body tissue is broken down during early lactation (live weight is lost), energy is available to the cow; one kg live weight lost saves 28 MJ ME from the ration. As aforementioned calculation reveal, 34 MJ of ME is required to put on 1 kg of live weight gain during lactation. It indicates there is a high level of efficiency of 0.82 involved in the energy transfer. NE from 1 kg body tissue lost multiplied by the efficiency of energy transfer provides 20 $\times$ 0.82 = 16.4 MJ to the cow.

Computation of Rations: Some Examples

1. Formulate a ration for the dairy cow weighing 600 kg producing 15 kg milk/day with 3.8% BF and 9.1% SNF in late lactation putting a live weight gain of 0.75 kg/day.

Calculation of requirements: Energy requirement

1. ME for maintenance, ME_m = 63 MJ/day (from the table)
2. ME requirement for each kg of milk with 3.8% BF and 9.1% SNF

$$\begin{aligned}
ME_1 \text{ (MJ)} &= \text{yield (kg)} \times 1.694 \ (0.386 \ BF + 0.205 \ SNF - 0.236) \\
&= \text{yield (kg)} \times 1.694 \ (0.386 \times 3.8) + 0.205 \times 9.1 - 0.236) \\
&= 15 \times 1.694 \times 3.0963 \\
&= 15 \times 5.24 \\
&= 78.6 \text{ MJ}
\end{aligned}$$

3. Allowance for live weight gain: $0.75 \times 34^* = 25.5$ MJ
   *ME required for 1 kg gain
   Therefore total energy required for the cow = 63 + 78.6 + 25.5
   $$= 167.1 \text{ MJ/day}$$

Protein requirement

TP: Tissue protein, which is the amount of protein needed to supply protein for retention in the body.

1. The tissue protein requirement for maintenance = 74 g (from the table)
2. The TP required for production of milk at 9.1% SNF
   $15 \times 35.1 = 526.5$ g (from the table)
3. The TP required for body weight gain:
   $0.75 \times 150^* = 112.5$ g

(*TP for live weight gain is 150 g per kg). Therefore total TP required for the cow = 74 + 526.5 + 112.5 = 713 g/day.

To meet this requirement of tissue protein, two further calculations are needed to arrive at the protein required in the feed.

1. Rumen degradable protein (RDP) g/day
   $$\begin{aligned}
   &= 7.8 \times ME \text{ required in MJ} \\
   &= 7.8 \times 167.1 \\
   &= 1303.4 \text{ g}
   \end{aligned}$$

2. Undegraded dietary protein (UDP) g/day or RUP
   $$\begin{aligned}
   &= 1.91 \times TP \text{ required} - 6.25 \times ME \text{ required} \\
   &= 1.91 \times 713 - 6.25 \times 167.1 \\
   &= 1361.8 - 1044.4 \\
   &= 317.4 \text{ g}
   \end{aligned}$$

Probable DM intake

From the table : 13.2 + 4.1 = 17.3 kg
From the formula : $(6 \times 2.5) + 1.5 = 15 + 1.5$
$$= 16.5 \text{ kg}$$

Energy concentration or energy density - M/D value

Energy density has been used in poultry and swine nutrition for a long time and it is a relatively new concept with ruminants.

$$M/D = \frac{\text{Total daily ME intake, MJ}}{\text{Total daily DMI, kg}} = \frac{167.1}{17.3} = 9.66$$

The M/D of a ration can vary from 7 for a ration of poor hay and straw, to about 13 for a ration containing a high energy concentrate mixture and a very good quality hay. A medium quality hay has 8.4 and a medium energy concentrate mixture has 12.5 MJ/kg.

Since 9.66 lies between 8.4 and 12.5 then a mixture of the two should provide a correct ration. It is possible by trial and error to get the weights of hay and concentrate mixture that will meet the requirements exactly. A more exact method is found in MAFF Technical Bulletin 33 for the rapid formulation of diet consisting of a single forage and a single concentrate mixture.

$$\text{Forage DM} = \frac{\text{DMI} \times (\text{compound feed ME} - \text{M/D})}{\text{Compound feed ME} - \text{forage ME}}$$

$$= \frac{17.3 \times 12.5 - 9.66}{12.5 - 8.4} = \frac{17.3 \times 2.84}{4.1} = 11.98 \text{ kg DM}$$

Therefore, the compound feed = 17.3 − 11.98 = 5.32 kg DM

$$\text{Forage, fresh hay} = \frac{11.98}{0.88} = 13.61 \text{ kg}$$

$$\text{Compound feed} = \frac{5.32}{0.90} = 5.91 \text{ kg}$$

2. Calculate the nutrient requirements of a 600 kg cow in early lactation and losing 0.25 kg weight per day. The cow is assumed to yield 40 kg milk with 3.8% BF and 8.8% SNF.

Energy requirement

1. $ME_m = 63$ MJ

2. $ME_l = 40 \times 5.14 = 206$ MJ

3. ME contributed from 0.25 kg

weight loss per day = $0.25 \times 28 = -7$ MJ

Total ME required = 63 + 206 − 7 = 262 MJ/day

Tissue protein requirement

1. for maintenance   = 74 g
2. for milk production   = $40 \times 33.1 = 1324$ g
3. from body weight loss = -112 g TP $\times 0.25$ kg = -28 g

Total tissue protein requirement = $74 + 1324 - 28 = 1370$ g

The amount of dietary protein in terms of RDP and UDP needed to meet the tissue protein requirement is calculated as follows.

$$RDP = 7.8 \times 260 = 2028 \text{ g/day}$$
$$UDP = (1.91 \times 1370) - (6.25 \times 262)$$
$$= 979.2 \text{ g/day}$$

Formulation of Diets Using Metabolisable Protein (MP) System and ME System

The Agricultural Research Council's Technical Review "The Nutrient Requirements of Ruminant Livestock" published in 1980 proposed certain minor revisions to the 'ME system of calculating requirements' of its earlier edition (ARC 1965), and proposed a new model for the calculation of the protein requirements of ruminants. In 1990 the AFRC TCORN Report No. 5, "Nutritive Requirements of Ruminant Animals: Energy", recommended, with only minor alterations, the adoption of the AFRC 1980 Review's full recommendations on energy requirements of ruminant animals.

TCORN Report No. 9, "Nutritive Requirements of Ruminant Animals: Protein" recommends the adoption of a system based on Metabolisable Protein (MP) as the unit. The AFRC TCORN prepared an advisory manual in 1993 to assist in the adoption of MP system of calculating protein allowances (replacing the DCP system) and ME system for energy for ruminants.

Metabolisable protein has two components digestible microbial true protein (DMTP) and digestible undegraded feed protein (DUP) (Look for greater details in Page No. 90). Microbial crude protein (MCP) is produced by the activities of the rumen microbes, which synthesise protein from fermentable metabolisable energy (FME) [ARC (1980, 1984) used digestible organic matter and AFRC (1992) used fermentable organic matter and later fermentable metabolisable energy] sources in the feed and amino acids or NPN from the breakdown of feed proteins in the rumen. About 0.25 of MCP is present as nucleic acids, which can not be used by the ruminant for the synthesis of body tissue, milk, etc. The microbial true protein (MTP) content is therefore 0.75 of the MCP, and MTP is 0.85 digestible in the intestines.

So DMTP (g/d) = 0.75 × 0.85 × MCP = 0.6375 MCP (g/d)

Digestible undegraded feed protein (DUP) is that fraction of the feed which has not been degraded during its passage through the rumen i.e. UDP, but which is digested and absorbed in the lower intestines of the animal. The digestibility of UDP can be predicted from the acid detergent insoluble nitrogen (ADIN) content of the feed or its modified ADF content.

DUP, g/kg DM = 0.9 (UDP − 6.25 ADIN)

MP (g/d) = 0.6375 MCP + DUP

[ERDP is used with an efficiency of 1.0 for MCP synthesis; MP (g/d) = 0.6375 ERDP + DUP]

UDP (g/d) = CP − RDP (ARC, 1980)

RDP = QDP + SDP

The cold water extracted fraction of the feed crude protein is called quickly degradable protein (QDP). Any urea added to the feed is to be included in the QDP fraction of the diet. The amount of QDP in a diet should be limited to less than 0.4 of the effective rumen degradable protein (ERDP). Urea is only utilised in the rumen with an efficiency of 0.8 and this value is assigned to the QDP fraction of feeds. The amount of the feed protein slowly degradable during the residence of the feed in the rumen is SDP. ERDP has been defined as a measure of the total nitrogen supply that is actually captured and utilised by the rumen microbes for growth and synthetic purposes.

ERDP, g/kg DM = 0.8 QDP + SDP

Now UDP, g/d = CP − (QDP + SDP) (AFRC, 1993)

Level of feeding (L) affects outflow rate (r) and this in turn affects degradability. As level of feeding increases ERDP decreases and DUP increases.

Computation of rations: Example: Formulate a diet using the combined ME and MP systems to a 600 kg cow giving 30 kg milk with 4.04% fat and 3.28% protein (4.5% lactose) and losing 0.5 kg/d.

Requirements:	Metabolisable energy (ME)	= 205 MJ
	Metabolisable protein (MP)	= 1625 g
	Level of feeding (L)	= 3.3
	Outflow rate (r)	= 0.08

* ME requirements are influenced by the ME concentration of the diet i.e. M/D value.
* MP = 0.6375 MCP + DUP = 0.6375 ERDP + DUP. Since ERDP and DUP are dependent on level of feeding, those values at an outflow rate of 0.08/ h are used while formulating the diet.
* Energy is always the first limiting factor. Adequate FME is important to achieve optimum MCP yield. For a feeding level (L) of 3.3, the MCP yield is 11.1 g/MJ FME. So an ERDP/FME ratio of at least 11.1 is required in the example.

Ration as given in AFRC (1993) pp. 51.

Feedstuff	Fresh wt. kg	DM kg	ME MJ	FME MJ	CP g	ERDP g	DUP g	MP g
Grass silage	40.0	10.0	110	81	1420	900	180	
Dried beet pulp	2.3	2.0	25	25	206	86	86	
Rolled barley	2.0	1.7	22	21	194	143	31	
Maize gluten feed	2.3	2.0	25	23	414	260	82	
Rapeseed meal	2.3	2.0	24	22	800	530	156	
Nutrients provided		17.7	206	171	3034	1919	535	1745
Requirements		18.3	205	173	–	1898	415	1625

MCP Yield at level of feeding 3.3 is 11.1 g/MJ FME

So ERDP requirement = 11.1 × FME
= 11.1 × 171
= 1898 g/d

MP = 0.6375 ERDP + DUP
1625 = 1210 + DUP

DUP requirement = 1625 -1210 = 415 g/d

Metabolisable protein supplied by the diet (1745 g/d) exceeds the requirement by 120 g/d and this may probably raise the milk protein level above the 3.28%.

Example of rations fed to high producing cows in a farm in The Netherlands

Holstein-Friesian dairy cows (18 pairs) were selected based on age, parity, daily milk production, body condition and average methane excretion per day. Cows from each pair were randomly assigned into two groups. Both groups were fed the same TMR *ad libitum* in the stable (two times a day) and the concentrate mixtures (MELK and VEM) were automatically supplied during the milking time based on the daily milk yield of individual cows (Tables 18, 19 and 20). This example has been added to give an idea on feeding of 32-kg milk yielding cows in advanced countries. Total dry matter intake is 23 kg, which comes to 3.5% of body weight.

TABLE 18   Ingredients of TMR and concentrate mixtures: MELK and VEM*

TMR (% of DM)		Concentrates (% of DM)		
			MELK	VEM
Grass silage	43.02	Sugar beet pulp	—	31.4
Maize silage	39.85	Palm kernel expeller	—	17.4
Grass seed hay	02.80	Citrus molasses	10.0	10.0
Brewery grain	07.30	Rapeseed expeller	—	09.1
Rapeseed meal and soya meal (50:50)	06.64	Soya hulls	14.8	08.1
Minerals and vitamin mix	00.26	Wheat	06.3	05.7
Calcium carbonate	00.13	Rapeseed meal	16.1	05.1
		Cane molasses	10.0	05.0
		Rapeseed meal	09.0	03.5
		Soya meal	—	02.6
		Premix	02.3	01.6
		Urea	00.3	00.3
		Vegetable oil	00.2	00.2
		Maize	31.1	—

* Haque, M.N., C. Cornou, and J. Madsen 2014

TABLE 19   Chemical composition and nutritive value (% DM) of total mixed ration and concentrate mixtures*

Attributes	TMR	MELK	VEM
Dry matter (% of fresh feed)	47.3	86.3	85.8
Crude protein	12.1	17.0	17.1
Crude fat	02.8	03.7	03.9
Crude fibre	25.3	11.2	14.4
Ash	06.2	06.5	06.9
Sugar	.05.8	07.6	11.9
Starch	11.48	29.66	6.27
ADF	26.0	16.0	22.0
NDF	45.1	20.7	30.8
Lignin	02.4	03.2	03.9
Calcium	00.48	00.84	00.81

Phosphorus	00.31	00.39	00.37
Enzyme solubility of organic matter (% of organic matter)	71.4	94.0	91.7
Buffer solubility (% of CP)	51.2	21.0	25.5
Digestible energy, MJ/kg DM	13.42	16.5	16.2
ME, MJ/kg DM (DE x 0.80)	10.74	13.2	13.0
Scandinavian Feed Unit, SFU/kg DM	00.87	01.22	01.19

* Haque, M.N., C. Cornou, and J. Madsen 2014

TABLE 20 Milk production and dry matter intake particulars (mean±SE) of cows*

Parameters	MELK	VEM	No of observations
Body weight, kg	647±19.2	674±15.9	18
Milk production, kg/day	31.8±0.56	31.6±0.54	270
Energy-corrected milk, kg/day	33.1±0.48	33.7±0.51	270
DM intake from TMR, kg/day	18.7±0.06	18.7±0.06	270
DM intake from concentrate, kg/day	04.5±0.12	04.8±0.12	270
Total dry matter intake, kg/day	23.2±0.14	23.5±0.14	270

* Haque, M.N., C. Cornou, and J. Madsen 2014

6

Unconventional Feeds: Characteristics and their Utilisation in Livestock and Poultry Feeding

The term nonconventional feed (NCF) or unconventional feed (UCF) is a relative term and may differ from country to country and region to region, and time to time in the same country. The nonconventional feed resources (NCFR) refer to all those feeds that have not been traditionally used for animal feeding either by farmers or by feed manufacturers in commercial feeds. These include the agricultural and industrial byproducts and wastes which have no value as human foods and could be used in animal feeds at certain percentages depending on their palatability, nutritional value and toxic factors/antinutritional factors.

Necessity of NCFR

India is endowed with a very large number of livestock with diversity in terms of species and breeds within the species. The world's best dairy buffaloes, draught cattle, carpet wool sheep and highly prolific goat breeds are found in this region. The large livestock numbers are both an asset and a liability. India has 2.4% of world's geographical area with 16% of world's human population and 15% of world's livestock and poultry population (Table 1a & 1b). Hence there is a stiff competition for food between humans and animals. Only 2% of rice and wheat, 5% of sorghum, 10% of barley and maize and 50% of bajra and ragi are diverted towards livestock and poultry feeding, the major chunk of which is fed to poultry and swine. Feed resources are a major limiting factor in exploiting the genetic potential of livestock.

As early as in 1976, National Commission on Agriculture indicated that there is a shortage of 44% concentrate, 38% green fodder and 40% dry fodder for meeting the nutritional requirements of livestock. A recent estimate (Ranjhan, 1994) shows a deficiency of 47, 25 and 40% respectively, in concentrates, green fodder and dry fodder. The area under fodder crops has been estimated to be 3.3% and 4.41% of total cultivable area as reported by two independent estimates. The trend in land utilization pattern is presented in Table 2. The area under green forage production is likely to be further reduced and most of the land would be used for cereal, pulses and oilseed crop cultivation. This would thus result in increased crop residues for animal consumption (Table 3). At some places, area under crops has been diverted to aquaculture as well. Major byproduct feeds from tree crops and field crops are furnished along with their extraction rates in Table 4.

Table 1a Livestock population in the year 2003 (in Million Numbers): India Vs World and the growth trends

Species	India*	Annual growth rates 1997–2003, %	World**	% of world of population
Cattle	185.18	−1.18	1350.9	13.7
Buffaloes	97.92	1.43	170.3	57.5
Yaks	0.06	1.52	–	–
Mithuns	0.28	–	–	–
Sheep	61.47	1.12	1038.7	5.9
Goats	124.36	0.22	771.5	16.1
Horse & ponies	0.75	−1.59	55.1	1.4
Mules	0.18	−3.74	12.9	1.4
Donkeys	0.65	−4.95	41.5	1.6
Camels	0.63	−5.92	19.2	3.3
Pigs	13.52	0.28	941.5	1.4
Total	485.00	–	4401.6	11.0

*   **Source:** 17th Livestock Census, Department of Animal Husbandry, Dairying & Fisheries, M/O Agriculture; Directorate of Economics & Statistics. M/O Agriculture - various census reports and Animal Husbandry Statistics Division,
** FAOSTAT - Website year 2006.

Population figures indicate that Indian cattle, buffalo, sheep and goats constitute to 14, 58, 6 and 16% of the world population, respectively (Table 1a & Table 1b). All this livestock and poultry have to be supported with only 2.4% of the world's geographical area and 4% of world's fresh water resources.

TABLE lb. Indian Livestock population in the year 2012 (in Million Numbers) and growth pattern*

Species	2007	2012	% Change
Cattle	199.08	190.90	−4.10
Buffaloes	105.34	108.70	3.19
Yaks	0.083	0.077	−7.64
Mithuns	0.264	0.298	12.88
Total bovines	304.76	299.98	−1.57
Sheep	71.56	65.07	−9.07
Goats	140.54	135.17	−3.82
Horse & ponies	0.612	0.625	2.12
Camels	0.517	0.400	−22.36
Pigs	11.133	10.294	−7.54
Mules	0.137	0.196	43.07
Donkeys	0.438	0.319	−27.17
Total livestock	529.696	512.057	−3.33
Poultry	648.829	729.209	12.39
Dogs	19.08	11.67	−38.85
Rabbits	0.424	0.592	39.55

* **Source:** 19th Livestock Census 2012 (15th October 2012 as the reference date); Animal Husbandry Statistics Division, Department of Animal Husbandry, Dairying & Fisheries, Ministry of Agriculture; elephant population increased from 1000 to 22000 during 2007 and 2012.

TABLE 2 Trend in Land Utilization in India.

Land	Million Hectares (1985 figures)
Geographical area	328.8
Land for use	297.3
Aerable land	164.8
Permanent crop	3.5
Permanent pasture	11.9
Forest land	67.4
Other land (including fallow and cultivable waste land)	49.6

To bridge the gap between the requirements and the availability of concentrates and roughages there is a need to use more and more nonconventional feeds. The use of NCFR has become essential in animal feeding due to limited availability of conventional food/feed ingredients, to minimise the competition of livestock with human beings for conventional food grains and for economic reasons.

TABLE 3 Yields (kg/ha) of Grain/Oilseed and Ratio of Byproduct to Grain/Oilseed of Crops in Different Seasons *.

S.No.	Crop	Kharif 1989	Rabi 1989	Summer 1990	Khariff 1990	Rabi 1990	Summer 1991	Average
1.	Groundnut	2412	3470	1352	2554	3769	1605	2527
		2.06	1.51	3.06	1.70	1.08	4.29	1.96
2.	Rice	4625	5856	5011	4859	5555	4587	5082
		1.29	1.36	1.48	1.47	1.07	1.47	1.36
3.	Fingermillet	3803	5156	2800	3038	3724	2110	3439
		1.59	1.10	2.77	1.60	1.46	4.14	1.86
4.	Pearlmillet	3274	-	2823	3400	-	2946	3111
		1.69		2.05	1.43		1.17	1.58
5.	Maize	3587	2420	2450	4183	3449	2286	3067
		1.46	1.76	2.93	1.59	1.51	2.25	1.83
6.	Greengram	943	1268	1749	1639	1912	1824	1555
		1.55	1.10	1.40	1.44	0.94	0.95	1.20
7.	Sunflower	1553	1667	1177	1754	1521	1032	1451
		1.05	0.99	1.12	1.02	1.63	1.41	1.20

* Reddy, D.V. (1992). Development of package of practices using crop byproducts based rations under Integrated Farming Systems. Annual Report (1992-93), Regional Agri. Research Station, A.P. A.U., Tirupati, pp. 88-100.

Efforts have been made to increase the animal feed resources in India by two ways. Firstly, ICAR has started an All India Coordinated Research Project on "Utilization of Agricultural Byproducts and Industrial Waste Materials for Evolving Economic Rations for livestock" during the year 1967. The coordinating unit has centres located in different parts of India. These centres identified new feed resources-agricultural, industrial and forest byproducts and conducted laboratory and animal experimentation for their feeding value.

Secondly several methods have been developed to improve the nutritional quality of the existing lignocellulosic crop residues for their increased utilization.

Continued and concerted efforts had been made through the years.

In the X Plan, the 3 network projects *viz*-Micronutrients in Animal Nutrition and Production, Agricultural byproducts as Animal Feed and Crop based Animal Production Systems had been converged into the ICAR - AICRP entitled **"Improvement of feed resources and nutrient utilization in raising animal production".** NIANP is the coordinating unit for this project with 22 participating centres including SAU's, sister ICAR institutes

TABLE 4 Major Byproduct Feeds from Trees and Field Crops.

Crop	Botanical name	Byproduct feed	Approximate extraction rate (%)
Field crops			
Rice	*Oryza sativa*	Broken rice	4-5
		Rice bran	10
		Rice husk	15-17
		Rice straw	100
Wheat	*Triticum aestivum*	Wheat bran	10
		Wheat straw	100
Maize	*Zea mays*	Maize bran	8-10
		Maize germ meal	16-18
		Maize stover	200
Groundnut	*Arachis hypogea*	Groundnut straw	125
		Groundnut meal	60
Sesame	*Sesamum indicum*	Sesame cake	60-70
Sunflower cake	*Helianthus annus*		70
Linseed/Flaxseed cake	*Linum usitatissimum*		70
Rapeseed cake	*Brassica campestris napus*		70
Safflower cake	*Carthamus tinctorius*		70
Clusterbean (Guar)	*Cyamopsis psoralioides/ Cyamopsis tetragonoloba*	Guar meal	70-80
Soybean	*Glycine max*	Soybean meal	70-75
Cotton	Gossypium spp.	Cotton seed meal	40-45
Sweet potato	*Ipomea batatas*	Sweet potato vines	25-35
Cassava	*Manihot esculenta*	Cassava leaves	6-8
Castor	*Ricinus communis*	Castor bean meal	45-50
Sugarcane	*Saccharum officinarum*	Green tops	15-20
		Molasses	3-4
		Bagasse	12-15
		Pressmud or filter cake	3-4 of sugarcane
Tree crops			
Neem	*Azadirachta indica*	Neemseed meal	45-50
Coconut	*Cocos nucifera*	Coconut meal	35-40
Oil palm	*Elaeis quineensis*	Oilpalm sludge (dry)	2
		Palm press fibre	12
		Palm kernel meal	2
Rubber	*Hevea brasiliensis*	Rubberseed meal	55-60
Mahua	*Madhuca indica*	Mahua meal	35-40
Mango	*Mangifera indica*	Mangoseed kernel	50-55
Karanj	*Pongomia pinnata/ P. glabra*	Karanj meal	55-60
Sal	*Shorea robusta*	Salseed meal	35-40
Tamarind	*Tamarindus indica*	Tamarind seed hulls	30-35
		T.S. kernel	60-65
Cocoa	*Theobroma cacao*	Cocoabean waste	5-10

and NGO's covering almost all parts of the country. The objectives and activities of this project are to address different farming systems and livestock production systems in the country through nutritional intervention in raising animal productivity and profitability.

Characteristics of NCFR

1. They are the byproducts of food production systems that have not been used, recycled or salvaged.
2. They are mainly organic and can be in a solid, slurry or liquid form.
3. Their economic value is often less than the cost of their collection and transportation for use and hence they are referred to as wastes. e.g. fallen tree leaves.
4. The field crops which generate valuable nonconventional feeds are excellent source of fermentable carbohydrates for ruminants. e.g. Tapioca, Sugarcane. Feeding these fermentable carbohydrates to ruminants is advantageous because of their ability to utilize NPN substances in the presence of fermentable energy.
5. Regarding the feeds of crop origin, the majority are bulky and of poor quality cellulosic materials with a high crude fibre and lignin content. These are suitable for ruminant feeding.
6. Some of the feeds contain toxic factors and have deleterious effect on animals. For example, castor bean meal, neem seed cake.
7. They have a considerable potential as feed materials. In case of some feeds, their value can be increased if processing techniques are employed.

Constraints in the Utilization of NCFR

1. Limited knowledge on the chemical composition and feeding value of residues: The present state of knowledge in most of these newer feeds is limited to proximate principles and usual calcium and phosphorus contents. Most of the NCFR contain certain toxic/ antinutritional factor(s). In case of some NCFR toxic/antinutritional factors have been identified, characterised, and quantified and detoxification methods have been developed; however, some of the detoxification methods are not cost effective while some are not easy for field application.

   Little is known about long range effects of these toxic factors on the animal health and productivity and hence NCFR have to be used in the livestock rations in limited quantities only.

2. Nonavailability of these materials in large quantities: Production of NCFR is scattered and in some cases the quantity produced is low especially for processing.
3. The availability is restricted to a season in the year. There is no sufficient storage facility during the season of availability.
4. Lack of managerial and technical skills to utilise the feeds *in situ*.
5. Processing difficulties: Difficulties in collection, handling, transportation and processing of these feeds such as high-moisture feeds, low-density feeds.

Nonconventional Feed Resources: Some Examples

1. **Concentates**
   - **Energy supplements:** Mango seed kernel, tamarind seed, tamarind seed kernel, tamarind seed hulls, dehulled tamarind seed, tapioca waste/cassava waste, salseed meal, deoiled salseed meal, spent tea waste, bamboo seed, prosopis pods, babul seeds and pods, rain tree pods, etc.

   - **Protein supplements**
     Vegetable protein supplements: Ambadi cake, castor bean meal, neemseed cake, guar meal, niger cake, karanja cake, rubber seed cake, kapok seed cake, sunnhemp seed, daincha seed, cassia tora seed, mahuaseed cake, tobacco seed cake, *water dammar seed cake*, bijada cake, water melon seed cake, safflowerseed cake/kardy cake, kosum cake, spent coffee seed cake,

     Animal protein supplements: Hatchery byproduct meal, poultry by product meal, liver residue meal, frog meal, prawn/shrimp waste, crab meal, hydrolysed feather meal, squilla meal

2. **Roughages**
   Top feed resources include forages available from trees and shrubs. These are conventional feeds for goats. During scarcity tree leaves serve as roughages for livestock.
   Tree leaves and fallen tree leaves: Banyan, pipal, mango, teak, bamboo, neem, gliricidia, banana, cassava, mulberry, khejri, etc.
   Other examples are groundnut shells, paddy husk/hull, coffee seed husk, cottonstraw, cottonseed hull bran, safflower straw, sunflower straw and heads, maize cobs, bajra cobs, *jower* cobs, cocoa pod husk, water hyacinth, legume pod husk-husks of bengalgram, blackgram, greengram, redgram, etc.

Nonconventional feeds fall largely into one of the four areas: Food-processing residues, crop residues, forest product residues and animal waste.

- **Sugar factory byproducts:** Sugarcane trash, sugarcane tops, bagasse, molasses, pressmud (is a byproduct of sugar industry during precipitation. It can be utilised as mineral supplement for large ruminants).

- **Starch Industry waste:** Maize germ, maize bran, maize gluten and maize oil meal

- **Brewery waste:** It is mostly the brewer's grains left after the extraction of malt required for the production of beer. Malted barley is the main ingredient. Dried brewer's grain is a very good source of protein and energy for the livestock.

- **Fruit and vegetable factory byproducts:** Mango peels and kernels, pineapple wastes, banana wastes, citrus peels, dried cocoa pod husk, oil plam byproducts (Palm press fibre, CP 4%; CF 36% (PPF), Plam kernel cake CP 19%; CF 16% (PKC), Palm oil sludge CP 10%; CF 18% (POS), Palm oil mill effluent), tomato processing wastes, potato processing wastes, vegetable wastes.

- **High moisture agroindustrial byproducts:** High moisture feedstuffs can deteriorate rapidly during warm weather, which will reduce palatability and quality. Vegetable and fruit processing residues such as apple pomace, tomato pomace, pineapple waste, citrus processing waste (Dried citrus pulp, citrus meal and fines, citrus molasses), Dairy whey, Pulp and papermill residues, Distillers grain, condensed molasses solubles, yeast sludge, Single cell protein.

- **Marine and aquatic waste:** Fish waste, Frog meal (leftovers of the frog leg industry), Seaweed Meal (agar-agar is being extracted from Sargussam sea weed and its byproduct can be used for livestock feeding. It contains 33% ash and 10% protein), Prawn waste.

- **Slaughterhouse byproducts:** Blood meal, meat meal, meat and bone meal, Tankage (a fat free product obtained by cooking of meat in water), Rumen contents.

- **Poultry industry byproducts:** Feather meal, offal meal/poultry waste meal, hatchery waste.

- **Animal wastes:** These are fallen and slaughtered animal wastes, animal organic wastes (excreta) and animal byproduct wastes. **Abattoir wastes** are blood meal, tankage, meat scrap, feather meal, horn and hoof meal. **Animal organic wastes** include poultry litter/

dried poultry waste, caged poultry droppings/dried poultry manure, cow manure, pig excreta,

Utilization of agroindustrial byproducts and agricultural wastes as animal feeds: Several agroindustrial byproducts (AIBP) and nonconventional feed resources (NCFR) have been assessed for their composition, potential toxic factors, nutritive value and per cent incorporation in ruminant and poultry rations. The Compound Livestock Feed Manufacturers Association (CLFMA) has been using these resources to formulate economic rations for livestock and poultry.

Optimum Level of Utilization of NCFR

The optimum level imply that inclusion of that ingredient beyond the level advocated is likely to reduce the performance of the animals, and may result

TABLE 5 Deleterious Factors Present in the More Common NCFR and AIBP

S. No	Name of the Feedstuff	Deleterious factor
1.	Ambadi cake (*Hibiscus cannabinus*)	Nil
2.	Banana waste, stems and leaves (Musa spp)	Tannins
3.	Babul seed powder (*Acacia arabica, A. nylotica*)	Tannins (5%)
4.	Vilayati babul pods (*P. juliflora*)	Tannins (0.7-1.5%)
5.	Cassava leaves, peelings and pomace	HCN (17.5 mg/ 100 g)
6.	Cassava/Tapioca starch waste	Nil
7.	Castor seed meal (*Ricinus communis*)	Ricin (0.2%)
8.	Cocoa seed husk (*Theobroma cacao*)	Theobromine (trace)
9.	Coconut pith (Coir waste)	Lignin (35-40%)
10.	Coffee seed hulls, pulp (*Coffea arabica*)	Caffeine and tannins (2.8%)
11.	Cottonseed cake	Gossypol (0.05 - 0.2%)
12.	Cowpea seed meal	Trypsin inhibitor
13.	Guar meal	Trypsin inhibitor and gum
14.	Kapok or silk cottonseed cake	Cycloponopenoid acid
15.	Karanj cake	Karanjine (10-15 mg/100 g)
16.	Mangoseed kernel	Tannins (5-10%)
17.	Neem seed cake	Nimbin, Tannins
18.	Mahua seed cake (*Madhuca indica*)	Mowrin
19.	Palm oil mill effluent	High ash (12-26%)
20.	Rubberseed meal (Hevea brasiliensis)	HCN (9 mg/100 g)
21.	Salseed meal (Shorea robusta)	Tannins (8-10%)
22.	Spent tea leaves (*Camellia sinensis*)	Tannins (12%)
23.	Sugarcane bagasse	Lignin (8-10%)
24.	Tamarind seed hulls	Tannins
25.	Water hyacinth (*Eichornia crassipes*) meal	Oxalic acid (2.4%)

in death if fed at higher levels. These levels are arrived by conducting feeding trials wherein graded levels of nonconventional feed ingredients are used; toxicological and histopathological studies are also included. The levels suggested would be influenced undoubtedly by component ingredients of the diet and the ability of the individual animal to utilise the material.

Some of the NCFR that have been tested are listed in the Table 6 along with nutritive value and the level of inclusion in the diet. Deleterious factors present in commonly used AIBP and NCFR are presented in Table 5. Now more and more NCFR are finding place in today's compound animal feeds and there is further scope as the availability of such feedstuffs increase. It is not uncommon to use 25 to 30 ingredients in the commercial feeds.

TABLE 6 Nutritive Value and Optimum Level of inclusion of NCFR in Ruminant Rations.

S. No.	Name of the ingredient	Nutritive value % on DMB		Optimum level of inclusion (%) in the concentrate mixture
		DCP	TDN	
1.	Ambadi cake	18.7	64.0	20
2.	Guar meal	23.0	65.0	10
3.	Karanj cake	25.5	62.0	15
4.	Mahua cake	8.0	60.0	20
5.	Rubber seed cake	18.6	66.0	25-30
6.	Spent anatto seeds	7.0	67.0	20
7.	Tapioca starch waste	1.8; 2.0	60.0; 64.7	25
8.	Salseed meal	1.6	57.8	10
9.	Babul seed powder	13.8	59.0	20
10.	Vilayati babul pods	10.0	75.0	30
11.	Tea waste	9.7	43.0	20
12.	Coconut pith (Coir waste)	-	62.7	25
13.	Poultry droppings	25.0	-	15
14.	Poultry litter	20.0	-	10
15.	Sunflower heads	6.0	55.0	20
16.	Cocoa pods husk[R]	6.6	63.5	20
17.	Castor bean meal	20.0	60.0	10
18.	Mangoseed kernel	6.0	70.0	10
19.	Water hyacinth meal	9.0	55.0	10-20
20.	Dehulled tamarind seed	10.0	70.0	30
21.	Tamarind seed hulls[R]	5.0	60.0	10
22.	Sugarcane bagasse[R]	1.1	49.2	-
23.	Palm oil mill effluent	-	-	40
24.	Palm press fibre[R]	-	-	30
25.	Palm oil sludge	-	-	10-15

R–Roughage

Because of this, the price of compound feeds never directly or proportionately increase when the prices of conventional raw materials go up.

However, when once a nonconventional feed finds place in the compound feeds, the price of such material goes up.

Processing to Complete Feeds or Total mixed ration (TMR)

In an effort to utilise the AIBP and NCFR in a more intensive way these are processed and complete rations have been developed for ruminants. All the feed ingredients inclusive of roughages are processed (chaffing, grinding (8 mm) and pelleting) and mixed into a uniform blend that discourages selection (Raj Reddy, 1987). These complete rations provide adequate and balanced nutrients in an optimum ratio of roughage to concentrates (Table 7).

TABLE 7 Ingredient Composition (%) of Complete Diets and their Nutritive Value.

Ingredients	Name of the crop residue				
	Dry forest grass	Sorghum straw	Wheat straw	Cotton straw	Sunflower straw
Dry forest grass	47.5	-	-	-	-
Sorghum straw	-	46.0	-	-	-
Wheat straw	-	-	50.0	-	-
Cotton straw	-	-	-	45.0	-
Sunflower straw	-	-	-	-	35.0
Tapioca chips	-	20.0	-	-	-
Groundnut cake	10.0	10.0	10.0	10.0	-
Maize grain	10.0	-	-	-	-
Cage layer droppings (dried)	-	10.0	15.0	-	-
Cottonseed cake	-	-	-	-	25.0
Molasses	10.0	12.0	13.0	15.0	8.5
Deoiled rice bran	-	-	10.0	-	10.0
Wheat bran	20.0	-	-	10.0	10.0
Rice polishings	-	-	-	17.0	10.0
Urea	-	0.5	0.5	1.5	-
Mineral mixture	1.8	1.0	1.0	1.0	1.0
Common salt	0.7	0.5	0.5	0.5	0.5
Nutritive value					
DCP (%)	7.7	7.0	7.3	9.5	5.3
TDN (%)	63.1	56.4	51.8	48.6	56.2

Complete feeds have a particular relevance and considerable future potential when viewed in the context of a shift towards more intensive systems of production of milk and mutton. The latter is distinctly likely, given the diminishing availability of land and the need to have more intensive feeding systems and efficient feed resource use.

The readers may refer Principles of Animal Nutrition and Feed Technology 2nd ed (page 344) for information on complete feed manufacturing machine and expander-extruder processing of complete feeds. The nutritive value of complete feeds could be further improved by expander-extruder technology. This is a system which combines the features of expanding (application of moisture, pressure and temperature to gelatinize the starch portion) and extruding (pressing the feed through constrictions under pressure).

Dr G.V. Narasa Reddy Principal Investigator, Team of Excellence on Feed Technology and Quality Assurance, NATP project of ICAR did pioneering work with his team of scientists, which culminated in conducting workshop at Veterinary College, Hyderabad during July 22-23, 2003. The project was aimed at providing appropriate solutions to improve the utilization of untapped feed resources and to develop package of practices for the supply of wholesome feed to the rural farmers. G.V.Narasa Reddy and his team of workers studied the processing behaviour of crop residues such as groundnut haulms, soybean straw, bajra straw, castor and palm press fibre when they were subjected to chopping, grinding, expander-extruder processing and steam pelleting. It was reported that expander-extruder processing and steam pelleting increased the nutritive value of crop residues.

Feeding of Livestock During Scarcity

Scarcity of feed is encountered during natural calamities such as drought, floods, etc. Under such conditions the feeding of animals become more important because of severe shortage of roughage, and roughage alone accounts for about 60-80% of supply of dry matter required. During such natural calamities animals are sometimes collected and fed in common places in groups. Sometimes feeds are offered to the farmers at subsidised rate.

Crop residues, dry grasses from forests, fallen tree leaves are to be collected from the places of their availability and transported to the place of scarcity. Since they are low density feeds, cost of transport is more, sometimes, than the cost of purchase. e.g. Rice straw. Cost of harvesting and collection in case of forest grasses and tree leaves is also considerable in addition to transporation cost. Hence, it is suggested that the crop residues, grasses and tree leaves are chaffed, densified with the addition of brans, molasses, minerals and compressed further at the place of availability. Such compressed feed blocks are to be transported to needy places to tide over the feed scarcity. These complete feed blocks meet the nutrient requirements for moderate growth and milk production.

The use of nonconventional feed resources and agroindustrial byproducts as well as drought resistant vegetation in combination with urea and molasses can be used for meeting the immediate nutritional requirement under conditions of scarcity.

Rations for Feeding during Scarcity

I. Complete Feeds

1. Ration with Groundnut straw or Groundnut haulms

Ingredient Composition	%	Nutrient Composition		
Groundnut straw	60	CP	:	12.5%
Maize grain	18	DCP	:	7.6%
Groundnut cake	8	TDN	:	60%
DORB	10.4			
Molasses	2.4			
Minerals + Salt	1.2			
Vitamin AD_2				

2. Compressed feed block (Reddy, 1990)

Ingredient Composition	%	Nutrient Composition		
		CP	:	8.4%
Urea ammoniated wheat straw	73	DCP	:	5.1%
Wheat bran	10	TDN	:	58.82%
Molasses	15	ME	:	2.07 Mcal/kg DM
Minerals + Salt	2			
Vitamin AD_2	10 g per 100 kg			

3. Ration with tree leaves

Ingredient Composition	%	Nutrient Composition		
Banyan tree leaves	50	CP	:	17%
Maize grain	27	DCP	:	8%
Groundnut cake	14	TDN	:	42%
DORB	7			
Minerals + Salt	2			
Vitamin AD_2				

II Concentrate Mixtures using Unconventional Feedstuffs
% Ingredient Composition

A.

	I	II
Maize	-	10
Tapioca chips	15	10
Babulseed powder	10	5
DORB	10	15
Deoiled mangoseed kernel	-	5
Decorticated tamarind seed waste	10	-
Deoiled salseed meal	-	5
Sunflower cake	10	5
Safflower cake	5	-
Niger cake (Sol. Extr.)	5	-
Niger cake (Exp.)	-	10
Tobacco seed cake	-	10
Dried poultry waste	10	-
Silk cottonseed cake	5	5
Cottonseed cake	10	10
Molasses	7	7
Mineral mixture	2	2
Salt	1	1

B.

Jowar	10
Mangoseed kernel	10
Deoiled rice bran	25
Deoiled salseed meal	5
Safflower cake	5
Silk cottonseed cake	15
Cottonseed cake	20
Molasses	7
Mineral mixture	2
Salt	1

7

Small Ruminant Nutrition

General Information on Goats and Sheep

Small ruminants, goats and sheep make a significant contribution to the rural income and employment, especially in arid, semi-arid and hilly regions of India where crop farming is difficult and where naturally available feed resoures are scarce. They are the major meat producers. The annual growth rates of 3.10% for goats and 3.87% for sheep are higher than for buffaloes and cattle.

India has 20 breeds of goats (Osmanabadi, Malabari, Beetal, Barbari, Jamunapari, Black bengal, Angora, Chegu, etc.) and 40 breeds of sheep (Deccani, Nellore, Mandya, Madras red, Muzaffarnagari, Marwari, Gaddi, etc.). In Black Bengal breed twinning and triplets are common. Chegu is a famous Pashmina goat in Kashmir. Exotic breeds are Saanen, Alpine, Anglo-Nubian, etc. Exotic breeds of sheep used for crossbreeding of local sheep to improve mutton production potential were Dorset and Suffolk, and for wool production were Merino, etc.

Comparative feeding behaviour and digestive physiology in goats and sheep are presented in Table 1. With moderate to high quality forages, digestion in goats, sheep and cattle is similar, but goats are more capable than sheep for using cell-wall rich and nitrogen poor forages. Goats retain the feed for longer time in the digestive tract, have a higher concentration of cellulolytic bacteria in the rumen and are more efficient in recycling of blood urea. In harsh conditions, goats consume less water and more dry matter than sheep.

Goats are among the most efficient domestic animals in the use of water, approaching the camel in the low rate of water turnover per unit of body weight. Goats appear to be less subject to high temperature stress than other species of domestic livestock and require less water evaporation to control

TABLE 1 Comparative Feeding Behaviour and Digestive Physiology in Goats and Sheep (Devendra, 1989).

	Characteristics	Goats	Sheep
1.	Activity	Bipedal stance and walk longer distances	Walk shorter distances
2.	Feeding pattern	Browser, more selective	Grazer, less selective
3.	Browse and tree leaves	Relished	Less relished
4.	Variety in feeds	Preference greater	Preference lesser
5.	Taste sensation	More discerning	Less discerning
6.	Salivary secretion rate	Greater	Moderate
7.	Recycling of urea in saliva	Greater	Lesser
8.	DMI for meat	3% of BW	3% of BW
	DMI for lactation	4-6% of BW	3% of BW
9.	Digestive efficiency with coarse roughages	Higher	Less efficient
10.	Retention time	Longer	Shorter
11.	Water intake/ Unit DMI	Lower	Higher
12.	Rumen ammonia concentration	Higher	Lower
13.	Water economy	More efficient	Less efficient
	Water turnover rate	Lower	Higher
14.	Nature of faeces	Less Water	Relatively higher
	Nature of urine	More concentrated	Less concentrated

body temperature. They also have the ability to conserve water by reducing losses in urine and faeces. Goats may get more water through forage because of their habit of browsing. Thus goats are less dependent on free water sources than other domestic animals.

NUTRIENT REQUIREMENTS AND FEEDING OF SHEEP

Nutrient Requirements of Sheep

Indian breeds of sheep have much lower adult weight (30-40 kg) and growth rate in comparison to many foreign sheep breeds (70 kg). Besides the genetic make-up, inadequate nutrition is the major factor responsible for such low growth rate and body weight. There is considerable scope for improvement of Indian sheep by feeding them according to the needs. Large scale crossbreeding work has been done from 4th five year plan period to 7th five year plan period involving exotic meat and fine wool type breeds and local indigenous sheep through All India Coordinated Research Projects (AICRP) on sheep for Mutton and AICRP on sheep for Wool located in different parts of the country with Coordinating Unit at Central Sheep Wool Research Institute (CSWRI), Avikanagar. The aim was to improve body weight, wool production and feed efficiency. However, with low nutrient intake regimen the survivability of crossbreds/synthetic breeds is relatively less compared to that of indigenous sheep.

Proper nutritional management is essential to exploit the full genetic potential of the crossbred sheep. Feed accounts for 55-60% in the total cost of rearing the sheep. Nutrient requirements of sheep NRC (1985), ARC (1980) and ICAR (1998) have been revised. The nutrient requirements presently available for small ruminants are NRC (2007), Feeding Standards for Australian Livestock (SCA, 1990) and ICAR (2013).

Energy: Insufficient energy probably limits performance of sheep and may result from inadequate amounts of feed or from feed of low quality. Supplies of feed may be inadequate as a result of overgrazing, drought, less availability of pasture lands.

Symptoms of energy deficiency: Energy deficiency, depending on severity, will cause slowing or cessation of growth, loss of weight, reduced fertility or reproductive failure, lowered milk production and shortened lactation period, reduced wool quantity and quality, including breaks in the fibre, and eventually increased mortality. Sheep suffering from energy deficiency have lowered resistance to infection by internal parasites. Energy deficiency may be complicated by protein, mineral and/or vitamin deficiencies.

Factors Affecting Energy Requirements

(a) Size, age, growth, pregnancy, lactation, season, parasitism, distance travelled during grazing and their relationship to protein which must be supplied in adequate amounts.
(b) Environment: temperature, humidity and wind may increase or decrease energy needs, depending upon relative values in relation to the zone of thermal neutrality.
(c) Shearing decreases insulation and may increase energy losses.
(d) Stress of any kind appears to increase energy requirements.

Symptoms of protein deficiency: Insufficient protein intake results in reduced appetite, lowered feed intake, and lowered efficiency in utilization of feed. Lower feed intake results in poor growth, poor muscular development, and loss of weight. The deficiency also reduces reproductive efficiency and wool production. Extreme deficiency results in severe digestive disturbances, anaemia and oedema.

Quality of protein: The protein produced by ruminal synthesis do not supply all the amino acids in quality or quantity needed by the host at the tissue level for maximal production. Postruminal administration of protein and/or amino acids has increased voluntary consumption of feed, weight gains, and wool growth. The sulfur containing amino acid, methionine, is the first limiting amino acid in microbial protein for both growth of wool and weight gain followed by lysine and threonine. Cystine apparently can replace methionine for growth.

Addition of 5% tallow in sheep ration increased the gain and reduced the cost of feed per kg gain. A minimum of 3% fat in sheep rations is essential.

Salt licks containing important major and minor minerals are kept in their shed as a free choice lick. Salt is added at 0.5% to complete diet or 1% to the concentrate mixture. They consume more salt per unit of body weight than the cattle.

Nutrient requirements of small ruminants

Feeding standards provide readers with the knowledge and means to adopt proper feeding practices. Nutrient requirements of small ruminants (sheep, goats, cervids, and new world camelids) published by NRC of the National Academies Press (USA) in 2007 combined the revisions of The Nutrient Requirements of Sheep (6th edition, 1985) and The Nutrient Requirements of Goats (1st edition, 1981) besides including information on cervids and alpacas and llamas. Requirements for energy, protein, minerals, vitamins, and water are furnished based on scientific evidence published in peer-reviewed technical sources.

After a thorough survey of all relevant information relating to goat nutrition in temperate zones, the Working Party established by AFRC Technical Committee for Responses to Nutrients (TCORN) provided the nutrient requirements of goats in 1998 in terms compatible with the current AFRC recommendations for cattle and sheep.

ICAR (2013) brought out 'Nutrient Requirements of Sheep, Goat and Rabbit' in a novel way based on current knowledge available in India and other countries and thus provide a comprehensive review of data on their requirements.

Fasting heat production and metabolizable energy required for maintenance (MEm) decreases as animal ages (NRC, 2007). Kearl (1982) suggested MEm of 92 kcal/kg $W^{0.75}$ for adult sheep. One of the factors that influence MEm is level of feed intake (NRC, 2007). Sheep cover long distances during grazing, so MEm requirements for grazing sheep will always be higher than for the restrained animals.

Tropical animal rearing at times depends much on tree / shrub leaves. Many of these contain condensed tannins, which can increase faecal nitrogen excretion and in turn decrease apparent digestibility of nitrogen. To maintain body growth in infected animals, protein requirement is increased due to loss or diversion of endogenous nitrogen. Therefore, in the event of infestation, animals would require a high feed energy intake, with a high ratio of amino acids to ME, higher rate of absorption of calcium and phosphorus.

Maintenance: The ICAR (1998) maintenance requirement values had been arrived at from several digestibility and balance trials in which animals maintained their body weight. DCP requirement was 2.73 g per kg metabolic body size while TDN and ME requirements were 27.3 g and 98 kcal per kg $W^{0.75}$. Paul et al (2003) analysed the performance and intake data of growing Indian sheep under tropical conditions obtained from feeding trials conducted in different research institutes. The estimated requirements for sheep of 7 - 15 kg BW are 37 g TDN, 560 kJ (134 kcal) MEm, 6.68 g CP and 4.43 g DCP per kg metabolic body size, while for 15.5 - 30 kg BW range the values are 35.3 g, 534 kJ (127.8 kcal), 6.98 g and 4.49 g, respectively. ME was calculated from TDN values using a factor of 1 kg TDN = 15.13 MJ ME (NRC, 1985). A mature sheep produces 2-6 g clean wool/d; therefore the DCP (Table 2) also covers the requirements for wool production. DM requirement as per cent of BW varies from 3.5 to 2.15 as the animal matures into adulthood.

TABLE 2 Nutrient requirements of Indian sheep (adult ewe, rams, yearlings) for maintenance, breeding, gestation and lactation (ICAR, 2013)

BW (kg)	Energy in Diet (ME, Mcal/kg)	DMI (g/d)	DMI (% BW)	Energy requirement		Protein requirement	
				TDN (g)	ME (Meal)	CP(g)	DCP (g)
Maintenance							
10	2.0	0.35	3.50	200	0.70	38	25
15	2.0	0.48	3.16	270	0.95	51	34
20	2.0	0.60	2.94	330	1.18	63	43
25	2.0	0.71	2.78	390	1.39	75	50
30	2.0	0.81	2.66	450	1.59	86	58
35	2.0	0.91	2.56	500	1.79	96	65
40	2.0	1.00	2.47	560	1.98	107	71
45	2.0	1.10	2.40	'610	2.16	116	78
50	2.0	1.19	2.34	660	2.34	126	84

55	2.0	1.27	2.28	710	2.51	135	91
60	2.0	1.36	2.23	750	2.68	145	97
65	2.0	1.44	2.19	800	2.85	153	103
70	2.0	1.53	2.15	850	3.01	162	107

Breeding

15	2.0	0.53	3.53	290	1.06	56	38
20	2.0	0.66	3.28	360	1.31	70	47
25	2.0	0.78	3.10	430	1.55	82	55
30	2.0	0.89	2.97	490	1.78	95	63
35	2.0	1.00	2.85	550	2.00	106	71
40	2.0	1.10	2.76	610	2.21	117	79
45	2.0	1.21	2.68	670	2.41	128	86
50	2.0	1.30	2.61	720	2.61	139	93
55	2.0	1.40	2.55	780	2.80	149	100
60	2.0	1.50	2.49	830	2.99	159	106
65	2.0	1.59	2.44	880	3.18	169	113
70	2.0	1.68	2.40	930	3.36	178	120

Gestation

15	2.4	0.60	4.01	400	1.44	77	51
20	2.4	0.75	3.73	500	1.79	95	64
25	2.4	0.88	3.53	590	2.12	112	75
30	2.4	1.01	3.37	670	2.43	129	86
35	2.4	1.13	3.24	750	2.72	145	97
40	2.4	1.25	3.14	'830	3.01	160	107
45	2.4	1.37	3.05	910	3.29	175	117
50	2.4	1.48	2.97	990	3.56	189	127
55	2.4	1.59	2.90	1060	3.82	203	136
60	2.4	1.70	2.83	1130	4.08	217	145
65	2.4	1.81	2.78	1200	4.33	230	154
70	2.4	1.91	2.73	1270	4.58	243	163

Lactation

15	2.4	0.72	4.81	480	1.73	92	62
20	2.4	0.90	4.48	600	2.15	114	76
25	2.4	1.06	4.23	700	2.54	135	90
30	2.4	1.21	4.04	810	2.91	155	104
35	2.4	1.36	3.89	910	3.27	174	116
40	2.4	1.51	3.76	1000	3.61	192	129
45	2.4	1.64	3.66	1090	3.95	210	140
50	2.4	1.78	3.56	1180	4.27	227	152
55	2.4	1.91	3.48	1270	4.59	244	163
60	2.4	2.04	3.40	1360	4.90	260	174
65	2.4	2.17	3.33	1440	5.20	276	185
70	2.4	2.29	3.27	1520	5.50	292	196

Sheep are seasonally polyestrus. Ewes need flushing ration just before and during the breeding season.

Flushing: The practice of increasing the nutrient intake of ewes and condition prior to and during breeding (for a month) is called flushing. Its purpose is to increase the ovulation rate and consequently the lambing rate. This special feeding of providing 25% more nutrients above the maintenance needs has to be given 2-3 weeks prior to breeding and continues into the breeding season.

Pregnancy: It is known that deficiency of one or more dietary nutrients may affect reproduction. A pregnant sheep need nutrients for foetus, uterus and mammary gland and related organ development. During the last trimester of gestation most of the energy is used by the foetus. Efficiency of energy use in pregnancy is low in comparison to growth or maintenance (NRC, 2007). To overcome the inevitable weight loss during early lactation, late gestation nutrition should be adequate enough to increase body weight or to ensure better body condition at lambing. Yearlings were assumed to be growing during gestation.

Nutrient requirements of ewes increase slowly during the first 15 weeks of pregnancy as the embryos grow and exert greater demands on the maternal tissue. Requirements during the final 6 weeks of pregnancy are greatly elevated.

Pregnancy (Table 2) and lactation (Table 2) requirements are presented (ICAR, 2013) for ewes of body weights ranging from 15 to 70 kg.

Breeding rams (during the breeding season) and pregnant ewes during the last 6 weeks of pregnancy should be provided with 50% more nutrients than the maintenance needs.

Nutrient requirements in sheep reach the highest levels during the first month of lactation. The peak milk production in ewes is achieved at around 21 days of lactation and high milk production levels are sustained for 6-8 weeks of lactation. Energy requirements for lactation vary with the amount and composition of milk produced.

Almost all the ewes lose weight during lactation, because energy intake is well below the requirement. Ewes must mobilize body reserves to sustain milk production. Hence, weight loss during early lactation is imminent. However, excess weight loss is not without its costs. Weight loss during lactation impacts protein requirements i.e. the more weight the ewes lose, the higher their protein need (ICAR, 2013). This situation is due to the ewe's ability to effectively mobilize body fat but having minimal ability to mobilize body protein for milk synthesis. At times it is economical to feed more energy rich grain to limit weight loss instead of feeding extra protein to balance energy from fat breakdown. It is also important to realize that fat conversion to milk is about 60% under protein and energy deficient rations whereas with adequate protein fed, fat conversion to milk is 80% (NRC, 2007).

Milk Production

Sheep are mainly raised for lamb and wool but not for milk production. However, high lactation performance is essential for the nutrition of the lamb during early age. This becomes all the more important if twins are nursed by the ewes. So the lactating sheep need (about) twice the maintenance requirements during the first 2 months of lactation followed by 1.5 times the maintenance during the remaining period. Requirements (Table 2) furnished are relevant to last 6 weeks of pregnancy in case of pregnant ewes and lactation requirements are relevant to first 2 months of the lactation.

Wool production: Requirements (Table 3) for wool production have been derived from the data on experiments conducted at the CSWRI, Avikanagar. Energy, protein and sulfur requirements are derived for Indian sheep.

Table 3 Daily nutrient requirement of sheep for wool production (Ranjhan, 1998)*

Live weight (LW), kg	DM, g % of LW	DM, g	DCP, g	TDN, Mcal	ME, g	Ca, g	P, g	S, g
20	730	3.1	40	330	1.19	1.5	1.0	1.7
25	870	3.5	47	390	1.41	1.7	1.1	2.1
30	1000	3.3	54	450	1.62	2.0	1.3	2.4
35	1100	3.1	60	500	1.80	2.2	1.5	2.6
40	1230	3.1	67	555	2.00	2.5	1.6	2.9
45	1350	3.0	73	610	2.20	2.7	1.8	3.2
50	1470	2.9	80	660	2.38	2.9	1.9	3.5
55	1580	2.9	85	710	2.56	3.2	2.1	3.8
60	1680	2.8	90	755	2.72	3.4	2.2	4.0

* Calcium and phosphorus requirements are based on NRC (1985).

Wool is a protein fibre composed of more than 20 amino acids. It also contains small amounts of fat. calcium and sodium. Nutrition plays an important role on its growth and quality parameters. Protein nutrition is important for wool growth and production, as wool is composed entirely of protein with very high level of cysteine and serine compared to other body tissues. Growth of wool requires more protein relative to energy, and draws amino acids, particularly methionine and cysteine, disproportionately from the body pool.

Staple length and diameter of fibre was reduced at low level of feeding, while crimps/cm increased. Chokla animals possessed high potential of wool production and the potential is exhibited at higher level of feeding, while in Avivastra sheep the capacity of wool production per unit body weight did not increase considerably with increased level of feeding (ICAR, 2013).

Growth: Nutrient requirements for growing lambs are presented in Table 4.

TABLE 4   Daily nutrient requirements of growing Indian sheep (ICAR, 2013)

BW (kg)	ADG (g/d)	ME level in diet (Mcal/kg)	DMI (kg/d)	DMI (% BW)	Energy requirement		Protein requirement	
					TDN (g)	ME (Meal)	CP(g)	DCP (g)
5	25	2.40	0.22	4.4	146	0.53	34	23
5	50	2.53	0.24	4.8	169	0.61	46	30
5	75	2.53	0.27	5.5	192	0.69	58	38
5	100	2.71	0.29	5.8	215	0.78	69	46
5	150	2.89	0.33	6.5	260	0.94	93	61
10	25	2.00	0.35	3.5	231	0.83	49	33
10	50	2.00	0.38	3.8	253	0.91	61	40
10	75	2.40	0.40	4.0	276	1.00	73	48
10	100	2.40	0.43	4.3	299	1.08	84	56
10	125	2.40	0.46	4.6	322	1.16	96	64
10	150	2.40	0.49	4.9	344	1.24	108	71
10	200	2.40	0.56	5.6	390	1.41	131	87
15	25	2.00	0.55	3.7	305	1.10	63	42
15	50	2.00	0.59	3.9	328	1.18	74	49
15	75	2.00	0.63	4.2	350	1.26	86	57
15	100	2.40	0.56	3.8	373	1.35	97	65
15	125	2.40	0.60	4.0	396	1.43	110	73
15	150	2.40	0.63	4.2	418	1.51	121	80
15	200	2.40	0.70	4.7	464	1.68	145	96
15	250	2.40	0.77	5.1	509	1.84	168	111
20	25	2.00	0.66	3.3	364	1.31	77	50
20	50	2.00	0.71	3.6	394	1.42	87	57
20	75	2.00	0.77	3.8	425	1.53	98	65
20	100	2.40	0.68	3.4	455	1.64	109	72
20	125	2.40	0.73	3.6	485	1.75	120	80
20	150	2.40	0.78	3.9	516	1.86	130	87
20	200	2.40	0.87	4.3	576	2.08	152	102
20	250	2.40	0.96	4.8	637	2.30	173	117
25	25	2.00	0.77	3.1	425	1.53	89	58
25	50	2.00	0.82	3.3	455	1.64	99	65
25	75	2.00	0.88	3.5	485	1.75	110	73
25	100	2.40	0.78	3.1	516	1.86	121	80
25	125	2.40	0.82	3.3	546	1.97	132	88
25	150	2.40	0.87	3.5	576	2.08	142	95
25	200	2.40	0.96	3.8	637	2.30	164	110

25	250	2.40	1.05	4.2	698	2.52	185	125
30	25	2.00	0.87	2.9	483	1.74	100	65
30	50	2.00	0.93	3.1	513	1.85	110	72
30	75	2.00	0.98	3.3	543	1.96	122	80
30	100	2.00	1.04	3.5	574	2.07	132	88
30	125	2.00	1.09	3.6	604	2.18	143	95
30	150	2.40	0.95	3.2	634	2.29	153	103
30	200	2.40	1.05	3.5	695	2.51	175	117
30	250	2.40	1.14	3.8	755	2.73	197	133
35	25	2.00	0.97	2.8	538	1.94	111	72
35	50	2.00	1.03	2.9	568	2.05	122	80
35	75	2.00	1.08	3.1	599	2.16	133	87
35	100	2.40	0.95	2.7	629	2.27	143	95
35	125	2.40	0.99	2.8	659	2.38	154	102
35	150	2.40	1.04	3.0	689	2.49	165	110
35	200	2.40	1.13	3.2	750	2.71	186	125
35	250	2.40	1.22	3.5	810	2.92	208	140

Newborn lambs (1–3 days old) require 117 kcal ME/kg $W^{0.75}$ for maintenance and 0.41 kcal ME/g weight gain (Kearl, 1982). The pre-weaning growth period is crucial. The maintenance requirements of growing sheep in 7-15 kg body weight range are 37g TDN, 6.68g CP and 4.43g DCP per kg $W^{0.75}$ and 35.3 g, 6.98g and 4.49g, respectively, for growing sheep of 15.5–30 kg range (Paul et al., 2003). The estimated the ME requirement for growth are 13.7 kJ (3.29 kcal) and 18.3 kJ (4.37 kcal) per g weight gain in 7–15 kg and 15.5–30 kg, respectively. The corresponding values for TDN requirements are 0.91 and 1.21g per g BW gain.

Minerals

Sheep need to be fed with adequate minerals in the diet depending on the season, level of feeding and physiological state. Dry season pasture contains less P than the green season pasture and tender leaves contain more P than older leaves. Iron and copper are generally lower in dry season fodders compared to rainy season fodders. Leguminous species are generally richer in macrominerals than the grasses growing under comparable conditions. Trace minerals such as iron, copper, zinc, cobalt and nickel are also generally higher in legume forages. Ruminants are more likely to suffer from Cu deficiency because of its low intestinal absorption (McDowell et al., 1984).

Vitamins

Among the fat soluble and water soluble vitamins, use of vitamin A and E has received much attention. A level of 1600–2000 RE (1 retinyl equivalent = 1 mg of all-trans retinol = 5.0 mg of all-trans beta carotene = 7.6 mg of other carotenoids) / kg DM in the diet can meet the requirements of the adult sheep for maintenance and for other physiological stages. However, the levels need to be enhanced by 50% for growing sheep. It is recommended at 10 IU vitamin E/kg BW as an aid to protect the sheep from infectious diseases and to extend quality of lamb meat and its shelf life. A level of 5–10 IU vitamin E per kg BW is suggested for Indian sheep (ICAR, 2013).

Feeds and Fodders for Sheep

Sheep have a special ability to survive on natural grasses, herbs, legumes, weeds, shrubs and farm wastes. They have a muzzle with a split upper lip and they can pick up tiny blades of herbage which are inaccessible to bigger animals. This also helps them to glean grains lost at harvest time. Sheep chew green material with less moisture in it.

Common property resources (CPRs) - the common grazing land, pasture and wastelands - provide large proportion of nutritional requirements of sheep and goats in India. The resource-poor farmers depend on CPRs as compared to the rich farmers.

The common leguminous feeds like cowpea, berseem, lucerne, siratro, *Stylosanthes*, sunhemp, horsegram, etc. and grasses such as *Cenchrus ciliaris, C. setigerus* are relished very much by sheep. Leafy leguminous hays and good grasses are valuable feeds for sheep. In India nearly 20% of the area is covered by forest which gives some pasture for sheep and goat raising. During monsoon, good quality pastures are available whereas during summer practically carrying capacity of these grasslands is less. So supplemental feeding of concentrate mixture is often recommended during dry season for better growth and production.

Systems of Sheep Rearing: They are

1. Extensive system
2. Intensive system
3. Semi-intensive system

Extensive Rearing of Sheep

The practical way to find out whether the non-producing animals are receiving sufficient nutrients from their grazing is to weigh them periodically. If the animals are maintaining their body weight or putting on a little weight to the extent of about 20 to 30 g per day, they can be stated to be on maintenance ration. If they are continually losing body weight, they need supplementation. On the other hand, if ewes are gaining weight more rapidly, it may be useful to reduce the grazing time.

Grazing the sheep in the entire pasture and leaving them there for the whole season is not conducive to making the best use of the grasses. Rotational grazing should be practised under which the pasture land should be divided by temporary fences into several sections. The animals are then moved from one section to another section. By the time the entire pasture is grazed, the first section will have sufficient grass cover to provide second grazing. Parasitic infestations can be controlled to a great extent. Further, it helps to provide quality fodder (immature) for most part of the year. Under rotational grazing system, it is advisable to graze the lambs first on a section and then bring in ewes to finish up the feed left by the lambs.

Semi-intensive and intensive system of rearing

Because of the decline in the quality and quantity of pasture from CPRs, now semi-intensive and intensive systems of rearing are also adopted. Under semi-intensive system, sheep are allowed to graze for 8 to 12 hours a day and then offered home-made / commercial concentrate mixture. Sometimes total mixed rations are offered including legume straws and gram pod husk. In peri-urban areas intensive system of rearing (stall feeding) is preferred.

Feeding of Preweaned Lambs from Birth to 90 Days Age

Sheep are superior to goats in their growth rate as young animals. The birth weights of lambs and kids are nearly the same, in the range between 2-3 kg. The development of lambs in the first four months is faster than the kids. Doubling and tripling of the birth weights is reached much earlier in lambs than by kids. The most critical period in the life of a lamb is during the first 48 hours. If a lamb is unable to nurse within half an hour after birth, it should be assisted to suckle to get the advantages of colostrum.

Creep Feeding: The creep is a small enclosure in a sheep pen having opening just wide enough for lambs to pass in, while the ewes are kept back. The practice of providing supplemental feed to nursing lambs is called creep feeding. Animal protein supplement is a must in creep feed. Lamb is to be fed creep feed of high quality according to appetite from 10 days of age to weaning at 90 days to promote growth during early age and rumen development. The amount of creep feed consumed is inversely proportional to the ewe's milk production.

Lambs below 30 days are functionally similar to non-ruminants. Therefore, quality of protein is important. Animal protein meals are to be fed because they are rich sources of lysine and methionine. Soybean meal is the preferred choice nowadays because of its assured good quality, palatability and protein content with rich lysine content while methionine is supplemented.

Feeding Schedule: Nellore brown lambs were allowed suckling thrice a day up to one month and thereafter twice a day. Creep feed was fed from 10th day onwards while sunnhemp hay (coarse ground) was fed from 15th day onwards. Feeding was continued up to 90 days age i.e. weaning.

Composition of Creep Feed: Maize 40, groundnut cake 30, wheat bran 10, deoiled rice bran 12, molasses, 5, mineral mixture 2 and salt one per cent fortified with vitamins A, B_2 and D_3 and antibiotic feed supplement. DCP is 17.4% and TDN is 73%. The performance of lambs is as follows.

Average weight at weaning = 14 kg

Average daily gain   = 130 g

Total creep feed consumed = 12.7 kg/lamb

Sunnhemp hay consumed   = 3.5 kg/lamb

Feeding of Growing—Finishing Lambs from Weaning to Slaughter

Extensive system of rearing will not meet the requirement of the growing-finishing ram lambs. Hence ram lambs should be given a concentrate mixture to supplement the nutrients obtained through grazing. Native breeds such as Nellore, Mandya, Madras red, etc. and their crosses need to be raised under semi-intensive/intensive system of rearing to exploit their genetic potential.

Concentrate Mixtures

1.			2.		
Maize/Jowar	25		Maize/Jowar	30	
Wheat bran	32		Groundnut cake	20	
Gram waste	26		Deoiled rice bran	40	
Groundnut cake	15		Molasses	8	
Mineral mixture	1		Mineral mixture	1	
Salt	1		Salt	1	
	100			100	
DCP	=	13%	DCP	=	13%
TDN	=	70%	TDN	=	70%

Feeding Schedule

BW kg	Concentrate mixture, g/d	Roughage* g/d	Remarks
12-15	200	400	8 hours grazing can be substituted in place of roughage
16-25	250	600	
26-35	300	700	

*Grasses such as *C. ciliaris*, *C. setigerus*; Legume pastures such as *S. hamata*, *S. scabra*, *Siratro;* Groundnut haulms, Grass-legume mixture may also be given.

It is better to keep the lambs in the stall for mutton production specially in the monsoon period because the animals do not relish to graze the wet grasses and are also prone to diseases. Free choice mineral block lick are to be provided in the sheds. Crossbred sheep should attain 30 kg body weight by 6 months of age while native breeds may take 9 months. In urban areas intensive dry lot feeding is practised and it is promising.

Diet and meat quality

Intramuscular fat (IMF) concentration is found to be a key element of eating quality of meat (tenderness). This depends to a large extent on a lamb's genotype (heritability of 0.48) as well as carcass weight and fatness. Processing factors obviously influence the myofibrillar components of shear force, but have no effect on the IMF component.

The composition of the fatty acids in meat is very sensitive to diet (Ponnampalam et al., 2014). A potential exception might be for the docosahexaenoic acid (DHA) content of muscle which is insensitive to diet, unlike the other omega 3 long chain fatty acids (Scollen et al., 2005). DHA had the highest heritability (0.22) of all the long chain fatty acids measured. Lamb meat can generally be regarded as good source of minerals (iron and zinc) and a source of omega 3 fatty acids when finished on green pastures.

Feeding of Pregnant Ewes during Last 6 Weeks of Gestation

During this time ewes need more energy, protein, minerals and vitamins to meet the increased requirements for foetal growth and the development of the potential for high milk production. Excessive energy intake may lead to fattening which results in birth difficulties in ewes. Low energy intakes can result in low birth weights with reduced viability in the lambs and perhaps pregnancy toxaemia in the ewe.

Since the pregnant ewe can not consume sufficient bulky roughages as the space in the abdomen is reduced due to the growth of foetus and its membranes, it has to be fed with good quality forage (cereal fodders 6% DCP and 60% TDN; grasses 6% DCP and 55% TDN) and a concentrate mixture supplement. Gliricidia leaf meal has 11–14% DCP and 53–60% TDN.

The practical way to find out whether the ewes in advanced pregnancy are receiving their quota of nutrients is to see their body weight gains. An average daily gain of 100 g for smaller breeds and 150 g for larger breeds is a fair measure of nutrient intake status at this stage of physiological function.

Feeding the Lactating/Suckling Ewe

After lambing, proper care should be taken while feeding mother ewes. Only a little grain mixture should be fed for the first two or three days and the ewe should have accessibility to good quality forage. As soon as the lamb(s) are able to take more milk, the ewe should be fed liberally with the good quality forages and concentrate mixture to take care of extra requirement of nutrients during lactation. Dry matter consumption may go up to 4% of BW.

The feeding of supplemental concentrate mixture can gradually be diminished after 8 to 10 weeks of lambing and can be stopped after 12-13 weeks of lambing as the lambs are weaned from the mother. The ewes may be maintained on grazing alone. This feeding system may continue until the next breeding season.

Feeding for Wool Production

Wool is a protein rich in sulfur containing amino acid, cysteine. Minerals play a very important role in wool production. Small quantities of selenium are essential; copper, cobalt, iodine, iron, etc. are all essential for the proper growth of wool.

Nutrition-Related Metabolic Disorders: Sheep

1. *Enterotoxaemia (overeating disease, pulpy kidney disease):* It is described in Section on Goats.

2. *Polio encephalamalacia (PEM) or Cerebrocortical necrosis (CCN):* This disease has been reported in most ages and classes of sheep, but it occurs most often in feedlot lambs. It may be due to

thiamin deficiency, probably associated with cofactors and antimetabolities, initiated by rumen produced thiaminases. It may be due to eating of certain plants. Affected animals are to be treated quickly with 200 to 500 mg of thiamin injected intravenously, intramuscularly, or subcutaneously.

3. *Pregnancy toxaemia (ketosis or acetonemia):* It occurs in ewes in late pregnancy and usually is restricted to those carrying twins. During late pregnancy there are high glucose demands (about 1.5 times maintenance levels) on the ewe by the rapidly growing foetus(es). The ewe mobilizes adipose tissue in an attempt to meet glucose needs, leading to metabolic acidosis and accumulation of ketone bodies in the blood. It can be prevented by ensuring adequate nutrient intake in the pregnancy so that increases in weight occurs. Propylene glycol or glycerol, 200 to 300 ml can be used orally as an energy source when ewes refuse to eat sufficient feed. The affected ewes show anorexia have a staggering gait and exhibit nervousness (See ketosis for more details).

4. *Urinary calculi (uroliths):* are mineral deposits occurring in the urinary tract and cause blockage of flow of urine. This generally occurs in male sheep, goats and bullocks and they may die due to consequential effects of rupture of urinary bladder.

Under intensive system of rearing, this disease appears to have a nutritional or metabolic origin; affected animals excrete alkaline urine that has a high phosphorus content. The incidence can be greatly reduced by preventing an excessive intake of phophorus and by maintaining a proper Ca to P ratio (2:1). Reducing the alkalinity of urine by feeding ammonium chloride at 0.5% of complete diet is also effective.

In grazing sheep, the disease is associated with the consumption of forages having a high silica content. Sodium chloride supplementation (at 4% or more of the total diet) helps to prevent urinary calculi in them.

Critical periods in development and production cycles in sheep

Reproduction: Some consequences of undernutrition during breeding and pregnancy are low conception, severe embryo wastage, pregnancy toxaemia, and low birth weights (poor lamb survival).

Hypoglycaemia (low blood sugar) results in pregnancy toxaemia and is usually fatal to the pregnant ewe.

Lactation

Ketosis, a metabolic state that is expressed during gestation as pregnancy toxaemia, may occur as a result of mobilization of fat to provide the elevated energy requirement. Concurrent with this ketotic state, hypocalcaemia may occur. The high demand for calcium in milk requires mobilization from the bone.

Feeding high levels of concentrates in early lactation can cause lactic acidosis, which is an intraruminal consequence of an accumulation of products of rapid carbohydrate fermentation.

Growth

Growing lambs encounter various acute nutritional disorders that result in an array of abnormal conditions. These include rickets, lactic acidosis, enterotoxaemia, urinary calculi (water belly), polioencephalomalacia.

Sheep, especially lambs, are more likely to suffer from copper toxicity compared to other animals.

NUTRIENT REQUIREMENTS AND FEEDING OF GOATS FOR MEAT AND MILK PRODUCTION

Goats are valued for economic milk production and as the main source for meat for a large section of populace. Some of the important dual purpose breeds (Meat and milk) are Jamunapari, Barbari, Beetal. Black Bengal is a meat purpose breed. Angora, Chegu (Pasmina) are of hair type breeds. Black Bengal, Barbari are examples of small breeds. Alpine and Saanen are examples of exotic dairy goats. A good, well-managed goat may produce as much milk at less cost as the ordinary cow. The average milk yield of a non-descript doe is 60 litres, while it is 100 and 250 litres for Barbari and Jamunapari breeds, respectively, per lactation of 120 days.

Nutrient Requirements of Goats

National Research Council of National Academy of Sciences, USA published nutrient requirements of goats in 1981. ICAR published the nutrient requirements of goats in 1985 in its Nutrient Requirements of Livestock and Poultry which was revised in 1998. Research on nutrition of goats in India has been conducted only at a few centres. ICAR established a Central Institute for Research on Goats (CIRG) at Makhdhum in U.P. The energy and protein requirements have been worked out on the basis of information available (Senger, 1992). The European association for animal production (EAAP) published a review of research work done between 1982 and 1990 summarised by group of experts under the programme of the FAO cooperative research Sub-network on goat production (EAAP Publication No. 46, 1991). Revised nutrient requirements presently available are NRC Nutrient requirements for small ruminants (2007), Feeding Standards for Australian Livestock (SCA, 1990) and ICAR (2013).

Different methods have been used to estimate the nutrient requirements of goats. One important method that used respiration calorimetry, though precise, is time consuming and quite expensive. Another approach is to use body weight gain as a measure of retention and relate it to energy intake based on regression equations. The advantage of this method is that the data can be collected under normal production conditions (Luo et al., 2004). In India, Mandal et al. (2005) also proposed a system based on regressions using data from 25 experiments conducted on 93 different dietary treatments.

ICAR second edition requirements (Ranjhan, 1998) are also retained (maintenance requirements, Table 5; pregnant does, Table 11; lactating does, Table 12) to facilitate easy grasp, comprehension and comparison.

The NRC (2007) nutrient requirements of milk goats (Table 7) and meat (Table 8) goats for maintenance only are presented to make the readers aware about the latest nutrient requirements.

TABLE 5 Daily Nutrient Requirements for Maintenance of Adult Goats (Ranjhan, 1998).

BW kg	DMI g	DM % BW	DCP g	TDN g	Ca g	P g
15	500	3.3	23	240	1.1	0.7
20	615	3.1	29	295	1.3	0.9
25	730	2.9	34	350	1.6	1.1
30	830	2.8	39	400	1.8	1.2
35	940	2.7	44	450	2.1	1.4
40	1040	2.6	48	500	2.3	1.5
45	1125	2.5	53	540	2.5	1.7
50	1230	2.4	57	590	2.7	1.8
55	1315	2.4	62	630	2.9	1.9
60	1410	2.3	66	675	3.1	2.1

The expression of protein intake in terms of DCP or CP does not provide substantial information with reference to the quantity of amino acids absorbed by the goats. However, relevant data for the development of feeding standards based on metabolizable protein system on Indian goats are

Table 6 Nutrient requirements of Mature does (Dairy) for maintenance only*

Body weight, kg	Daily DMI		Energy requirements		Protein requirements**					Mineral requirements		Vitamin requirements	
kg	kg	% BW	TDN kg/d	ME Mcal /d	CP @20% UIP g/d	CP @40% UIP g/d	CP @60% UIP g/d	MP g/d	DIP g/d	Ca g/d	P g/d	A RE/d	E IU/d
20	0.59	2.96	0.31	1.13	40	38	36	27	28	1.3	0.9	628	106
30	0.80	2.68	0.43	1.54	54	51	49	36	38	1.6	1.2	942	159
40	1.00	2.49	0.53	1.91	67	64	61	45	48	1.9	1.5	1256	212
50	1.18	2.36	0.62	2.25	79	75	72	53	56	2.1	1.7	1570	265
60	1.35	2.25	0.72	2.58	90	86	82	61	64	2.4	2.0	1884	318
70	1.52	2.17	0.80	2.90	101	97	92	68	72	2.6	2.2	2198	371
80	1.68	2.10	0.89	3.20	112	107	102	75	80	2.8	2.4	2512	424
90	1.83	2.03	0.97	3.50	122	116	111	82	87	3.0	2.6	2826	477

*Energy concentration 1.91Mcal /kg diet; **Protein requirements expressed as crude protein (CP), metabolizable protein (MP), and degradable intake protein (DIP). The CP requirement differs with the proportion of undegradable intake protein (UIP) because of the required minimum DIP; RE=retinal equivalent: 1.0 µg of all-trans retinol, 5.0 µg of all-trans betacarotene, 7.6 µg of other carotenoids.

Table 7 Nutrient requirements of Mature does (nondairy) for maintenance only*

Body weight, kg	Daily DMI		Energy requirements		Protein requirements**					Mineral requirements		Vitamin requirements	
	kg	% BW	TDN kg/d	ME Mcal /d	CP @20% UIP g/d	CP @40% UIP g/d	CP @60% UIP g/d	MP g/d	DIP g/d	Ca g/d	P g/d	A RE/d	E IU/d
20	0.50	2.50	0.26	0.96	36	35	33	24	24	1.2	0.8	628	106
30	0.68	2.26	0.36	1.30	49	47	45	33	32	1.4	1.0	942	159
40	0.84	2.10	0.45	1.61	61	58	55	41	40	1.7	1.3	1256	212
50	0.99	1.99	0.53	1.90	71	68	65	48	47	1.9	1.5	1570	265
60	1.14	1.90	0.60	2.18	82	78	75	55	54	2.1	1.7	1884	318
70	1.28	1.83	0.68	2.44	92	88	84	62	61	2.3	1.9	2198	371
80	1.41	1.77	0.75	2.70	101	97	93	68	67	2.5	2.0	2512	424
90	1.54	1.72	0.82	2.95	111	106	101	74	74	2.6	2.2	2826	477

*Energy concentration 1.91Mcal /kg diet; **Protein requirements expressed as crude protein (CP), metabolizable protein (MP), and degradable intake protein (DIP). The CP requirement differs with the proportion of undegradable intake protein (UIP) because of the required minimum DIP; NRC (2007)

TABLE 8 Daily nutrient requirements of growing male goats under tropical conditions*

Body weight (kg)	Body weight gain (g/d)	Daily Dry Matter Intake kg	Daily Dry Matter Intake % BW	Energy Requirements TDN kg/d	Energy Requirements ME Mcal/d	Protein Requirements CP g/d	Protein Requirements DCP g/d	Mineral Requirements Ca g/d	Mineral Requirements P g/d	Vitamin Requirements Vit A 10000 IU	Vitamin Requirements Vit D IU
5	0	-	-	0.101	0.36	19	11	-	-	-	-
5	25	0.20	4	0.141	0.51	31	20	0.8	0.6	0.4	78
5	50	0.21	4.2	0.181	0.66	42	28	1.1	0.9	0.5	105
5	75	-	-	0.221	0.80	53	37	-	-	-	-
5	100	-	-	0.262	0.95	65	45	-	-	-	-
10	0	-	-	0.169	0.61	33	19	1.2	0.9	0.5	112
10	25	0.36	3.6	0.21	0.76	44	27	1.2	0.9	0.5	112
10	50	0.37	3.7	0.25	0.90	55	36	1.5	1.2	0.6	139
10	75	0.35	3.5	0.29	1.05	67	44	1.9	1.5	0.8	162
10	100	-	-	0.33	1.19	78	53	-	-	-	-
10	125	-	-	0.371	1.34	89	61	-	-	-	-
10	150	-	-	0.411	1.48	100	70	-	-	-	-
15	0	-	-	0.229	0.83	44	25	-	-	-	-
15	25	0.45	3	0.27	0.98	56	34	1.5	1.1	0.7	142
15	50	0.5	3.3	0.31	1.12	67	42	1.9	1.4	0.8	169
15	75	0.5	3.3	0.35	1.26	78	51	2.2	1.7	1	192
15	100	-	-	0.39	1.41	89	59	-	-	-	-
15	125	-	-	0.431	1.56	101	68	-	-	-	-
15	150	-	-	0.471	1.70	112	76	-	-	-	-
20	0	-	-	0.285	1.03	55	31	-	-	-	-
20	25	0.58	2.9	0.325	1.17	66	40	1.8	1.3	0.8	172
20	50	0.60	3.0	0.365	1.32	78	48	2.1	1.6	0.9	199
20	75	0.62	3.1	0.405	1.47	89	57	2.4	1.9	1.1	232
20	100	0.62	3.1	0.446	1.61	100	65	2.8	2.1	1.2	254
20	125	-	-	0.486	1.76	111	74	-	-	-	-
20	150	-	-	0.526	1.90	123	82	-	-	-	-
25	0	-	-	0.337	1.22	65	37	-	-	-	-
25	25	0.68	2.7	0.377	1.36	76	46	2.1	1.5	0.9	197
25	50	0.71	2.8	0.417	1.51	88	54	2.4	1.8	1	224
25	75	0.73	2.9	0.457	1.65	99	63	2.7	2.1	1.2	247
25	100	0.74	3.0	0.498	1.80	110	71	3.1	2.3	1.3	279
25	125	0.71	2.8	0.538	1.94	121	80	3.4	2.5	1.4	307
25	150	-	-	0.578	2.09	133	88	-	-	-	-
30	0	-	-	0.386	1.39	75	43	-	-	-	-
30	25	0.77	2.6	0.426	1.54	86	51	2.4	1.7	1.0	223
30	50	0.80	2.7	0.466	1.69	97	60	2.7	2.0	1.1	250
30	75	0.83	2.8	0.507	1.83	108	68	3.1	2.3	1.3	273
30	100	0.84	2.8	0.547	1.98	120	77	3.4	2.5	1.4	305
30	125	-	-	0.587	2.12	131	85	-	-	-	-
30	150	-	-	0.627	2.27	142	94	-	-	-	-

* TDN. ME, CP and DCP requirement calculations: from the published values of Mandal et al. (2005); DMI, Ca, P, Vitamin A and D values: as recommended by Kearl (1982) Source: ICAR (2013)

not available. Hence, Mandal et al. (2005) derived and presented protein requirements in terms of CP and DCP (Table 8).

Dry Matter Intake

Dry matter intake vary from 35 to 80 g per kg metabolic body size for different Indian breeds of goats with a 70 g as average (3.2% of BW). The DMI for the smaller breeds (Barbari and Black Bengal) is higher than the larger breeds (Jamunapari, beetal). DMI varies according to the energy density of the diet and the physical character of the roughage. DMI in the growing kids (pre-ruminant and early growth) ranges between 35-50 g per kg metabolic body size whereas in lactating Jamunapari goats ranges from 120 to 140 g. DMI of goats is higher in comparison to large farm animals.

Meat goats : 4% of BW
Dairy goats : 4-6% of BW

Maintenance: The nutrient requirements per kg metabolic body size are DCP 3.0 g and TDN 30 g (Table 5) for maintenance as per the second revised edition (Ranjhan 1998). ICAR (2013) nutrient requirements (Table 8) provide a satisfactory guideline for the formulation of rations and for developing supplementary feeding strategy for animals reared under semi-intensive system. In deriving these requirements of goats, primary data obtained from the results of research studies conducted in India were used (Mandal et al., 2005). However, the requirements of DM, Ca, P, vitamins A and D have been included as recommended by Kearl (1982).

Growth: The daily nutrient requirement values of goats for different, body weights and growth rate functions are presented in Table 8 as recommended by ICAR (2013) vis a vis with ICAR second edition requirements (Ranjhan, 1998) in Table 9. The requirements for growth have been given for body weights ranging from 5 to 30 kg and at each body weight for different rates of growth (Table 8).

Sengar (1980) reviewed two decades of Indian research on protein and energy requirements of goats based on metabolism studies conducted in nitrogen-free and low-nitrogen-containing diets. The maintenance requirements of energy and protein were 125 kcal DE and 3.13 g DCP / kg $W^{0.75}$, respectively. The consolidated requirements of energy and protein for growth, irrespective of stage of growth were 7.55 kcal DE and 0.195 g DCP / g gain.

The energy requirement for 1 g of average daily gain (ADG) was estimated to be 1.61 g TDN (Mandal et al., 2005). This value is comparable to the value (1.85 g TDN/g gain) adopted in the feeding standards of Kearl

TABLE 9 Daily Nutrient Requirements of Growing Kids (Ranjhan, 1998).

BW kg	ADG g	DMI g	DM % BW	DCP g	TDN g	Ca g	P g
10	50	380	3.8	27	265	2.0	1.4
	100	510	5.1	37	355	2.7	1.8
	150	635	6.3	47	445	3.4	2.3
15	50	510	3.4	33	330	2.7	1.8
	100	645	4.3	43	420	3.5	2.3
	150	785	5.2	53	510	4.2	2.8
20	50	640	3.2	39	385	3.3	2.2
	100	790	3.9	49	475	4.1	2.7
	150	985	4.9	59	590	5.1	3.4
25	50	760	3.0	44	440	3.8	2.5
	100	915	3.7	54	530	4.6	3.0
	150	1070	4.3	64	620	5.3	3.6

(1982) and ICAR (1998). Mandal et al. (2005) reported maintenance requirement of TDN to be 30.1 g/kgW$^{0.75}$. TDN requirements for maintenance and different production traits were calculated using the derived prediction equations and these are presented in Table 10.

Pregnancy and Lactation

The lactation requirements (Table 12) are given on a production level of 0.5 to 1.0 kg milk per day and these include the maintenance requirements at different body weights.

Energy and protein requirements of mature does during breeding and rams pre-breeding are 10 % greater than at other times. Flushing is a strategy for increasing ovulation rate in females by feeding high-energy feeds just before and during the breeding period.

Once conception has occurred, providing nutrients at a level only slightly above that of maintenance is sufficient. The later stage of pregnancy is very critical in goats. Substantial increases in nutrient (Table 11) levels are required during the last trimester of gestation, especially in litter-bearing females, to prevent pregnancy toxaemia and provide for normal fetal development.

The DMI in case of Alpine breed during lactation in temperate conditions is 3.6 kg/day or 6.8% of BW or 181 g per kg metabolic body size. The voluntary DMI rises just after parturition and reaches a maximum between 6 and 10 weeks of lactation and thereafter decreased.

Decreased dry matter intake has been reported with the advancement of pregnancy due to the reduction in the volume of abdominal cavity, limiting the distension of digestive tract and ultimately the food intake.

The recommended requirements include the maintenance requirement at different body weights (Table 12 and 13). On an average the lactation requirement is 345 g TDN and 45 g DCP per kg of 4% FCM over and above the maintenance requirement (Ranjhan 1998).

The nutrient requirements of goats in general are relatively higher presumably due to their higher activity, higher twinning rate and comparatively more milk yield. The productivity of a goat depends on how it has been fed during its pregnancy and lactation (Rajpoot, 1978). A comprehensive study was conducted involving Jamnapari, Beetal, Barbari and Black Bengal breeds of goats and their crosses on *ad lib feeding* (Table 10). The DE, ME and NE values estimated for gain in body weight are 8.22, 6.71 and 3.78 kcal/g, respectively. The corresponding values for combined requirement for maintenance and growth were 233.8, 190.7 and 107.7 kcal /kg $W^{0.75}$.

Rajpoot (1978) reported the maintenance requirements of lactating does as 191, 156 and 88 kcal, respectively, as DE, ME and NE. The combined requirements for lactation (maintenance +milk production) were 313 kcal DE, 256 kcal ME and 144 kcal NE / doe of 30 kg average body weight and producing 1 kg with 4% FCM/day (Rajpoot, 1978). Sengar (1980) reported the requirements of energy and protein for milk production of goats as 1520 kcal DE (1246 kcal ME) and 46.6 g DCP/kg 4% FCM in native goats.

The total DCP requirements for maintenance and gain (Table 10) are much higher (19-35%) than the values recommended by NRC (1981), Kearl (1982) or ICAR (1998). Both the feeding standards currently being used in India (Kearl, 1982; ICAR, 1998) were based on a few reports on Indian goats and utilized protein requirement values derived from nitrogen balance trials or from studies involving non-producing animals.

TABLE 10 Energy requirements (per kg $W^{0.75}$) of goat breeds for maintenance and different production traits

Parameter	Requirement (k cal)		
	DE	ME*	NE*
Maintenance (adult non-producing)	125	102	58
Maintenance plus gain	234	191	108
Pregnancy	227	185	104
Maintenance of dairy does	191	156	88
Maintenance plus lactation	313	256	144

* ME = DE x 0.82; NE = ME x 0.56; Adapted from ICAR (2013)

TABLE 11 Daily Nutrient Requirements of Pregnant Does (Ranjhan, 1998).

BW kg	DMI g	DM % BW	DCP g	TDN g	Ca g	P g
15	700	4.7	42	385	2.1	1.4
20	865	4.3	52	475	2.6	1.7
25	1025	4.1	62	564	3.1	2.1
30	1170	3.9	71	645	3.5	2.3
35	1320	3.8	80	725	4.0	2.7
40	1460	3.6	88	802	4.4	2.9
45	1590	3.5	96	875	4.8	3.2
50	1725	3.4	104	984	5.2	3.5
55	1850	3.4	112	1018	5.5	3.7
60	1975	3.6	120	1086	5.9	3.9

TABLE 12 Daily Nutrient Requirements of Lactating Does (Ranjhan, 1998).

BW kg	MILK yield, kg	DMI g	DM % BW	DCP g	TDN g	Ca g	P g
20	0.5	865	4.3	51	468	4.3	2.9
	1.0	1185	5.9	74	640	5.9	3.9
25	0.5	968	3.9	56	523	4.8	3.2
	1.0	1290	5.2	79	695	6.4	4.3
30	0.5	1060	3.5	61	573	5.3	3.5
	1.0	1380	4.6	84	745	6.9	4.6
35	0.5	1155	3.3	66	623	5.8	3.9
	1.0	1470	4.2	89	795	7.3	4.9
40	0.5	1245	3.1	70	673	6.2	4.1
	1.0	1565	3.9	93	845	7.8	5.2
45	0.5	1320	2.9	75	713	6.6	4.4
	1.0	1640	3.6	98	885	8.2	5.3
50	0.5	1410	2.8	79	763	7.0	4.7
	1.0	1730	3.5	102	935	8.6	5.7
55	0.5	1490	2.7	84	803	7.4	4.9
	1.0	1805	3.3	107	975	9.0	6.0
60	0.5	1570	2.6	88	848	7.8	5.2
	1.0	1890	3.1	111	1020	9.4	6.3

The maintenance requirement of CP was estimated to be 5.83 g/ kg $W^{0.75}$. The CP requirement for live weight gain was 0.45 g/ g BW gain. The maintenance requirement of DCP was 3.32 g/ kg $W^{0.75}$ and requirement for live weight gain was 0.34 g/ g BW gain.

Sengar (1980) reported the total requirements (maintenance + pregnancy) of goats as 221.8 kcal DE and 5.55 g DCP / $kgW^{0.75}$ of does with a mean weight of 30.4 kg and gaining 61.8 g/d at pregnancy during the last two months of gestation.

Mineral and trace element research in goats

Professor Manfred Anke and his team from Germany did extensive and significant mineral and trace element research with goats since 1960 and the contributions were published in mostly in German. To have a wider global audience and appreciation, G.F.W.Haenlein and M.Anke reviewed the long term studies with dairy goats (from 1975 until 2010) on the effects of feeding deficient semi-synthetic rations in one of 16 elements.

Criteria for establishing nutritional essentiality of an element: The seven criteria are retardation of growth, reduced reproductive performance, reduced longevity, participation of the element in an essential tissue or organ, development of disorders, reproducibility of results in other species and removal of deficiency effects with nutritional supplements (Anke et al.. 1984).

Semi-synthetic rations: The development of the complex semi-synthetic ration system was important as it enabled to produce significant deficiencies of single elements in long term replicated studies and their interactions with other elements. Interrelationships between minerals were investigated for Cu with Zn, Cu with Cr, Cu with S, Cu with Cd, Cu with Fe, and Cu with P, using a semi-synthetic ration (Table 13) developed in

TABLE 13 Composition of the semi-synthetic control ration[a] for goats (Anke et al., 1987a)

	kg/100 kg		g/l00kg		mg/l00kg
Potato starch	48.3	NaCl	350.0	$Cr_2(SO_4)_3.18H_2O$	600
Beet sugar	32.0	$Al_2(SO4)3$ 60%	200.0	$(NH_4)VO_3$	460
Casein	10.0	MgO	220.0	NaF	220
Urea	3.0	K_2SO_4	350.0	$NaWO_4.H_2O$	180
Sunflower oil	3.0	$ZnSO_4.7H_2O$	50.0	KJ	100
KH_2PO_4	1.34	$FeSO_4.7H_2O$	45.0	$(NH_4)_6Mo_7 O_{24}.4H_2O$	92
$CaCO_3$	1.0	$MnSO_4.4H_2O$	40.0	SeO_2	80
		S	35.0	$CoSO_4.7H_2O$	80
		$LiCO_3$	10.6	$As_2 O_3$	40
		$CuSO_4.5H_2O$	4.0	$CdCl_2.H_2O$	36
		KBr	3.0	Vitamin A	2000
		$Ni_2SO_4.7H_2O$	3.4	Vitamin D_3	400
				Vitamin E	2000

[a]Protein content 18.5% on DMB

1970 for determining essentiality of different trace elements, and effects of deficient rations (Anke et al., 1987). This semi-synthetic ration was expanded from the original 24 elements to 57 elements in 1989 by adding small amounts of salts of trace elements. The use of the semi-synthetic ration had the advantage of providing a constant supply of nutrients, minerals and trace elements in the studies which lasted many years.

Indicator tissues for the detection of deficiency status in ruminants: The concept of indicator tissues for a deficiency status, especially hair was Professor Anke's early pioneering contribution. It was determined that the value of an indicator tissue (Table 14) for mineral deficiencies differs in reliability by the kind of minerals involved. Extensive analyses shows that deficiencies in Mo, Se and I can be detected reliably by analyzing blood serum or hair samples, while this is not true for deficiencies in Cu, Mn, Zn, Cd and Pb, for which liver analyses are best, except for Zn that requires analyses of ribs.

TABLE 14 Indicator tissues[a] for the detection of deficiency status in ruminants (Anke et al., 1988)

Tissue	Cu	Mn	Zn	Mo	Se	I	Cd	Pb	As	Ni	Li
Liver	***	***	0	***	**	***	**	***	***	*	*
Kidneys	0	*	0	**	*	***	***	***	***	**	0
Brain	***	0	0	*	0	0	0	0	*	*	0
Ribs	0	0	***	*	0	0	0	***	0	0	*
Blood serum	*	0	0	***	***	***	0	*	*	*	***
Hair	*	*	*	***	**	***	*	*	**	**	**

[a]Indicator tissues with (***) best, (**) medium, (*) low or (0) no reliability for detection of deficiency.

Effects of deficiency of trace minerals and interactions

Bentonite clay is high in **iron (Fe)** contents. Addition of bentonite clay to a normal goat ration caused significant decreases in **copper (Cu)** contents in liver and **zinc (Zn)** contents in ribs of the experimental goats; decreased Cu contents of tissues and milk by 10% in the presence of 5 ppm Cd, also observed.

Molybdenum (Mo) excess or deficiency in certain soils and regions has caused considerable nutritional interest, especially because of its antagonistic interrelationship with Cu.

Selenium deficiency in ruminants leads to "white muscle disease" and other less specific problems such as weak newborns, abortion, retained placenta, with considerable economic losses. A 9-month long Se deficiency study showed a significant decrease of GSHPx (glutathione peroxidase enzyme) and significant increases of the enzymes creatine kinase, aldolase, lactate dehydrogenase, hydroxybutyrate dehydrogenase, aspartate aminotransferase and alanine aminotransferase. The increase in creatine kinase activity is related to the occurrence of muscular dystrophy and the increase of aspartate amino transferase to liver damage in the Se-deficient goats.

Fluorine has been known to strengthen the enamel in teeth of humans and dogs for many years, but evidence of it being an essential nutritional mineral was missing until this was demonstrated in extensive studies from 1985 to 1989 by Anke and Groppel.

Long term research on **phosphorus (P)**-deficient nutrition with large numbers of dairy goats of the native Alpine-type breed showed statistically significant effects. Clearly conception rates were decreased, abortion rates increased, low birth weight was more frequent, feed consumption and milk yield was less and kid mortality was greatly increased.

Under field conditions the bioavailability of **Zn** is influenced by interactions with Ca, Cd, Ni and phytic acid, which can induce a secondary Zn-deficiency if their intake is high.

Long term experiments lasting 10-22 months in dairy goats on low levels of **iodine** in the semisynthetic ration revealed that efficiency of first insemination of goats and body weight gain of their kids was significantly reduced, while abortion rate and kid mortality was very high and length of pregnancy increased. The I-deficient goats as well- as their newborn kids had greatly hypertrophied thyroid glands.

Aluminum (Al) has been mainly associated with toxicological effects due to industrial pollution and side effects of medications, but publications around 1975 suggested that Al could also be an essential element. The Al-deficient ration caused a high abortion rate and mortality of the goats. Male kids in the 4th year (from 9 years of repeated studies) showed distinct weakness of coordinated movement of their hind legs. Feed intake was significantly greater for pregnant and lactating goats, which may be related to the increased milk yield by the Al-deficient goats. Birth weight and weight gain were not affected. There was a tendency for more male kids with lighter weights in the Al-deficient group.

It was concluded, that although Al-deficiency caused definite changes in goats, they were only sufficient to establish a "possible" essentiality of Al nutritionally according to the 7 criteria set forth by Anke et al in 1984. It was also stated that under practical field conditions a nutritional Al-deficiency is not expected because of the ubiquity of the element in the feed chain.

For a long time **arsenic** (As) was known principally as very toxic or in small dosages to have medicinal benefits. Based on the extensive research studies, it was concluded, that As is a nutritionally essential element, but four levels must be distinguished. (1) Deficiency at <50 ug/kg ration DM, (2) normal supply at 100-500 u.g/kg DM depending on animal species and chemical form of As salt, (3) therapeutic treatment at 3.5-5.0 mg/kg DM, and (4) above that the toxic level of As supply.

Bromine (Br) is found in soils and in vegetation in relatively high amounts. Sea plants accumulate much more Br and so do fish. Bromine has been used in the treatment of epilepsy and sleeplessness. No Br deficiency symptoms in animals or humans were known at the time because of the rich supply in the biosphere. Studies into the* possible essentiality of Br were initiated in 1986 and continued until 1995 (Anke and his team 1993). Br-deficient nutrition of pregnant and lactating goats and their kids caused reduced feed intake, less growth, decreased reproduction efficiency, much higher abortion rate and mortality, increases in milk fat content and blood contents of triglycerides, but significantly lower hemoglobin and hematocrit.

Cadmium (Cd) is one of the most dangerous heavy metals in the food chain, especially because of its carcinogenicity, and it has been spread widely through industrial pollution. Like As and Pb, only cadmium toxicity had been known for a long time, until the experimental findings of Anke and his team demonstrated its essentiality in 1970s. Reproductive efficiency, birth weight of kids and milk production of the Cd-deficient goats were significantly reduced, while abortion rate and mortality of kids were greatly increased.

Cd deficiency symptoms are not expected in farm animals, since their normal Cd intake in feeds is considerably above the level of a deficiency ration. Bentonite is a soil component rich in montmorillonite and absorbs minerals. It has been observed that addition of 3% bentonite resulted in significant decreases of Cd contents in the organs of goats. It also affected organ and milk contents of Ca, P, Mg, Na, K, Cu, Zn, Mn and Li. Therefore, bentonite is a useful supplement to reduce the health dangers of Cd pollution in the feed chain.

Lithium (Li) had been known for its therapeutic role in the treatment of people with manic-depressive psychosis, but its nutritional essentiality was not studied in animals until the 1970s. Li-deficient goats had significantly reduced reproductive efficiency, lower birth weights and body weight gains, less male than female kids born and decreased milk production than the controls, but severely higher abortion rate and mortality. Significant morphological signs of Li deficiency are the atrophy of the thymus in contrast to Br deficiency, which showed thymomegaly. Both conditions are related to reduced immunological resistance.

Nickel (Ni) is known as a nutritionally essential element in goats in the 1970s. Ni deficiency causes growth depression and increases mortality of kids. Blood hemoglobin and hematocrit levels were reduced by Ni deficiency, as were GOT and P-lipoprotein levels, while a-lipoprotein was increased. This was interpreted to indicate restricted fat synthesis and glucose shortage due to Ni deficiency (Anke et al., 1980). The higher a-lipoprotein content and the lower ^-lipoprotein content are part of normal cholesterol metabolism and disturbed triglyceride synthesis. It was concluded that Ni deficiency produced deficiencies in Zn and hemoglobin, which caused the high mortality in newborn kids and lactating goats. Parakeratosis-like changes of skin and hair were also noted in Ni-deficient goats.

Vanadium (V) is widely used in industrial plant operations and its concentration in soil and plants including vegetables are known to' increase near industrial operations. However, no detrimental effects have been observed in animals or humans. As analog to phosphorus (P), it interferes with P metabolism, mimics growth factors and plays -a role in cell proliferation, repair and angiogenesis. It is used in diabetes therapy as it has insulin-like effects. By 1980 any nutritional essentiality of V for animals was still unclear and no specific deficiency symptoms had been reported. Thus long term deficiency experiments with growing, pregnant and lactating goats over 15 generations using the semi-synthetic feed ration were initiated by the University Jena team (Anke and his team) and repeated for 15 years.

Consistently significant reduction in reproduction efficiency was found with high abortion rate and mortality of goats and their kids. The sex ratio of the newborn kids showed a strong decrease of male kids. Kids were born with deformed forefoot tarsal joints and forelegs, and the symptoms were similar to those occurring with P, Mn or vitamin D deficiencies. There were no effects of V deficiency on blood hemoglobin. Feed intake was less and so was milk yield. Blood analyses showed an increase in P-lipoprotein, triglycerides and creatinine, and the enzymes of the citrate cycle whereas those of the amino acid metabolism (AST, ALT) were not affected by V deficiency (Anke et al., 1986). Vanadium deficiency reduced the life expectancy of goats by 50%. It was concluded that V is a nutritionally essential element for goats and other animals, but no deficiency is expected to occur under normal farm conditions.

Titanium (Ti) has become important because of its strength, lightness and corrosion resistance in industrial applications of the space industry, for surgical implants, prostheses, and the paint and food industry (Anke and seifert, 2004). Its essentiality in plant nutrition was studied in the 1970s and in animal nutrition by the University Jena team during the 1990s (Arnhold et al., 2006). Feed intake by Ti-deficient kids was significantly reduced as was growth. It was concluded that Ti is an essential element in animal nutrition, but deficiencies are not expected under normal farm conditions.

Deficiency levels and sufficiency levels of minerals and trace elements in goats are presented in Table 15. To conclude, trace element deficiencies may lead to various disorders of biochemical aetiology (Braun et al., 2010). Balancing diets with trace elements is important for optimum nutrition of small ruminants (Dove, 2010).

TABLE 15 Deficiency levels and sufficiency levels of minerals and trace elements in goats*

Element	Deficiency level in ration	Sufficiency level in ration
Al	162 µg/kg DM ($n = 21$)	25.0 mg/kg DM ($n = 24$)
As	10.0 µg/kg DM($n = 113$)	350 µg/kg DM ($n = 131$)
Br	0.8 mg/kg DM ($n = 30$)	20.0 mg/kg DM ($n = 32$)
Ca	–	3.3 g/kg DM ($n = 26$)
Cd	68 µ.g/kg DM ($n = 79$)	300 µg/kg DM ($n = 71$)
Cu	2.0 mg/kg DM ($n = 22$)	8.0 mg/kg DM ($n = 31$)
Cr	0.36 mg/kg DM ($n = 4$)	1.4 mg/kg DM ($n = 4$)
F	0.3 mg/kg DM ($n = 29$)	2.0 mg/kg DM ($n = 31$)
Fe	–	50 mg/kg DM ($n = 26$)
I	0.04 mg/kg DM ($n = 19$)	0.4 mg/kg DM ($n = 18$)
Li	1.0 mg/kg DM ($n = 19$)	24.0 mg/kg DM ($n = 29$)
Mg	–	1.0 g/kg DM ($n = 26$)
Mn	–	60.0 mg/kg DM ($n = 26$)
Mo	24 µg/kg DM ($n = 98$)	533 µg/kg DM ($n = 139$)
Ni	0.1 mg/kg DM ($n = 30$)	4.4 mg/kg DM ($n = 37$)
P	2.5 g/kg DM($n = 11$)	4 g/kg DM ($n = 14$)
Se	0.04 mg/kg DM ($n = 43$)	0.56 mg/kg DM ($n = 97$)
Ti	170 µg/kg DM	1750 ug/kg DM
V	25.0 µg/kg DM ($n = 53$)	2.0 mg/kg DM ($n = 48$)
Zn	5.0 mg/kg DM ($n = 22$)	90 mg/kg DM ($n = 31$)

Data were derived from several published articles. Data for goats for Co, K, Na, S, Rb, Wo were not presented in the reviewed proceedings.
*G.F.W.Haenlein and M.Anke (2011) Mineral and trace element research in goats: A review, Small Ruminant Research 95: 2-19

Feeding Habits of Goats

Basically goats are browsers; standing on their hind limbs (bipedal stance), they always like to pluck the tender leafy twigs of herbs, shrubs, small trees. Goats have special feeding habits on account of their small mouth, prehensile tongue and movable upper lip. In comparison to other domestic animals, goats have unique preferences for shrubs and tree leaves. Goats select from a wider array of plants, particularly woody plants. The goat is acknowledged as a mobile pruning machine that modified bushy shrubs and thereby increased the accessibility of cattle to more nutritious forage. This observation of synergistic effects between animal species has led to widespread acceptance of combination grazing.

Goats consume approximately the same weight of forage DM as do sheep of similar size. It was suggested that goats will eat more forage if they have access to the more preferred species. Field observations indicate that goats under browse conditions perform better. Devendra (1975) found that voluntary intake by goats decreased as the forage matured. The effect is overcome partially by chopping and pelleting the forage.

Browse (leaves and twigs of trees and shrubs) generally contain higher levels of CP and P during the growing season than do grasses. However, many of these contain one or more inhibitors that may bind or otherwise prevent utilization of nutrient contained in the plants, e.g. lignin, silica, tannin. Essential oils (terpene-based organic compounds) are present at relatively high levels in some range shrubs and apparently inhibit growth of rumen bacteria. There is growing evidence that many of the grasses, shrubs and tree leaves selected by goats are of high nutritional value.

Goats are reported to be less sensitive than other ruminants to the toxic effects of tannic acid.

Common Feeds and Fodders

Tree leaves: Babul, neem, pipal, mango, prosopis, gliricidia, mulbery, subabul, banyan, etc. These tree leaves are also called as top feed.
Grasses: *Cenchrus ciliaris, C. setigerus*, Para, guinea, napier, etc.
Legume pastures: Stylosanthes hamata, S. scabra, siratro, butterfly pea, etc.
Legume fodders: Berseem, lucerne, cowpea, etc.
Cereal fodders: Maize, jowar, oats, etc.
Dry feeds: Dry pods of babul (acacia), *Prosopis juliflora*, rain tree, subabul; cereal straws, legumes straws (groundnut haulms, gram straw), gram husk and gram waste.

A free choice lick of mineral mixture has to be kept in goat sheds.

Feeding of Kids

The kid should be allowed to suck its dam for the first three or four days so that they can get good amount of colostrum. Colostrum feeding is a main factor in limiting kid losses. The effectiveness of the transfer of immunoglobulins from colostrum to kid's plasma, is a function of antibody concentration, level of colostrum intake by the kid and time of consumption in relation to birth. Kids may loose the ability to absorb immunoglobulins from colostrum 20-28 hours after birth, but there is an evidence that the ability persists longer in starved kids. It has been reported that colostrum can be stored in a deep freezer for up to two years and remain immunologically effective; Further, cow colostrum is also efficient for lambs and kids. Colostrum is given at the rate of 100 ml per kg live weight. Immunoglobulins are thermosensitive. Therefore, during thawing, the temperature of colostrum should not be raised above 50°C. Colostrum can be preserved with 1 to 1.5% (vol/wt) propionic acid or 0.1% formaldehyde. Propionic acid is preferred for preservation as it keeps the pH value low. The chemically treated colostrum is kept at cool place to ensure better quality.

After 3 or 4 days of age they should be suckled only for a brief period to let the milk down. The final stripping should be done by keeping the kids with their mothers for an hour or so after milking. The number of offsprings produced by goats is higher than sheep. In some breeds of goats like Black Bengal twinning and triplets are quite common. The non-descript breeds of goats may produce just sufficient milk for the offspring only under the average condition of feed supply. These goats produce between 0.3-0.4 kg of milk daily.

The kids start nibbling the grasses from 15 days of age. Creep feed is also introduced at the same time. These help rapid growth of the kids and hasten the development of the rumen.

Feeding Schedule for a Kid from Birth to 90 Days

Age of kids	Dam's milk or cow milk* ml	Creep feed g	Forage, green/day g
1-3 days	Colostrum 300 ml, 3 feedings	-	-
4-14 days	350 ml, 3 feedings	-	-
15-30 days	350 ml, 3 feedings	A little	A little
31-60 days	400 ml, 2 feedings	100-150	Free choice
61-90 days	200 ml, 2 feedings	200-250	Free choice

*If milk is fed by the bottle, then it should be fed at the body temperature of the kid.

Two types of creep mixtures can be offered depending on the type of the roughage available. If grasses and cereal fodders are available, a creep feed with 18% DCP and 75% TDN has to be offered. If leguminous fodders are available, a creep feed with 12% DCP and 70% TDN has to be offered.

Feeding of Goats

Male kids are castrated at 3 to 4 months of age. This improves the growth rate and carcass quality. The expected growth rate is between 70 to 100 g per day from weaning to slaughter. The slaughter weight is 25 to 35 kg for smaller and larger breeds. But they are slaughtered at lesser weights.

Feeding of goats for different physiological functions, such as reproduction and lactation has to be done. Good quality fodders containing 6% DCP and 62% TDN are needed to feed gestating and lactating does. Goats under intensive system of feeding stall feeding of goats may be undertaken profitably with complete feeds. Poor quality straws such as jowar stover/maize stover are ammoniated (by urea hydrolysis) and such treated straws are blended with concentrates. Goats are considered to be better converter of fibrous feeds into chevon (goat meat) and milk of high biological value. Several unconventional roughages and concentrates are incorporated in complete feeds and efficiently used for economic meat and milk production.

Tree Foliage and Hybrid Napier Fodder Based Feeding

Where other livestock fails, the goats are able to serve the mankind even under very harsh ecological conditions. Both sheep and goats help the smallholder livestock farmers to gain livelihoods against several odds. Crop residues are the most important feed for ruminants in smallholder crop-livestock production systems. The tree leaves are classed as emergency fodder for livestock in general, but they form an integral part of sheep and goat feeding. These tree foliages - subabul (*Leucaena leucocephala*), sesbania (*Sesbania grandiflora*), acacia (*Acacia auriculiformis*), jack (*Artocarpus heterophyllus*), yellow gold mohur (*Peltophorum ferrugineum*) and cashew (*Anacardium occidentale*) foliage were offered at supplementary level to goats fed on NB green fodder feeding (Reddy et al., 2009). Each tree foliage (i.e., leaves and tender twigs) was offered at the rate of 300 g per day per goat, as freshly harvested daily, as first feed and once it was completely consumed, chopped (2-4cm) NB hybrid green fodder was offered at *ad libitum* level. It was concluded that tree foliage from sesbania, jack, subabul and acacia had high potential- while yellow gold mohur and cashew had moderate potential-supplementary effect in goats fed on Napier Bajra hybrid green fodder in meeting their nutrient requirements for a moderate growth.

Moringa leaves

Moringa oleifera (drumstick tree) is a promising pantropical multipurpose tree, with high CP (23.3%) and negligible tannins content (Makkar and Becker, 1996). The plants are cut at about 30-40 cm above the ground 60 days after planting or re-growth. The sun dried leaves and less lignified part of the branches are then ground and mixed in an industrial mixer to obtain a homogenous meal.

Protection of protein from rumen degradation

Groundnut cake and mustard cake are the two most commonly used protein sources in the diet of ruminants in India. However, their degradability in rumen is very high, resulting in the depreciation of protein value for ruminants. Protection of protein from rumen degradation increases outflow of dietary amino acids to the small intestine.

Different methods: Different methods have been evolved to reduce the protein degradability in rumen. These include heat treatment, tannic acid treatment, formaldehyde treatment, coating of protein by fat, lignosulfonate treatment. Good method should reduce the ruminal CP degradability without affecting the post ruminal protein digestibility. But consumer preference for natural and sustainable methods enlarged our search for alternative things.

Condensed tannins present in certain tree leaves may be used since they protect the protein from rumen degradation without affecting its digestibility later in the tract. Manish Dubey et al. (2007) from IVRI, Izatnagar reported that supplementation of condensed tannin (1-3%) from *Psidium guajava* leaves could be used as natural protectant of protein without any adverse effect on the efficiency of microbial protein synthesis.

Nutrition-related Metabolic Disorders

Enterotoxaemia

Enterotoxaemia caused by *Clostridium perfringens* is a common economically important devastating disease of sheep and goats throughout the world, and is probably the most important cause of sudden death in goats of different ages. There are significant differences between sheep and goats in terms of pathogenesis, epidemiology, clinical presentation and management of enterotoxaemia (Sumithra et al., 2013). The Gram-positive, spore-forming, anaerobic bacterium *C. perfringens* is an important cause of various histotoxic and enteric diseases of human and domestic animals. *Clostridium perfringens* type D, C and B are the main organisms involved in caprine enterotoxaemia while pathological role of type A is equivocal. Epsilon toxin is considered to be the principal toxin involved although potential effects of other toxins are unknown. Peracute form of enterotoxaemia with sudden death is more common in kids.

In general, morbidity does not exceed 10% of the herd but its lethality is high and usually kills 100% of the affected animals (Miyashiro et al., 2007). Symptoms are diarrhoea, depression, lack of coordination, digestive upsets, coma, and death.

Predisposing factors: *C. perfringens* is normally present in soil and intestinal tract of animals in relatively small numbers. Under certain conditions which provide an ideal environment for bacterial proliferation or which slow down peristalsis, these organisms proliferate in intestine and produce toxin in lethal quantities (Songer, 1996). These include high carbohydrate intake (high grain diet, high milk intake, etc.) wherein the causative bacteria multiply and produce a toxin. Thus it is a disease that afflicts suckling lambs, creep-fed lambs, growing-finishing lambs, and ewes fed high levels of grain.

But many well understood predisposing factors in sheep cannot be strictly applied to goats (Ayers, 1984). For example, the disease usually occurs in single lambs of high milk producing ewes but type of birth is not a predisposing factor in goats (Ayers, 1984). Another is that the greatest loss by enterotoxaemia occurs in growing lambs on concentrate rations in feed lots but this management condition is rarely encountered among goats (Smith and Sherman, 2011).

Sudden exposure to grain and garden greens, large increase in quantity of milk consumed without gradually increasing the amount over several days (Ayers, 1984), a heavy worm burden (both tapeworms and lung worms), changes from poor to lush pasture, feeding of bread or other bakery goods and feeding of a bran/molasses mash (King, 1980) are mentioned as the predisposing factors in goats. But some outbreaks of enterotoxaemia type D have been reported by Uzai et al. (1994) in goats under extensive grazing systems without known diet change. Uzalet al. (1994) suggested that environmental stress, heavy infestations with coccidia, and an anthelmintic over dose might be the possible predisposing factors for this outbreak.

Prevention: Vaccination is the major prophylactic measure used to reduce the losses or minimize the severity of enterotoxaemia in all species. Since there is no specific vaccine against caprine enterotoxaemia, ovine vaccines are generally used in goats (Blackwell et al., 1983). After the initial double immunization, booster dose is generally recommended in every 3 or 4 months (Uzal and Kelly, 1996). In addition, vaccination at 2-3 weeks before parturition is required to increase the protective effect of colostrum. In case of kids, the first dose is given at 4-6 weeks of age (Smith and Sherman, 2011).

Management practices: Additional measures such as avoidance of excessive feeding of carbohydrates, reduction of feed volume with intermittent feeding schedule and exercise are recommended to prevent enterotoxaemia (Miyashiro et al., 2007). The best prevention in stable-fed goats is frequent feeding of milk, grain, and forage in small amounts. Changes of concentrates and forages in the ration should be introduced gradually over several days.

Though the use of heterologous bovine colostrum is recommended as a prophylactic measure against caprine arthritis and encephalitis, Veschi et al. (2008) realized that this approach has no value against caprine enterotoxaemia. Once diagnosis is established in a herd, excessive feeding of carbohydrates must be stopped immediately and a booster dose should be given to previously vaccinated animals. Non-vaccinated animals must receive two doses of vaccine at 2-3 weeks' interval (Smith and Sherman, 2011). Recently Elizondo et al. (2010) showed that vegetable tannins can inhibit the *in vitro* growth of *C. perfringens* in a dose-dependent manner. These results suggest that tannin-supplemented diet can be useful to prevent enterotoxaemia although further studies are required (Sumithra et al., 2013).

Critical periods in development and production cycles in goats

Reproduction: Ovulation, conception, gestation, and parturition all are important events in the reproductive process. The period surrounding the breeding event determines the potential for reproductive rate and is influenced by nutritional status and strategy.

Lactation: Nutrient requirements in goats are highest during lactation compared with the other periods of the production cycle. The assumed milk fat and protein concentrations are 4% (approximately 0.74 Mcal/kg) for goats other than Angora. For Angoras, milk fat and protein concentrations were assumed as 5 and 4%, respectively.

Ketosis, hypocalcaemia, lactic acidosis are the metabolic disorders. Ketosis and hypocalcaemia together result in milk fever (parturient paresis).

Growth: The developing kid has high levels of requirements for all nutrients. Lactic acidosis, enterotoxaemia, urolithiasis may be observed. Several conditions can occur as a result of vitamin deficiencies. Polioencephalomalacia occurs due to thiamin deficiency.

Toxicities affecting small ruminants

Excess copper, urea, toxic plants, and nitrates may be present in feeds and fodder.

The total diet dry matter copper requirement for goats and sheep is 7 to 10 ppm. The maximum tolerable level of copper for sheep and goats (unofficially adopted) is 25 ppm. More recent research has shown that goats may be able to tolerate much more copper than previously thought. Care should be taken to keep total diet copper at no more than 18 ppm, when sheep and goats are housed and fed together (NRC, 2007).

Urea toxicity may occur if urea is fed at high levels. Most cases of urea poisoning are due to poor mixing of feed or errors in calculating the amount of urea to add to the ration. Accidental over-consumption of urea-containing supplements also has resulted in some cases of urea toxicity. Proper level of urea, uniform mixing in the feed, sufficient energy from carbohydrate sources need to be followed to avoid toxicity.

Nitrate accumulation occurs in forages when the uptake of soil nitrates continues even as plant photosynthesis and carbohydrate and protein synthesis cease. Factors that contribute to the accumulation of nitrates in plants include drought, frost, low light intensities, low temperatures, soil nutrient deficiencies, excess nitrogen fertilization, and some plant diseases. Nitrate will accumulate to varying levels within the plant with the lower portions generally containing the highest concentrations. When conditions exist that may lead to accumulations of nitrate in forages, they should be tested for nitrate concentrations. Some concentrations of nitrates are acceptable to be fed to certain classes of livestock. In general forages with nitrate levels of less than 4400 ppm are safe to feed to all livestock.

Problems Anticipated due to abrupt change of diet

Abrupt change of diet in amounts and ratio of concentrate and roughage or ingredients of diets is a recurring cause of health problems in animals. Small ruminants have relatively fast metabolism compared to larger ruminant livestock and tend to eat more frequently. Therefore, a large meal once or twice daily consisting of a large concentration of grain is somewhat unnatural and makes small ruminants susceptible to metabolic diseases. Digestive systems of small ruminants are sensitive and require time to adapt to changes in rations. When dietary changes are made over a time, it allows the microbial populations in the rumen to shift and adapt to the type of feedstuff being offered.

A rapid shift to a high grain ration may cause enterotoxaemia, cause animals to refuse feed, or induce diarrhoea or other digestive upset. Similarly, when a small ruminant that is accustomed to consuming a high grain ration is suddenly introduced to forage only diet, the rumen microbes are unable to digest the fibrous portions of the diet effectively. Changing rations gradually and allowing time for adaptation is important for good health of the animal and assures continued productivity.

8

Poultry Nutrition
Formulation of Poultry Diets

Poultry birds that are reared in India include commercial chickens (white and coloured broilers and laying hens), improved chickens for low-input rural poultry production (Vanaraja, Giriraja, Gramapriya, Nadanam-99, Gramalakshmi, CARI-Nirbeek, etc), native and exotic ducks, Japanese quails, turkeys, guinea fowls and emus.

The term poultry includes birds reared for economic gains like chickens, ducks, ostriches, emus, quails, turkey, etc.

Improvement in growth rate and Feed efficiency are vital

Improvement in growth rate and efficiency of the broiler chicken production has been attributed as a major factor that contributes to its higher per capita consumption. In USA between 1950 and 2005 consumption of chicken meat increased from 9.4 kg to 39.2 kg/day (USDA, Economic Research Service, 2014), and it is primarily due to availability of poultry products at affordable prices, which has been made possible via intentional genetic selection through traditional quantitative techniques (Hunton, 2006). From 1957 to 2005, broiler growth rates increased by over 400%, with a concurrent 50% reduction in feed conversion ratio (FCR). The rate of increase in 42-d live BW during the period was 3.30% per year, compounded for 48yr (Zuidhof et al., 2014). Similarly, FCR to 42 d of age has decreased by 2.55% per year, also in a compounding manner. Simply put, the amount of feed required to produce chicken meat and breast meat is reduced by one-half and 67%, respectively. Because feed accounts for approximately 67% of the cost of producing chicken, the US consumer price index for poultry products increased at half the rate of all other products (USDA, Economic Research Service, 2014)

Digestive system and Digestion of feed

The avian gastrointestinal tract has a greater number of organs than their mammalian counterparts. The avian digestive tract (Fig. 1) starts with the beak, followed by a toothless mouth, tongue, pharynx, esophagus, crop, proventriculus, ventriculus or gizzard, small intestine, caeca, rectum, cloaca and vent. Accessory organs include the salivary glands, biliary system, pancreas. Peyer's patches, and bursa. The digestive tract is lined with a continuous mucous membrane from the mouth to the vent. This provides protection from abrasion by the food as it passes through and prevents the entry of microorganisms. The intestines are attached to a mesenteric membrane, which contains the blood vessels that perfuse the region of the digestive tract.

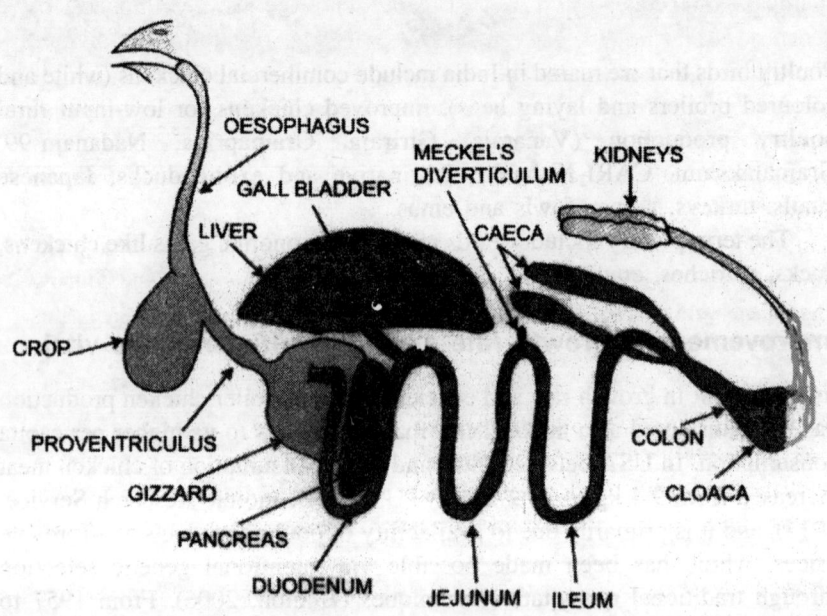

FIGURE 1   Avian digestive tract

Birds pick up feed by the beak on the basis of feel and appearance rather than taste or smell. Birds generally have poorer taste acuity than mammals. This is probably due to the rapid transit of food through the mouth, lack of mastication, and relatively low saliva addition to the food. Low taste acuity is reflected in very low numbers of taste receptors: 62 in Japanese quail, 350 in parrots, compared with 9000 in humans and 17,000 in rabbits. The tongue, oral cavity, and beak of birds have a rich supply of touch receptors, and they augment the bird's relatively poor gustatory capacity with a strong tactile sense. It can be generally concluded that birds can taste the same four primary flavours (sour, sweet, bitter, salty) as humans but with considerably less acuity.

Esophagus and crop

The esophagus extends from pharynx along the neck into the thoracic cavity and terminates in the proventriculus. It has a relatively greater diameter than that found in mammals in order to accommodate food that has not been reduced in size by chewing. To aid in swallowing large food items, the esophagus is expandable and is enriched with mucous glands to provide lubrication. The epithelial lining is thick and cornified for protection against mechanical damage as a result of swallowing whole-foods. The thickness of this cornified layer and the size of mucous glands are greatest in granivores and herbivores (Ziswiler, 1985).

The main function of the esophagus is to pass food from the mouth to the proventriculus. In some species, the storage function of the esophagus is enhanced by its widening just prior to entering the thoracic cavity to give one or more clearly partitioned diverticula, known as a crop. Crops are particularly well developed in granivores. A crop also permits 'tanking up' in the evening so that food can be slowly released to supply nutrient's during the nighttime. An additional function of the crop in granivores and herbivores is the provision of a moist environment where food begins to soften, permitting more efficient digestion. However, in chickens and quail, mucous glands are only present near the entrance of the crop, so most of the water needed for softening must be consumed with the meal. There are no enzymes secreted into the crop but those present in the food may provide some digestion while residing in the crop.

Stomach

The stomach of most birds consists of two parts: the proventriculus (glandular stomach) and the gizzard (muscular stomach), which is sometimes called the ventriculus. In granivores and herbivores, the gizzard is very muscular and dominates the proventriculus in size. The feed passes quickly through the oesophagus to the crop. Next, the feed passes to the proventriculus, where feed is acted upon by enzymes, particularly pepsin, and further acidified by hydrochloric acid. Feed is crushed in the gizzard with the help of insoluble grit by rhythmic contractions. The gizzard has a number of important functions, such as aiding digestion by particle size reduction, chemical degradation of nutrients and regulation of feed flow, and responds rapidly to changes in the coarseness of the diet (Svihus, 2011). It may be recommended to include at least 20 to 30% cereal particles larger than 1 mm in size, or to include at least 3% coarse fibres such as oat hulls, in the diet.

Small intestine

The small intestine functions in enzymatic digestion and absorption of the end products of digestion. The small intestine consists of a duodenum, jejunum, and ileum, although these segments are not clearly demarcated in most birds. The bile and pancreatic ducts enter the duodenum. The duodenum originates from the gizzard and forms a loop around the pancreas. The duodenum ends at the point where the small intestine leaves its association with the pancreas. Posterior to the duodenal loop is the jejunum, followed by the ileum. The jejunum extends from the end of the duodenum to the vitelline diverticulum (Meckel's diverticulum), which is the remnant of the yolk sac. The ileum extends from the vitelline diverticulum to the caecal junction.

The intestinal mucosa contains villi and crypts of Lieberkuhn. Epithelial cells of the villi have about 1O3 microvilli per square millimeter on their apical surface, increasing the absorbing surface area 15-fold. The avian mucosal epithelium does not contain an equivalent of mammalian Brunner's glands, but numerous goblet cells. They secrete copious mucus, which protects the epithelium from digestive enzymes and abrasion by the digesta. The mucus is particularly thick along the anterior duodenum, where it protects the villi from the excessive acidity of the digesta leaving the gizzard.

Caeca

The caeca originate from the rectum at a location immediately posterior to the junction of the small intestine and the rectum. The caeca are highly developed in herbivores and omnivores, where they serve as a site for microbial fermentation of complex carbohydrates that resist digestion in the small intestine. In some species they may serve water- and nitrogen-absorption or immunosurveillance functions.

Rectum

The length of intestine between the ileocaecal junction and the cloaca is called the rectum. A frequently used synonym for the avian rectum is 'colon'.

Cloaca

The rectum empties into the cloaca, which has a much larger diameter than the return. The cloaca serves as a storage area for urine and faeces and it receives the ureters and the exit ducts of the reproductive system.

The bursa of Fabricius is a prominent diverticulum of the dorsal cloaca. It serves as location for the differentiation of B lymphocytes in the immature chick and becomes a secondary lymphoid organ involved in immunosurveillance of the lower gastrointestinal tract later in life.

Duck and Goose: The digestive system of the duck is similar to that of the fowl. The bill of the duck is much larger than that of the fowl but the crop is smaller. When feeding from a trough ducks tend to push feed out of it and onto the ground causing considerable wastage. Fibre can be fermented in the caecae of ducks to produce volatile fatty acids. The goose has no crop. But there is an enlargement at the end of the gullet that serves as a temporary feed storage organ.

Accessory organs

The liver, gallbladder, and pancreas are important accessory organs of the digestive system. The colour of liver changes from yellow at hatching to dark red over the next two weeks but becomes yellowish again in laying hens. The primary nutritional role of the liver is metabolism of absorbed nutrients and the production of bile acids and bile salts.

Bile acids are usually conjugated to taurine, but glycine conjugation occurs in some species. Bile salts, along with cholesterol and phospholipids, are secreted into the bile canaliculi and collected by the bile ducts. Depending on the species, the duct from the right side of the liver may enlarge into or branch into a gallbladder. In some species, a gallbladder is absent (e.g., Ostrich, hummingbirds, and many species of passerines, doves, pigeons, and parrots). In ducks, bile from the left side of the liver can reach the gallbladder through a common sinus. In the chicken, bile from the left duct drains directly into the duodenum without being stored in the gallbladder.

The pancreas lies within the duodenal loop. The digestive enzymes produced are collected into one, two or three ducts that enter the duodenum, usually near the entrance of the bile duct. Avian pancreatic juice contains enzymes similar to those of mammals, including amylase, lipases, trypsin, chymotrypsin, carboxypeptidases A, B, and C, deoxyribonucleases, ribonucleases, and elastases. The pancreas also produces bicarbonate (HCO_3), which buffers the intestinal pH.

Digestion of food in the birds

Retrograde movement of digesta

The uptake of nutrients is dependent on their prehension, digestion and absorption from the gastrointestinal tract and requires the coordinated effort of all digestive organs. As the digesta moves from mouth, esophagus, stomach, intestines, towards vent, the food is denatured and hydrolyzed. This posterior flow of digesta is often interrupted in birds by reflexes in the opposite direction, which is known as retrograde flow. Retrograde movement of digesta occurs between the proventriculus and the gizzard; the small intestine and the gizzard; the rectum and the caeca; and the cloaca and the rectum.

Two types of digestion may occur as feed passes the gastrointestinal tract. (1) **Autoenzymatic digestion** is due to the action of enzymes of bird origin, which are produced in the proventriculus, small intestine, pancreas, and possibly other organs of the digestive tract. (2) **Alloenzymatic digestion** is due to enzymes of microbial origin (fermentative digestion), usually in the lumen of caeca or rectum. Species that consume large amounts of plant fibre may extensively utilize alloenzymatic digestion.

Alloenzymatic digestion

Because of low oxygen tension in these areas, fermentation is the primary activity, and fermentation and alloenzymatic digestion are often used synonymously. It is now recognized that digestion in birds involves the movement of digesta back and forth between the stomach and small intestine, one cannot use the mere presence of an enzyme in stomach contents as an indicator of its origin. The reversible flow of digesta between the stomach and small intestine in birds maximizes digestive efficiency while minimizing intestinal weight and length.

Microbial fermentation may occur in the crop of some species. Hoatzin has a very large crop with rich microbial flora that makes a substantial contribution to the digestion of foliage. A limited amount of pregastric fermentation may also occur in less specialized species such as pigeons, quails and chickens. The contribution of this microbial action to digestion of the feed is minor.

The major contribution of microbial action to the digestive process occurs in the caeca, although some fermentation may also occur in the posterior ileum. The large intestine of the ostrich has a high concentration of facultative anaerobes, which resemble the flora of mammalian ruminants in microbial ecology. The contribution of microbial fermentation to the nutrition of a bird is a function of the volume of digesta present in the fermentation area and the length of time it spends there. High volumes and slow rates of passage (caeca are blind-ended) favour microbial fermentation. In most birds, the caeca are the primary area in the digestive tract. In emu and possibly geese, the posterior small intestine may retain digesta long enough to make a significant contribution to total fermentation. In ostrich, the rectum is a major site for fermentation. The microbial contribution to the energy requirements of ostrich may approach 50%. In omnivorous chicken, caecal fermentation only contributes about 3-4% of the energy needs.

Symbiotic relation between microflora and the host: Uric acid arriving from the retrograde flow of urine can be utilized by caecal anaerobes to meet their nitrogen requirement while other nutrients are present in the contents. Caecal flora provides volatile fatty acids as fermentation end products. Some birds consume part of their faeces, especially the caecotropes, permitting the digestion and absorption of microbial protein and other nutrients by the host enzymes.

Digestion of nutrients

Digestion of nutrients in the gastrointestinal tract of avian omnivores is generally very similar to that in their mammalian counterparts. The complement of enzymes secreted by GIT and the pancreas is similar. Carbohydrate and protein digestion begins in the lumen of the GIT due largely to the action of pancreatic enzymes and is completed by enzymes attached to the intestinal villi. Lipid digestion is largely a luminal event and requires enzymes from the pancreas and bile acids from the liver.

About 30 percent of the free fatty acids are absorbed into the blood stream without further metabolism. The rest are resynthesized into triglycerides in the endoplasmic reticulum, utilizing both the monoglyceride and the glycerol-3-phosphate pathways. The newly synthesized triglycerides and phospholipids coalesce with apoproteins to form lipoproteins. These lipoproteins enter into the interstitial fluid and further diffuse through spaces between cells of the lamina propria and enter the capillaries. Thus, the lipoproteins absorbed in the chicken's small intestine enter the portal blood and not the lymphatics as in mammals. Hence the lipoproteins in the chickens are called portomicrons rather than chylomicrons as in mammals.

Ratites - Digestive System and Digestion

Ratites (ostriches, emus, kiwis, rheas and cassowaries) do not have crop. In ostriches and emus, some of the crop storage function is provided by a large proventriculus. The ostrich has a very large, comparatively thin walled, proventriculus that is prone to impaction. Ostriches lack gall bladder while emus and rheas have it. Ratites are capable of fermentation, making their digestive system similar to that of the ruminant. The volatile fatty acids (VFAs) measured in the proventriculus and ventriculus (Mackie, 1987) were of acetate primarily, which was suggestive of foregut fermentation. Because of hindgut fermentation, ratites may be able to extract more dietary energy from high fibre feed.

The large intestine of the ostrich is about three times as long as-the small intestine. In relation to body size, the caeca in the ostrich are no large than those in other poultry. VFA production in the ostrich large intestine and caeca approach levels similar to those in the forestomach of ruminants. Rate of passage of feed through the digestive tract is about 39 hours and 48 hours, respectively, in ostrich of 6.75 kg and 45 kg live weight.

The gastrointestinal tract of the emu is anatomically different from that of the ostrich. Rate of passage in adult emus is 5.5 hours (Herd and Dawson, 1984). Emus have been shown to digest 35-45% of the NDF in the feed. The ostrich has the ability to digest more than 50% of the dietary NDF as early as 10 weeks of age. This means that the ostrich was 40% more efficient than poultry in deriving energy from high fibre feed. Ostrich chicks that are less than 10 weeks-old cannot utilize fibre as well as older birds. However, fibre should be present in the feed to promote healthy microflora development in the hindgut.

Young ostriches, like other young animals, are not able to digest fat very well. However, by 10 weeks of age, the ostrich can digest as efficiently as a 12-week only turkey. Though ostriches lack gallbladder, fat digestibility is not impaired in later ages. The total fat content be limited to 6-8% in young ostriches. The digestibility of NDF and fat increases as the age advances, respectively, from 3 weeks to 120 weeks, which are 6.5% and 61.6% for NDF and 44.]% and 92.9%) for fat (Schneideler and Angel, 1994). Obesity is a problem in adult ostriches.

Feeding systems and Feed formulation

Poultry birds are generally reared either under intensive, semi-intensive or extensive systems. The commercial broilers, layers, breeders and Japanese quails are reared under intensive production system. In intensive system of production, birds may be reared either on deep litter or cage system. Commercially, the broilers are reared on deep litter system mainly due to low investment and labour cost. Layer chickens can be reared under both deep litter and cage systems; the usual practice is the cage system.

The cage system of rearing layer chickens has been considered as a super-intensive system with 1-4 birds in a cage, arranged in single or double or triple rows (California cage system). The major disadvantages include incidence of leg problem, cage layer fatigue, fatty liver syndrome, flies and increased obnoxious gases due to improper ventilation.

Improved native chickens, guinea fowls and ducks are reared in extensive or semi-intensive system. Emu and Turkey are reared in either of these systems based on the flock size.

Feed formulation involves the judicious use of feed ingredients to supply the nutrients required by poultry in adequate amounts and proportions. While choosing the feed ingredients a consideration is also given to their current price to formulate least cost diets.

Feeding of the Chicken

The following information is needed for feed formulation:

1. Nutrient requirements for chicken feeds
2. Information on feed ingredients

Nutrient Requirements for Chicken Feeds

Chicken are reared for meat and egg production. Chicken reared for meat are called broilers and those reared for eggs are called layers. The nutrient requirements of chicken depend upon the species, breed and its genetic make up, age, production status and environmental conditions.

Determining Nutrient Requirements

Several different methods have been used to estimate the nutrient requirements. (1). **Empirical methods**: Often the requirements are determined by empirical methods, in which experimental diets containing graded nutrient levels are fed and the minimal level that optimizes the bird's health care and performance is set as the requirement. (2). **Factorial method** of determining requirements: The requirement may be calculated by factorial summation of the energy used for specific metabolic processes inherent in that function (e.g., ME expended for basal metabolism + energy for activity + ME for thermoregulation + ME for egg production). (3). **A combination of empirical and factorial-summation methods** has been used to estimate the requirements of chickens, turkeys, quails, ducks, geese and pheasants in several physiological states. These are published by the US National

Academy of Sciences (NRC, 1994). The ninth revised edition of the NRC Nutrient Requirements of Poultry has been a benchmark publication for the research, judicial and regulatory communities and the poultry scientific community has looked to this publication for benchmark diet formulation.

These (NRC, 1994) requirements are for an average bird in a population and do not make allowances for genetic variation or environmental influences. A margin of safety is added to provide for uncertainties since nutrient requirements are minimal levels established under optimal conditions. This margin of safety permits the building up of nutrient storage pools that buffer 'the periods' of infectious diseases, environmental stresses, etc. Large margin of safety are employed for some nutrients, for example many vitamins and some trace minerals, where digestibility is highly variable across the feeds and the danger of toxicity is relatively low. Cost or toxicity considerations may limit the amount of nutrient (for other nutrients) included in the formulated diets to levels very near to the bird's minimum requirement.

Expression of nutrient requirements

Nutrient requirements are expressed in two ways: on an intake basis per day (g per day or g per kg body weight) or on a concentration basis, i.e., % of the diet or g per kg diet. Poultry are fed in groups. In practice, requirements are typically expressed as concentrations, because it is more convenient to formulate practical diets from a collection of individual ingredients. Further, requirements expressed on a percentage basis change slowly and linearly throughout a bird's life cycle (Fig. 2). This is because a bird's feed intake usually changes proportionally with changes in its nutrient needs, minimizing the change in the concentration of the nutrient that is required in the diet.

Birds actually require a specific quantity of a nutrient each day and the daily requirement (kcal ME per day or mg per day) is the most accurate form of expression. In practice, this form of expression is useful if a bird's daily requirements are relatively constant, as in adult birds that are not reproducing. But in growing birds the daily requirements change very rapidly, making this form of expression severely cumbersome in application. Correction of the daily requirement for metabolic body size ($BW^{0.75}$) eliminates-part of this volatility and is especially useful for comparison of maintenance energy needs across species.

Further refinements in nutrient requirements include expression on a digestible or metabolizable nutrient basis. Amino acid requirements are often expressed on a digestible basis while vitamin and mineral requirements are expressed on a bioavailable basis.

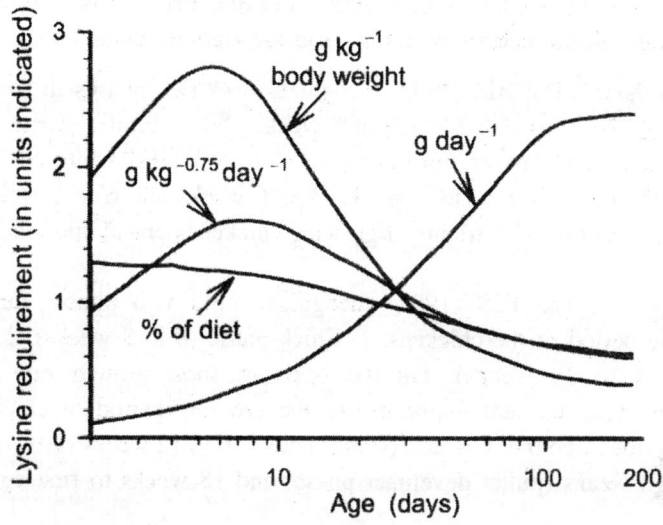

FIGURE 2 The expression of a dietary requirement on a g 100 g⁻¹ basis (%) gives the most consistent values over the period of growth of broiler chickens. Expressed as %, the requirement gradually declines by about half with age; when expressed as mg lysine day⁻¹, the requirement increases by about 25-fold with age.

The latest feeding standards available are 'Poultry Nutrient Requirements by Bureau of Indian Standards (2007), Nutrient Requirements of Poultry (1994) by the NRC of the National Academy of Sciences (USA) and similar requirements proposed by the ARC (UK).

Requirements need to be updated

Nutritional requirements are not static but dynamic. Therefore, with change in genetic makeup, feeding system and feeding management, there is a need for verification, updating and fine-tuning of nutritional requirements on a continuous basis. Applegate and Angel (2014) made a case for revision of the NRC 1994 poultry requirements in view of the substantial amounts of published data and change in perception and definition of a nutrient requirement. First it was a requirement, as a percent of diet, to preventing a nutrient deficiency, to now being a requirement to optimize growth or egg production response per unit of nutrient intake. As economics becomes an increasingly more important driver for the implications of research, the scientific community has begun to embrace the concept of return on investment of nutrient used for compositional growth or egg production.

For optimum growth of young chickens, they should be fed diets containing all the necessary nutrients in the right amounts.

Broilers: The BIS (1992) recognizes only two phases in the broilers from day old to marketable age of 8 weeks, that is broiler starter phase (0 to 5 weeks) and broiler finisher phase (5 to 8 weeks) while NRC (1994) divide the period into 0 to 3 weeks, 3 to 6 weeks and 6 to 8 weeks since the requirements for nutrients of growing chickens depend upon their rate of growth.

Layers: The BIS (1992) recognizes only two phases during the growing period of the chickens, 1. Chick phase (0 to 8 weeks), 2. Grower phase (8 to 20 weeks). On the basis of their growth rate and the accompanying nutrient requirements, the growing period of chickens has been divided into 0 to 6 weeks (starter phase), 6 to 12 weeks (grower phase), 12 to 18 weeks (pullet developer phase) and 18 weeks to first egg (NRC, 1994).

Types of chicken feeds according to BIS (2007) are as follows. Requirements are presented in Tables 1 to 12.

1. Broiler pre-starter feed: 1 - 7 days
2. Broiler starter feed: 8 - 21 days (earlier 0 to 5 weeks; 0 to 6 weeks)
3. Broiler finisher feed: 22 - finish (42 days) (earlier after 5 weeks; 6 to 8 weeks)
4. Broiler breeder chick feed
5. Broiler breeder grower feed
6. Broiler breeder layer feed
7. Broiler breeder male feed
8. Layer chick feed
9. Layer grower feed
10. Layer phase-I feed
11. Layer phase-II feed
12. Layer breeder chick feed
13. Layer breeder grower feed
14. Layer breeder layer feed
15. Layer breeder male feed

ICAR (2013) Requirements of Poultry

Use of ARC and NRC standards under Indian conditions may not be appropriate as the requirements differ due to several factors such as genetic makeup, environmental temperature, managemental practices, metabolic characteristics, feedstuff qualities and dietary variables. Substantial differences also exist in the estimates of nutritional requirements for chicken and other poultry species of tropical countries from that of temperate climate. Studies conducted in India on nutritional requirements of chicken have been reviewed (Reddy, 1996; Mandal et al., 2005a) and are incorporated in ICAR (2013) requirements; similarly for other categories of poultry birds.

Commercial white broilers are generally reared for 6 weeks under three phases, *viz.* pre-starter, starter and finisher. Under special circumstances these birds are reared up to 8 weeks of age to produce larger broilers (roasters), suitable for production of different value-added products. The basic purpose of phasing out is to provide nutrients as per the need depending upon the growth rate and type of growth.

Coloured broilers grow comparatively at slower rate than white broilers but have high survivability. Therefore, their nutritional requirements are less than the commercial white broilers.

Nutrient requirements of broiler breeders (Table 13) and layer chicken including cockerels and breeder males (Table 14 and 15) as given by ICAR in its 3rd revised edition (ICAR, 2013) are furnished for a comparative study with BIS (2007) for broiler breeder feed (Table 4, 5 and 6) and layer feeds (Tables 7 to 12).

Requirement of Broiler Chicken Feeds

Table 1 Requirement of chicken feeds: IS 1374: 2007 (Clauses 4.1.2 ,7.1, E-4.2 and E-5)

Sl. No.	Characteristics	Requirements for Broiler feed		
		Pre-starter	**Starter**	**Finisher**
1	Moisture, percent by mass, Max	11	11	11
2	Crude protein (N X 6.25), percent by mass, Min	23	22	20
3	Ether extract, percent by mass, Min	3.0	3.5	4.0
4	Crude fibre percent by mass, Max	5.0	5.0	5.0
5	Acid insoluble ash, percent by mass, Max	2.5	2.5	2.5
6	Salt (as NaCl), percent by mass, Max	0.5	0.5	0.5

Note: The values specified for characteristics at Sl.No. 2 to 6 are on dry matter basis.
Pre-starter:1 to 7 days; Starter: 8 to 21 days; Finisher: from 22 days to finish (42days).

Table 2 Requirement of chicken feeds: IS 1374: 2007 (Clauses 4.1.2 and 7.1)

Sl. No.	Characteristics	Requirements for Broiler feed		
		Pre-starter	Starter	Finisher
1	Calcium (as Ca) percent by mass, Min	1.0	1.0	1.0
2	Total phosphorus, percent by mass, Min	0.7	0.7	0.7
3	Available phosphorus, percent by mass, Min	0.45	0.45	0.45
4	Lysine, percent by mass, Min	1.3	1.2	1.0
5	Methionine, percent by mass, Min	0.5	0.5	0.45
6	Methionine + cystine, percent, Min	0.9	0.9	0.85
7	Metabolizable energy (kcal/kg), Min	3000	3100	3200
8	Aflatoxin B_1(ppb), Max	20	20	20

Notes:
1. The energy value may also be declared as productive energy value; 1.6 calories of metabolizable energy is equal to 1 calorie productive energy.
2. The values specified for characteristics at Sl.No. 1 to 8 are on dry matter basis.
3. Pre-starter:1 to 7 days; Starter: 8 to 21 days; Finisher: from 22 days to finish (42 days).

Table 3 Requirements for Minerals, Vitamins, Amino Acids and Fatty Acids per kg Chicken Feed (Clause 4.1.3 and 7.1)

Sl. No.	Characteristics	Requirements for Broiler feed		
		Pre-starter	Starter	Finisher
1	Manganese, mg/kg, Min.	100	100	100
2	Iodine, mg/kg, Min	1.2	1.2	1.2
3	Iron, mg/kg, Min	80	80	80
4	Zinc, mg/kg, Min	80	80	80
5	Copper, mg/kg, Min	12	12	12
6	Selenium, mg/kg, Min	0.15	0.15	0.15
7	Vitamin A, IU/kg, Min	11000	11000	10000
8	Vitamin D_3, IU/kg, Min	3000	3000	3000
9	Thiamin, mg/kg, Min	2.5	2.5	2.5
10	Riboflavin, mg/kg, Min	6.0	6.0	6.0
11	Pantothenic acid, mg/kg, Min	15.0	15.0	15.0
12	Nicotinic acid, mg/kg, Min	40.0	40.0	40.0
13	Biotin, mg/kg, Min	0.15	0.15	0.15
14	Vitamin B_{12}, mg/kg, Min	0.015	0.015	0.015
15	Folic acid, mg/kg, Min	1.0	1.0	1.0
16	Choline, mg/kg, Min	500	500	500
17	Vitamin E, mg/kg, Min	30	30	30

18	Vitamin K, mg/kg, Min	1.5	1.5	1.5
19	Pyridoxine, mg/kg, Min	5.0	5.0	5.0
20	Linoleic acid, g/100g, Min	1.1	1.1	1.1

Note: Pre-starter:1 to 7 days; Starter: 8 to 21 days; Finisher: from 22 days to finish (42 days).

Table 4 Requirement of chicken feeds: IS 1374: 2007 (Clauses 4.1.2 ,7.1, E-4.2 and E-5)

Sr. No.	Characteristics	Requirements for Broiler breeder feed			
		Chick	Grower	Layer	Male
1	Moisture, percent by mass, Max	11	11	11	11
2	Crude protein (N X 6.25), percent by mass, Min	20	16	16	15
3	Ether extract, percent by mass, Min	2.5	2.5	2.5	2.5
4	Crude fibre percent by mass, Max	7.0	9.0	9.0	9.0
5	Acid insoluble ash, percent by mass, Max	4.0	4.0	4.0	4.0
6	Salt (as NaCl), percent by mass, Max	0.5	0.5	0.5	0.5

Notes: The values specified for characteristics at Sl.No. 2 to 6 are on dry matter basis.

Table 5 Requirement of chicken feeds: IS 1374: 2007 (Clauses 4.1.2 and 7.1)

Sr. No.	Characteristics	Requirements for Broiler breeder feed			
		Chick	Grower	Layer	Male
1	Calcium (as Ca) percent by mass, Min	1.0	1.0	3.5	1.0
2	Total phosphorus, percent by mass, Min	0.7	0.7	0.7	0.7
3	Available phosphorus, percent by mass, Min	0.45	0.45	0.40	0.40
4	Lysine, percent by mass, Min	1.0	0.80	0.85	0.8
5	Methionine, percent by mass, Min	0.45	0.40	0.45	0.4
6	Methionine + cystine, percent, Min	0.7	0.7	0.7	0.7
7	Metabolizable energy (kcal/kg), Min	2800	2750	2800	2750
8	Aflatoxin B_1(ppb), Max	20	20	20	20

Notes: 1. The energy value may also be declared as productive energy value; 1.6 calories of metabolizable energy is equal to 1 calorie productive energy.
2. The values specified for characteristics at Sl. No. 1 to 8 are on dry matter basis.

Table 6 Requirements for Minerals, Vitamins, Amino Acids and Fatty Acids per kg Chicken Feed (Clause 4.1.3 and 7.1)

Sr. No.	Characteristics	Requirements for Broiler breeder feed			
		Chick	Grower	Layer	Male
1	Manganese, mg/kg, Min.	100	100	100	100
2	Iodine, mg/kg, Min	1.5	1.5	1.5	1.5
3	Iron, mg/kg, Min	80.0	80.0	80.0	80.0
4	Zinc, mg/kg, Min	80.0	80.0	80.0	80.0
5	Copper, mg/kg, Min	12	12	12	12
6	Selenium, mg/kg, Min	0.15	0.15	0.20	0.15
7	Vitamin A, IU/kg, Min	12000	12000	15000	12000
8	Vitamin D_3, IU/kg, Min	2500	2500	3000	2500
9	Thiamin, mg/kg, Min	2.0	2.0	3.0	2.0
10	Riboflavin, mg/kg, Min	5.0	5.0	6.0	5.0
11	Pantothenic acid, mg/kg, Min	15.0	15.0	25.0	15.0
12	Nicotinic acid, mg/kg, Min	40.0	40.0	50.0	40.0
13	Biotin, mg/kg, Min	0.20	0.20	0.20	0.20
14	Vitamin B_{12}, mg/kg, Min	0.025	0.025	0.030	0.025
15	Folic acid, mg/kg, Min	3.0	3.0	4.0	3.0
16	Choline, mg/kg, Min	850	850	700	500
17	Vitamin E, mg/kg, Min	20.0	20.0	50.0	20.0
18	Vitamin K, mg/kg, Min	2.0	2.0	3.0	2.0
19	Pyridoxine, mg/kg, Min	5.0	5.0	6.0	5.0
20	Linoleic acid, g/100g, Min	1.0	1.0	1.0	1.0

Requirement of Layer Chicken Feeds

Table 7 Requirement of chicken feeds: IS 1374: 2007 (Clauses 4.1.2 ,7.1, E-4.2 and E-5)

Sr. No.	Characteristics	Requirements for Layer feed			
		Chick	Grower	Layer phase-I	Layer phase-II
1	Moisture, percent by mass, Max	11	11	11	11
2	Crude protein (N X 6.25), percent by mass, Min	20	16	18	16

3	Ether extract, percent by mass, Min	2.0	2.0	2.0	2.0
4	Crude fibre percent by mass, Max	7.0	9.0	9.0	10
5	Acid insoluble ash, percent by mass, Max	4.0	4.0	4.0	4.5
6	Salt (as NaCl), percent by mass, Max	0.5	0.5	0.5	0.5

Notes: The values specified for characteristics at Sl.No. 2 to 6 are on dry matter basis.

Table 8 Requirement of chicken feeds: IS 1374: 2007 (Clauses 4.1.2 and 7.1)

Sr. No.	Characteristics	Requirements for Layer feed			
		Chick	Grower	Layer phase-I	Layer phase-II
1	Calcium (as Ca) percent by mass, Min	1.0	1.0	3.0	3.5
2	Total phosphorus, percent by mass, Min	0.7	0.65	0.65	0.65
3	Available phosphorus, percent by mass, Min	0.45	0.4	0.4	0.4
4	Lysine, percent by mass, Min	1.0	0.7	0.7	0.65
5	Methionine, percent by mass, Min	0.4	0.35	0.35	0.3
6	Methionine + cystine, percent, Min	0.7	0.6	0.6	0.55
7	Metabolizable energy (kcal/kg), Min	2800	2500	2600	2400
8	Aflatoxin B_1(ppb), Max	20	20	20	20

Notes: 1. The energy value may also be declared as productive energy value; 1.6 calories of metabolizable energy is equal to 1 calorie productive energy.

2. The values specified for characteristics at Sl.No. 1 to 8 are on dry matter basis.

Table 9   Requirements for Minerals, Vitamins, Amino Acids and Fatty Acids per kg Chicken Feed (Clause 4.1.3 and 7.1)

Sr. No.	Characteristics	Requirements for Layer feed			
		Chick	Grower	Layer phase-I	Layer phase-II
1	Manganese, mg/kg, Min.	70	60	60	60
2	Iodine, mg/kg, Min	1.0	1.0	1.0	1.0
3	Iron, mg/kg, Min	70	60	60	60
4	Zinc, mg/kg, Min	60	60	60	60
5	Copper, mg/kg, Min	12	9	9	9
6	Selenium, mg/kg, Min	0.15	0.15	0.15	0.15
7	Vitamin A, IU/kg, Min	9000	8000	8000	8000
8	Vitamin D_3, IU/kg, Min	1800	1600	1600	1600
9	Thiamin, mg/kg, Min	2	1.5	1	1
10	Riboflavin, mg/kg, Min	6	5	5	5
11	Pantothenic acid, mg/kg, Min	10	9	7	7
12	Nicotinic acid, mg/kg, Min	40	20	20	20
13	Biotin, mg/kg, Min	0.10	0.10	0.10	0.10
14	Vitamin B_{12}, mg/kg, Min	0.010	0.008	0.008	0.008
15	Folic acid, mg/kg, Min	1.0	0.50	0.50	0.50
16	Choline, mg/kg, Min	500	200	400	400
17	Vitamin E, mg/kg, Min	15	10	10	10
18	Vitamin K, mg/kg, Min	1.5	1.5	1.5	1.5
19	Pyridoxine, mg/kg, Min	3.0	3.0	3.0	3.0
20	Linoleic acid, g/100g, Min	1.0	1.0	1.0	1.0

Table 10   Requirement of chicken feeds: IS 1374: 2007 (Clauses 4.1.2 ,7.1, E-4.2 and E-5)

Sr. No	Characteristics	Requirements for Layer breeder feed			
		Chick	Grower	Layer	Male
1	Moisture, percent by mass, Max	11	11	11	11
2	Crude protein (N X 6.25), percent by mass, Min	20	16	17	16
3	Ether extract, percent by mass, Min	2.0	2.0	2.0	2.0

4	Crude fibre percent by mass, Max	7.0	9.0	9.0	9.0
5	Acid insoluble ash, percent by mass, Max	2.5	2.5	2.5	2.5
6	Salt (as NaCl), percent by mass, Max	0.5	0.5	0.5	0.5

Note: The values specified for characteristics at Sl.No. 2 to 6 are on dry matter basis.

Table 11 Requirement of chicken feeds: IS 1374: 2007 (Clauses 4.1.2 and 7.1)

Sr. No	Characteristics	Requirements for Layer breeder feed			
		Chick	Grower	Layer	Male
1	Calcium (as Ca) percent by mass, Min	1.0	1.0	3.5	1.0
2	Total phosphorus, percent by mass, Min	0.65	0.60	0.60	0.60
3	Available phosphorus, percent by mass, Min	0.45	0.4	0.4	0.4
4	Lysine, percent by mass, Min	0.95	0.7	0.70	0.80
5	Methionine, percent by mass, Min	0.4	0.4	0.4	0.4
6	Methionine + cystine, percent, Min	0.7	0.6	0.6	0.6
7	Metabolizable energy (kcal/kg), Min	2800	2600	2600	2600
8	Aflatoxin B_1(ppb), Max	20	20	20	20

Notes: 1. The energy value may also be declared as productive energy value; 1.6 calories of metabolizable energy is equal to 1 calorie productive energy.
2. The values specified for characteristics at Sl.No. 1 to 8 are on dry matter basis.

Table 12 Requirements for Minerals, Vitamins, Amino Acids and Fatty Acids per kg Chicken Feed (Clause 4.1.3 and 7.1)

Sr. No	Characteristics	Requirements for Layer breeder feed			
		Chick	Grower	Layer	Male
1	Manganese, mg/kg, Min.	100	100	100	100
2	Iodine, mg/kg, Min	1.5	1.5	1.5	1.5
3	Iron, mg/kg, Min	80.0	80.0	80.0	80.0
4	Zinc, mg/kg, Min	80.0	80.0	80.0	80.0

5	Copper, mg/kg, Min	12	12	12	12
6	Selenium, mg/kg, Min	0.15	0.15	0.20	0.15
7	Vitamin A, IU/kg, Min	12000	12000	15000	12000
8	Vitamin D_3, IU/kg, Min	2500	2500	3000	2500
9	Thiamin, mg/kg, Min	2.0	2.0	3.0	2.0
10	Riboflavin, mg/kg, Min	5.0	5.0	6.0	5.0
11	Pantothenic acid, mg/kg, Min	15.0	15.0	25.0	15.0
12	Nicotinic acid, mg/kg, Min	40.0	40.0	50.0	40.0
13	Biotin, mg/kg, Min	0.20	0.20	0.20	0.20
14	Vitamin B_{12}, mg/kg, Min	0.025	0.025	0.030	0.025
15	Folic acid, mg/kg, Min	3.0	3.0	4.0	3.0
16	Choline, mg/kg, Min	850	850	700	500
17	Vitamin E, mg/kg, Min	20.0	20.0	50.0	20.0
18	Vitamin K, mg/kg, Min	2.0	2.0	3.0	2.0
19	Pyridoxine, mg/kg, Min	5.0	5.0	6.0	5.0
20	Linoleic acid, g/100g, Min	1.0	1.0	1.0	1.0

NRC (1994) gave the energy requirements in terms of nitrogen corrected ME (ME_n).

Table 13 Nutrient requirements of broiler breeders (as fed basis)*

Nutrients	Chicks (0-4 wk)	Growers (5-18 wk)	Pre-breeder (19-23 wk)	Breeder (24 wk onwards)	Males (24 wk onwards)
ME (kcal/kg)	2,800	2,650	2,700	2,700	2,750
Crude protein (%)	20.0	16.0	16.5	16.0	14.0
Calcium (%)	1.0	1.0	1.5	3.0	0.90
Available phosphorus (%)	0.45	0.45	0.38	0.35	0.30
Lysine (%)	1.1	0.80	0.80	0.75	0.60
Dig. Lysine (%)	0.99	0.66	0.68	0.67	0.57
Methionine (%)	0.45	0.40	0.36	0.35	0.30
Dig. Methionine (%)	0.41	0.33	0.30	0.31	0.26
Arginine (%)	1.1	0.85	0.87	0.90	0.80
Dig. Arginine (%)	0.99	0.71	0.74	0.79	0.70
Tryptophan (%)	0.20	0.16	0.17	0.16	0.14
Dig. Tryptophan (%)	0.18	0.13	0.14	0.14	0.12
Threonine (%)	0.70	0.60	0.52	0.52	0.48
Dig. Threonine (%)	0.63	0.50	0.44	0.45	0.42
Vitamin A (IU/kg)	12,000	20,000	18,000	15,000	12,000
Vitamin D_3 (ICU/kg)	3,000	4,500	4,000	3,500	2,000
Vitamin E (IU/kg)	80	100	100	100	200
Vitamin K (mg/kg)	3	5	5	5	5
Pyridoxine (mg/kg)	5	8	6	6	6
Thiamin (mg/kg)	4	5	5	4	4.4
Riboflavin (mg/kg)	20	20	20	20	20

Pantothenic acid (mg/kg)	30	30	30	30	25
Niacin (mg/kg)	60	80	75	66	60
Choline (mg/kg)	1,200	1,200	1,200	1,200	1,200
Folic acid (mg/kg)	4	4	4.8	4	4
Biotin (mg/kg)	0.25	0.30	0.30	0.25	0.25
Vitamin B_{12} (mg/kg)	0.03	0.03	0.04	0.03	0.03
Manganese (mg/kg)	100	120	120	100	120
Zinc (mg/kg)	100	100	120	100	100
Iron (mg/kg)	80	80	80	80	80
Copper (mg/kg)	20	20	20	20	20
Iodine (mg/kg)	2.0	3.0	3.0	2.5	2.5
Selenium (mg/kg)	0.3	0.3	0.3	0.3	0.35

* Source: ICAR (2013)

Table 14 Nutrient requirements (as fed basis) of starting and growing egg type pullets and cockerels*

Nutrients	Laying pullets			Cockerels	
	0-8 wk	8-16 wk	16-18 wk	0-4 wk	4-10 wk
ME (kcal/kg)	2,600	2,600	2,700	2,600	2,600
Crude protein (%)	18.5	15.5	15.0	19	17.5
Lysine (%)	0.85	0.65	0.50	0.98	0.90
Methionine (%)	0.32	0.29	0.27	0.35	0.33
Methionine + Cysteine (%)	0.65	0.59	0.54	0.70	0.67
Threonine (%)	0.68	0.58	0.50	0.78	0.70
Linoleic acid (%)	1.0	0.8	0.8	1.0	0.8
Calcium (%)	1.0	0.80	2.0	.0	0.85
Available phosphorus (%)	0.4	0.35	0.32	0.41	0.38
Sodium (%)	0.15	0.15	0.15	0.15	0.15
Chloride (%)	0.15	0.12	0.12	0.15	0.15
Copper (mg/kg)	8.0	5.0	5.0	8.0	8.0
Iodine (mg/kg)	0.35	0.35	0.35	0.35	0.35
Iron (mg/kg)	60	60	60	60	60
Manganese (mg/kg)	50	40	40	50	45
Selenium (mg/kg)	0.15	0.10	0.10	0.15	0.15
Zinc (mg/kg)	40	35	35	40	40
Vitamin A (IU/kg)	3,000	2,500	3,000	3,000	2,500
D_3 (IU/kg)	300	250	300	300	250
E (IU/kg)	10	10	10	10	10
K (mg/kg)	0.5	0.5	0.5	0.5	0.5
Thiamin (mg/kg)	1.0	1.0	1.0	1.0	1.0
Riboflavin (mg/kg)	3.6	1.8	1.8	3.6	3.0
Pyridoxine (mg/kg)	3.0	3.0	3.0	3.0	3.0
Vitamin B_{12} (mg/kg)	0.009	0.003	0.003	0.009	0.005
Biotin (mg/kg)	0.15	0.10	0.10	0.15	0.15
Folic acid (mg/kg)	0.55	0.25	0.25	0.55	0.55
Niacin (mg/kg)	25.0	11.0	11.0	25.0	25.0
Pantothenic acid (mg/kg)	10.0	10.0	10.0	10.0	10.0
Choline (mg)	1,300"	900	500	1,300	1,000

* Source: ICAR (2013)

Table 15 Nutrient requirements (as fed basis) of Leghorn type hens and breeder males*

Description	Age (wk) 18-30	18-30	Age (wk) >30	>30	Breeder male >20 wk
Live wt. (g)	1,300	1,400	1,400	1,500	-
Egg Mass (g)	42.5	45	45	50	-
Shed temp. (°C)	25	25	25	25	-
Feed intake (g)	90	100	100	110	-
Nutrient					
ME (kcal/kg)	2,750	2,600	2,600	2,550	2,600
Crude protein (%)	20.0	18.0	16.5	15.0	16.5
Lysine (%)	0.90	0.82	0.76	0.68	0.76
Methionine (%)	0.40	0.36	0.34	0.32	0.34
Methionine + Cysteine (%)	0.78	0.70	0.65	0.60	0.65
Threonine (%)	0.63	0.56	0.52	0.47	0.52
Arginine (%)	0.93	0.84	0.77	0.70	0.77
Tryptophan (%)	0.21	0.19	0.18	0.16	0.18
Linoleic acid (%)	1.10	1.00	1.0	0.85	1.0
Calcium (%)	3.80	3.61	3.60	3.40	1.00
Available phosphorus (%)	0.36	0.28	0.32	0.30	0.32
Sodium (%)	0.17	0.15	0.15	0.14	0.15
Iodine (mg/kg)	0.040	0.035	0.035	0.032	0.035
Iron (mg/kg)	55	50	50	45	50
Manganese (mg/kg)	50	45	45	40	45
Selenium (mg/kg)	0.08	0.06	0.06	0.05	0.06
Zinc (mg/kg)	50	45	45	40	45
Vitamin A (IU/kg)	5,000	4,500	4,500	4,000	4,500
D_3 (IU/kg)	500	o 450	450	400	450
E (IU/kg)	15	10	10	10	10
K (mg/kg)	0.6	0.5	0.5	0.45	0.5
Thiamin (mg/kg)	0.85	0.70	0.70	0.65	0.70
Riboflavin (mg/kg)	3.5	3.0	3.0	2.8	3.0
Pyridoxine (mg/kg)	3.5	3.0	3.0	2.8	3.0
Vitamin B_{12} (mg/kg)	0.004	0.004	0.004	0.004	0.004
Biotin (mg/kg)	0.12	0.10	0.10	0.09	0.10
Folic acid (mg/kg)	0.30	0.28	0.28	0.25	0.28
Niacin (mg/kg)	12.0	10.0	10.0	9.0	10.0
Pantothenic acid (mg/kg)	2.5	2.0	2.0	1.80	2.0
Choline (mg)	1,200	1,050	1,050	950	1,000

* Source: ICAR (2013)

Energy

Metabolizable energy is considered. The usefulness of ME values in formulating poultry feed from a practical view point is based on the following: ME is the energy available to the bird for transformation in the body.

1. Determination of ME value of feeds is easy in poultry.

2. ME value of an ingredient is independent of other dietary components, and

3. The ME value remains relatively constant regardless of age, type or nature of production of the bird.

ENERGY UTILIZATION BY A LAYING HEN

Faeces	Urine	HI	Maintenance	Eggs & Tissue
800	300	600	1500	800

←——————————————— 4000 Kcal GE ————————————→
←——————————— 3200 Kcal DE ————————→
←————————— 2900 Kcal ME ————————→
2300 Kcal NE_m + p ————————→

This illustrates that of 4000 Kcal of gross energy consumed from 1 kg of diet, the hen is capable of metabolizing 2900 Kcal and 2300 Kcal are available for maintenance and transfer into body tissue and egg. The relative amounts of energy voided or used at various stages will, of course, vary with the composition of the diet, species, genetic makeup and age of poultry, as well as the environmental conditions.

Metabolizable energy is determined by measuring feed intake and excreta output over a 2 to 5-day test period. Apparent ME is most commonly determined through actual measurement of feed intake and excreta output. In case of indicator method, (through use of an inert dietary marker, such as chromic oxide (Cr_2O_3)), quantitative collection of excreta is not necessary; only a representative sample is required. Total collection of excreta method eliminates the sometimes troublesome chromic oxide determination, but requires very accurate measurement of feed consumed and the accurate collection of excreta. Method of determination of TME is described in Chapter 14 of *Principles of Animal Nutrition and Feed Technology.*

The use of **TME** is particularly important at low levels of dietary intake and for foods high in fibre or plant secondary products. A further refinement in measurement of food energy content is to correct for the loss or retention of body protein, so that values derived from birds that are growing or losing weight are comparable. Use of nitrogen-corrected ME (ME_n) is especially important for foodstuffs that have poor amino acid balance or levels and foods that have toxins (Sibbald, 1989).

A bird's daily ME requirement is equal to the amount of energy expended through the oxidation of nutrients (heat production) plus energy retained in tissues. The amount of energy retained in body tissues, eggs, or feathers is determined by bomb calorimetry. The rate of heat production is commonly determined in birds by either direct or indirect calorimetry. Direct calorimetry measures ME expenditure by the rate at which heat is released from a bird. Indirect calorimetry measures the rate of O_2 consumption and CO_2 release, which can be used to calculate the rate of ME expenditure.

ME value of a feed will vary according to whether amino acids it supplies are retained or are deaminated with their N excreted in the urine as urea/uric acid. Since the extent of N differs with age, a correction factor is essential. Hence, ME values are corrected to zero N balance by deducting for each gram of N retained or by adding for each gram of N catabolized.

Nitrogen - Corrected ME

For convenience, all computations are adjusted to a condition of zero nitrogen retention (AME_n).

AME per gram diet = GE per gram diet - (Excreta energy per g diet − 8.22 × g N retained per g diet).

If, during an ME determination, nitrogen is retained by the animal, the excreta will contain less urinary nitrogen and hence less energy would be excreted as compared with an animal that is not retaining N. Assuming that if nitrogen is not retained it will appear as uric acid, a correction value of 8.22 Kcal/g nitrogen retained (8.1 kcal is taken as equivalent to 34 KJ) was added because this is the energy obtained when uric acid is completely oxidized.

True ME for poultry is the gross energy of the feed consumed minus the gross energy of the excreta of feed origin. A correction for nitrogen retention may be applied to give TME_n value. ME_n and TME_n values of certain feedstuffs (as fed basis, NRC 1994) are furnished below to make the readers aware about them.

Feedstuff	ME_n	TME_n
	← Kcal/kg →	
Corn grain	3350	3470
Barley grain	2640	2900
Oats grain	2550	2625
Rice bran	2980	3085
Wheat bran	1300	1725
Sorghum grain	3288	3376

TME_n = GE per gram diet - (Excreta energy − Endogenous energy loss) − 8.22 × gN retained per g diet

TME is always higher than AME but both are highly correlated.

Protein and Amino Acids

The total protein requirement for poultry can be met easily. However, it is difficult to meet the requirement for essential amino acids. Ideal protein concept is followed and ideal ratios of EAAs to lysine are developed. A protein that contains a perfect balance of amino acids, both among the essential and between essential amino acids and nonessential amino acids, has been described as an ideal protein.

Amino acid requirements for maximum growth are lower than that for immunity. Antibodies are proteins, therefore any deficiency of essential amino acids particularly during the growing chicken results in poor immunocompetence.

The dietary limitations of lysine gave rise to only a slight depression of immune response. Moderate reduction of threonine in the diet produced profound depression of humoral immune response (Lotan et al, 1980). Methionine is known for its cellular immunity (Bhanja et al., 2004ab). Konashi et al. (2000) reported that the branched chain amino acids (isoleucine, leucine and valine) affect the humoral and cell-mediated immune response by affecting antibody production.

Commercial layers that produce around 320 eggs annually require higher levels of lysine, methionine, total sulphur amino acid and tryptophan, branched chain amino acids (isoleucine, leucine and valine), arginine.

Essential amino acids for poultry: Essential amino acids are ten in number. Birds require glycine also. Its requirement is relatively larger because glycine is needed for the biosynthesis of uric acid (an end product of the nitrogen metabolism in birds). Glycine may be synthesized from creatine and serine as long as folic acid, vitamin B_{12} and pyridoxine are not deficient.

Cysteine and tyrosine are semiessential amino acids, which can be obtained from methionine and phenylalanine, respectively. Serine, in the same way, can be obtained from glycine. Arginine is essential for poultry and yields urea and ornithine on metabolism. Ornithine and glycine are used for detoxification of aromatic compounds in the liver.

Limiting amino acids: Among the EAA, the amino acids that are likely to be low in practical diets (critical amino acids) are arginine, isoleucine, threonine, lysine, methionine and tryptophan. Threonine and tryptophan are only marginally deficient and a careful ingredient selection will avoid their deficiency. Arginine deficiency is usually not a problem because groundnut cake is a popular vegetable protein supplement and groundnut is rich in arginine. Therefore, the limiting amino acids in poultry nutrition depend on the source of protein used in the diet. Lysine is the first limiting amino acid in most of the soya-free diets while methionine has been the most limiting one in diets based on soybean meal.

The amino acid in a feed that is most deficient relative to a bird's requirement is referred to as the first limiting amino acid. The limiting amino acid concept may also be explained as follows. The ratio between the amount of amino acid present in a protein supplement and its requirement gives an idea. The lowest ratio gives the first limiting amino acid. The next lowest ratio gives the second most limiting amino acid. It has been reported that methionine is the only limiting amino acid in soybean meal and lysine is the limiting one in sesame (gingilly or til) cake.

Lysine requirement as a per cent of protein is less for egg production than for growth, and a deficiency in diets for egg production is not usual. In general, all amino acids must be present in the diet at the same time for their efficient utilization. The needed amino acids can be supplemented in the practical diets. Synthetic L-lysine and DL-methionine are available commercially at a reasonable price for use in feeds. Threonine is the costliest synthetic amino acid. Threonine is limiting amino acid in sorghum, wheat, etc.

Threonine is the third limiting amino acid for broilers, second limiting amino acid in growing Japanese quails and first limiting amino acid in starting egg-type pullets. Threonine is closely associated with the digestive enzymes and mucus in the digestive tract.

Optimizing amino acid nutrition – early protein nutrition impacts on the development of broiler chicks

Protein metabolism is considered to be regulated by amino acids, with major consequences on tissue development. Tesseraud et al. (2011) in their review reported that lysine greatly affects carcass composition and muscle growth particularly breast muscle development and breast muscle quality in chickens; increasing lysine improves breast muscle quality by increasing its ultimate pH and water holding capacity. Other essential amino acids, such as threonine and valine, do not have as pronounced an effect as lysine on body composition.

Amino acids act as modulators of signal transduction pathways that control metabolism and cell functions, in addition to being substrates for protein synthesis. Enhanced responses to amino acids have been reported during the neonatal period, suggesting that early protein nutrition impacts on the development of broiler chicks.

Methionine and cysteine have a very significant place among amino acids because they have several additional roles. They are precursors of essential molecules: cysteine is used for the synthesis of glutathione, and thus participates in the control of oxidative status; methionine is a source of methyl groups needed for all biological methylation reactions, including methylation of DNA and histones, etc.

Supplementary action between different proteins

Blood meal and corn gluten meal: Blood meal is rich in lysine and tryptophan but deficient in isoleucine while corn gluten meal is deficient in lysine and tryptophan but rich in isoleucine. One part of blood meal to 4 parts of corn gluten meal mixture is more effective in promoting chick growth.

Soybean and sesame meal: Soybean meal is rich in lysine but less in methionine while sesame meal is deficient in lysine but rich in methionine.

Excesses of amino acids: Methionine is the most growth depressing when added at 40 g per kg diet. Excess threonine depress growth in chicks. Excesses of amino acids are also deleterious because an excess of one amino acid may create an increased demand for another one. For example, a toxicity of dietary lysine is overcome by increasing the levels of arginine or glycine; threonine alleviates the toxic effect of an excess of tryptophan; glycine reduces the toxic effects of an excess of methionine; similarly the toxic effects of an excess leucine or valine are alleviated by isoleucine. These are the established interactions among the amino acids. In practical feeding situations when several feed ingredients are used in formulating balanced diets moderate excesses are generally ignored.

Amino acid interactions

Amino acid interactions may exist. These interactions may be due to amino acid imbalance, amino acid antagonism or amino acid toxicity. Amino acid interactions lower amino acid utilization i.e. the nitrogen retention in the body.

Amino acid imbalance: Amino acid imbalance may be caused in diets formulated with feed ingredients without supplemental amino acids. In such diets, protein content is high with excess levels of some amino acids. The utilization of the first limiting amino acid is reduced in poultry. Amino acid in excess competes with the dietary limiting amino acid for transport to the brain, causing reduced feed intake and consequent reduced performance.

From a practical point of view, it is suggested to keep each amino acid at a level above the minimum requirement but not exceeding 1.5 times the requirement.

Amino acid antagonism: Amino acid antagonism is an interaction between structurally similar amino acids resulting in the precipitation of adverse effects. Example: lysine-arginine antagonism - Excess dietary lysine specifically impairs the utilization of arginine, due to increased renal arginase activity, resulting in increased oxidation of arginine. Thus, high levels of dietary lysine increase the requirement for arginine. The ratio of lysine to arginine may be 1: 0.9-1.5. Excess arginine is not a problem to be considered in practical feed formulation. Fortunately, situations of excess lysine are unlikely unless attempted deliberately or done by a mistake.

Another example: High dietary levels of leucine or valine reduce the utilization of isoleucine (Calvert et al., 1982). Surplus leucine or valine induces the enzymes that cataboize all three branched-chain amino acids, causing greater loss of isoleucine and exacerbating its deficiency. The result is high dietary level of one branched-chain amino acid increases the requirement for the other two.

Toxicity: Amino acid toxicity is due to an individual amino acid. In practical diets, it is not encountered. Methionine is the most toxic of the amino acids, depressing growth and feed intake at levels of about three to four times the requirement. Higher levels of dietary protein (higher levels of methionine and cysteine results in the production of sulfate; two moles of acid are produced per mole of amino acid oxidized) cause a metabolic acidosis and may contribute to a variety of problems in birds, including poor bone mineralization, thinning of egg shells and poor growth.

Birds excrete most of their waste nitrogen as uric acid rather than urea or ammonia. Because of disposal of excess amino acid nitrogen by the uric acid synthetic pathway, birds require higher amounts of arginine, methionine and glycine relative to mammals.

How to avoid amino acid interactions?

Ideal ratios of essential amino acids to one reference amino acid, i.e., ideal protein or ideal amino acid profile, are calculated for each category of birds. Lysine is chosen as the reference amino acid. Such ratios of amino acids are rather stable and thus amino acid interactions are avoided.

Digestibility of amino acids is variable as like the digestibility of other nutrients. Hence, it is obvious that feeds are to be formulated on the basis of digestible amino acids rather than on total amino acids.

Factors Affecting Amino Acid Requirement

1. Energy content of the diet: As the energy content of the diet increases the requirement of all essential amino acids also increase.
2. Content of polyunsaturated fats: Polyunsaturated fats upon peroxidation produce aldehydes which may bind lysine.
3. Raw soybeans cause hypertrophy of pancreas. The eventual increased production of trypsinogen (It is high in methionine) increases dietary methionine requirement.
4. Certain antibiotics spare amino acids by reducing their destruction.
5. It has been reported that lasalocid (a coccidiostat) reduced the sulfur amino acid requirement by as much as 0.1%.
6. Excessive levels of one or more of the essential amino acids will increase the requirement for the first limiting amino acid.

Calorie-Protein Ratio

It is defined as the metabolizable energy (Kcal) per kilogram divided by the percentage of crude protein in the ration. The ratio varies with the age of the bird. Calorie-protein ratio is maintained for effective utilization of protein as well as amino acids. The concentrations of essential amino acids are more important than protein as such. Faster growth is achieved when the protein level is increased, i.e. at lower calorie to protein ratio. Calorie protein ratios for BIS requirements are presented here.

	Type	Calorie - Protein ratio	
		BIS (1992)	BIS (2007)
1.	Broiler starter feed	122	141
2.	Broiler finisher feed	145	160
3.	Chick feed	130	140
4.	Growing chicken feed	156	156
5.	Laying chicken feed	144	144 to 150

Calorie protein ratio is of paramount importance in poultry, swine as well as ruminants for efficient feed utilization. Sometimes it is reported as nutrient to calorie ratio. The energy need of animals and their requirements of several nutrients are correlated. It was found logical to express nutrients in weight per unit of energy needed. For example, protein to calorie ratio may be expressed as g protein/1000 Kcal ME or g protein/1000 Kcal ME_n. Similarly g Ca/1000 Kcal ME or mg riboflavin/1000 Kcal ME or available lysine per 1000 Kcal ME.

Energy Requirements of Chicken

Experimental studies have shown that the ME requirements are approximately 18% higher than the NE requirements. This is due to the specific dynamic action of nutrients; consumption of protein causes about 30% increase in heat production while consumption of carbohydrate and fat yield 15 and 10% heat increment, respectively. In a well balanced diet containing 20% protein, 5% fat and 65% carbohydrate, the average heat increment is 18%. Thus the NE_m requirements are approximately 82% of the ME_m requirements. Since the chicken has a higher body temperature than mammals, its energy expenditure for maintenance is greater. (Also see estimates of energy and protein requirements p. 49)

1. Energy requirement for maintenance of layers

The basal metabolism studies indicate that the
NE_m requirement of adult hen = $83 \times BW$ kg$^{0.75}$ Kcal/day
NE_m requirement of 1.75 kg adult hen = $83 \times 1.75^{0.75}$
$$= 83 \times 1.52 = 126 \text{ Kcal/day}$$
$$ME_m \text{ requirement} = 126 \times 82\% = \frac{126}{0.82} = 154 \text{ Kcal/day}$$

Activity allowance is 50% of the energy for hens kept in deep litter needed for basal metabolism and 37% for caged hens.

Therefore, total ME requirements for non-laying hens = 154 + 57
 (kept in cages)
$$= 211 \text{ Kcal/day}$$
The energy content of a large egg = 86 Kcal
Then the total ME requirement of a laying hen
(W Leghorn) (in 100% production at 21°C) $\quad$ = 297 Kcal/day

2. Energy for growth

The energy for growth ranges from approximately 1.5 to 3.0 Kcal per gram of body gain. This depends upon the amount of fat in relation to protein in the body gains. The requirements of growing cockerels are higher than that of pullets.

Growth rates, basal metabolism, type of tissue deposited, and efficiency of feed utilization all to some extent are determined by the levels of various hormone secretions, particularly growth hormone, thyroxine and the sex hormones.

3. Calculation of energy requirement of broilers

Weight of the broiler breeder : 2.5 kg

Age	:	25 Weeks
NE_m	:	$83 \times 2.5^{0.75} = 83 \times 1.99 = 165$ Kcal/day.
ME_m	:	$165/0.82 = 201$ Kcal/day.
Activity	:	50% of $ME_m = 101$ Kcal/day.
$ME_m \cdot$ Activity	:	302 Kcal/day.

Egg production is 85%

ME_m egg $= 86$ Kcal $\times 0.85 = 73$ Kcal/day.

These pullets are still growing and body gain is approximately 500 g over 10 week period.

i.e. $= 7.14$ g gain/day.

Energy requirement for gain: 18% protein and 15% fat are present.

1.285 g Protein $\times 4.0$ Kcal $= 5.14$
1.05 g Fat $\times 9.0$ Kcal $\quad = 9.45$
$\underline{}$
14.60 say 15 Kcal.

Total ME required $= ME_m + ME_{activity} + ME_{egg} + ME_{gain}$
(for the period $= 201 + 101 + 73 + 15$
25 - 30 weeks of age) $= 390$ Kcal/hen/day.

Protein Requirements of Chicken

1. The protein requirements of growing chickens may be calculated as follows: Growing white leghorn chicken has 61% of efficiency in utilization of protein. That is of the daily protein consumed about 61% is only retained in the body.

    (a) Maintenance requirement $= 250$ mg N/kg BW/day
    $ = 1600$ mg Protein/kg BW/day.

    (b) Tissue growth (Tissues contain 18% protein)
    Daily gain in g $\times 0.18$.

    (c) Feather growth: Feathers contain 82% protein and
    feathers comprise 7% body weight at 4 weeks of age.
    Daily protein requirement for a growing chicken
    $= [(BW)$ in g $\times 1.6/1000) + ($Daily gain in g $\times 0.18) +$
    (Daily gain in g $\times 0.07 \times 0.82)] \div \%$ efficiency of protein utilization.

2. Calculation of protein requirement for egg production:
   Maintenance requirement of WLH hen = 3 g/day
   Protein content in one egg = 6 g/day
   Total requirement = 9 g/day.
   Efficiency of protein utilization
   for maintenance and egg production = 55%
   Therefore, the protein requirement of the hen

$$= 9 \times \frac{100}{55} = 16.36 \ \text{g/day}$$

If hen eats 120 g diet per day, then the protein content of the diet should be 13.6%. If hens eats 100 g diet only, then the protein content of the diet should be 16.4%.

BROILERS

The growth of (meat) birds depends upon the level of a balanced protein in their diet along with other nutrients. In absence of optimum level of protein and amino acids, the growth is retarded and birds may need a longer time to reach the marketable weight. Higher protein diets are fed during the first two weeks as pre-starter phase. Growing broiler strains of chickens are approximately 67% efficient in the retention of dietary protein. Feeding of the high protein pre-starter diets is beneficial since it gives a stimulus for the early growth of the broilers and it does not cost much because of very small feed intake during the first two weeks.

Breast meat is the major part of edible meat and contains high concentration of lysine. Lysine requirement for optimum FCR is higher than that for optimum body weight gain. This may be the probable reason for the controversy on the level of dietary lysine for optimum body weight gain, FCR and breast muscle development. Methionine is the first limiting amino acid in broilers on conventional maize-soya diets. Methionine supplementation improves dietary amino acid balance and promotes greater protein build up, increases breast muscle yield and decreases fat deposition.

Enhancement of energy level of the diet in the finishing stage, accompanied with a decrease in protein content causes the broiler chicken to consume more calories than it can use for growth. This excess energy will be coverted into body fat, thereby producing the desired body finish for the market broiler.

Essential Fatty acids (EFA): The absolute requirement for linoleic acid is considerably greater than that for α-linolenic acid. Quantitatively, the primary need for EFA is for the synthesis of phospholipids, which are incorporated into cell membranes and yolk lipids. Thus, nutritional needs are driven by the rate of growth and egg production. NRC (1994) stated 1% requirement in practical diet formulation for linoleic acid. This level is adequate for reproduction. Almost all natural foods that meet the energy requirement of birds meet the requirement for these two fatty acids, and frank deficiencies are rare.

Deficiencies of linoleic acid are most readily identified by a slow rate of growth and the accumulation of fat in the liver. Biochemically enriched eicosatrienoic acid (20:3 n-9) is noted. In reproductively active birds, a deficiency is expressed as impaired spermatogenesis in the male, and the production of fewer and smaller eggs in the female. Fertilized eggs often have higher embryonic mortality.

L-carnitine: Adabi et al. (2011) reviewed the functional effects of L-carnitine in poultry nutrition. L-carnitine is synthesized endogenously and it is also received from exogenous sources. It has been suggested that the requirement of L-carnitine may be increased under certain circumstances such as via higher performance, various stress conditions and where the diet is deficient in animal protein sources. It plays an obligate role in fatty acid metabolism by directing fatty acids into the mitochondrial oxidative pathway through the action of specialized acytransferases.

Minerals: Minerals to be supplied in diet are known as critical minerals. They are calcium, nonphytin phosphorus, sodium, chlorine, manganese, zinc, iron, copper, iodine, selenium (magnesium, potassium and sulphur are not deficient in practical diet). The use of organic sources can potentially improve intestinal absorption of trace elements as they reduce the interference from agents that form insoluble complexes with the ionic state elements. It is well known that the requirements of trace minerals for immunity are higher than that for maximum production.

Vitamins: The vitamins A, B_2, D_3. K and B_{12} are to be supplemented in the feed (and water) for broilers and layers disregarding their contribution from the feedstuffs. Usually, thiamin, riboflavin, niacin, pyridoxine, pantothenic acid, choline and vitamin E are supplemented in diets of broiler chicken and chicks. Vitamins C and E improve immunity. Hence supplementation is beneficial under stress conditions. Feedstuffs supply sufficient biotin and folic acid for growth and egg production.

Diets deficient in B_2 have more effect on early embryonic mortality and hatchability than reduced egg production and fertility. Severely affected chicks and embryos (that failed to hatch because of riboflavin deficiency) are oedematous and dwarf. Hatched and surviving chicks show 'clubbed down' condition. This 'clubbed down' results from failure of down feathers to rupture the sheaths, thus causing them to coil. Riboflavin deficient chicks develop 'curled toe paralyses'. Toes are curled inwards and body weight is supported on the hocks. The sciatic and brachial nerves undergo marked swelling and softening.

Some common sources of Ca and P

Source	% Element			Biological availability of P %
	Ca	P	F	
Calcite grit	34	-	-	-
Calcium carbonate	38	-	-	-
Limestone, ground	36	-	-	-
Oyster shell	38	-	-	-
Steamed bone meal	29	12.6	0.05	82-100
Monosodium phosphate	-	22.5	-	100
Dicalcium phosphate (DCP)	21	18.5	0.14	85-92
Defluorinated rock phosphate	32	18	0.16	85-95
Tricalcium phosphate	38.7	20	-	72-90
Soft rock phosphate	17	9	1.2	50-65
Phosphoric acid	-	31.6	-	100

A Trace Mineral Mix

Element	mg/kg diet	Salt	mg/kg diet
Zinc	80	ZnO	99.7
Manganese	60	$Mn\,SO_4$	164.7
Copper	5	$CuSO_4 \cdot 5H_2O$	19.69
Iodine	0.5	KIO_3	0.84
Selenium	0.1	$Na_2SeO_3 \cdot 5H_2O$	0.33
Iron	20.0	$FeSO_4$	20.0

A Vitamin Supplement for General Use

	Units/kg diet
Vitamin A, IU	6000
" D₃, IU	1500
" E, IU	10
" K, mg	2
" B₁₂, mg	0.01
Choline chloride, mg	1000
Folacin, mg	0.5
Niacin, mg	30
Pantothenic acid, mg	15
Pyridoxine, mg	2
Thiamin, mg	2
Riboflavin, mg	4
Antioxidant, mg	100

Selenium in poultry breeder nutrition

Selenium (Se) is shown to be an essential element for poultry and farm animal nutrition. Severe Se deficiency is related to the decreased production and reproduction performance of poultry. The importance of Se nutrition of poultry males is related to the high proportion of polyunsaturated fatty acids (PUFAs) in avian semen and its susceptibility to lipid peroxidation. It is generally accepted that the hatching process is an oxidative stress and improvement in antioxidant defences of the embryo can increase hatchability.

Antioxidant systems in the chicks: Maternal diet plays a role in determining the development of the antioxidant system in the chick during embryogenesis and in early postnatal development (Surai, 2002a). The antioxidant system of the newly hatched chick includes the fat-soluble antioxidants (vitamin E and carotenoids), water-soluble antioxidants (ascorbic acid and glutathione) as well as antioxidant enzymes (superoxide dismutase (SOD), GSH-Px and catalase) and selenium as a part of various selenoproteins (Surai, 2006).

Requirements of selenium: NRC (1994) requirements for Se are quite low, varying from 0.06 ppm (laying hen) up to 0.2 ppm (turkey, duck). However in commercial conditions, with their associated stresses, the Se requirement increases substantially. The natural form of selenium in plant-based feed ingredients consists of various seleno amino acids with selenomethionine (SeMet) being the major form. Generally speaking, there are two major Se sources for poultry, namely inorganic selenium (mainly sodium selenite (SS) or selenate) and organic selenium in the form of selenomethionine (SeMet; mainly as Se-Yeast or SeMet preparations). It seems likely that the level of SeMet in the yeast is the major determinant of its value as a Se source (Surai and Fisinin, 2014).

Research work and commercial applications clearly showed that organic Se is more efficiently transferred from the feed to the egg and further to the developing embryos providing an effective amount of Se for selenocysteine (SeCys) synthesis and formation of active selenoproteins. A range of selenoproteins (at least 25) participate in regulation of various functions of the body, including redox balance maintenance and antioxidant defences. An analysis of published research and commercial data indicates that 0.2-0.3 ppm of selenium in organic form would be the recommended level for supplementation in breeders (Surai, 2006).

Distribution in the egg contents: Vitamin E and carotenoids are transferred from feed into egg yolk and further to embryonic tissues. Se content of the egg also depends on its concentration in the hen's diet, and also on the form of dietary Se used, since organic Se is more efficiently deposited in the egg albumen and at higher supplementation (0.3 ppm) in the egg yolk. In general Se almost equally distributed between egg yolk (58%) and egg albumin (42%). Recently it has been shown that SeMet comprised 53-71% of total Se in the egg albumen and 12-19% in the egg yolk (Lipiec et al., 2010). SeMet is non-specifically incorporated into the egg proteins in place of methionine and its level would depend on the ratio SeMet/Met in the feed. Since SeMet is not synthesised by animals, only plant material or supplements could provide this amino-acid in the chicken diet. Therefore, one could expect that an inclusion of SeMet sources would affect mainly Se level in the albumen and to lesser extent in the egg yolk.

Maternal effects of selenium: It is generally accepted that the quality of newly hatched chicks depends on the egg composition. However, recent developments in the areas of maternal programming and gene expression, indicate that maternal affects can be seen further into the postnatal development of chicks, than previously thought. Taking into account an existence of specific selenoproteins (iodothyronine deiodinases) responsible for thyroid hormone metabolism (Surai, 2006) and effects of Se on gene expression, one can expect specific effects of maternal Se on progeny (Surai and Fisinin, 2014).

Nutritional Deficiencies and Imbalances

Deficiencies of nutrients, imbalances and interactions among nutrients are reflected in the performance of the birds. They also end up in disorders in bones, blood, muscles, nervous system and skin and feather abnormalities.

An attempt has been made to compile this information in a nutshell for the benefit of students in the diagnosis of nutritional problems.

Nutritional disorder/deficiency Symptoms observed	Causative nutrient
1. Reduced feed intake, general malnutrition.	Amino acid deficiencies and imbalances
2. Reduced growth, lack of vigour, general malnutrition	Amino acid, mineral or vitamin deficiencies or imbalances
3. Diarrhoea in chicks, ducks, poult, quail	A deficiency of niacin, riboflavin or biotin; excess of lactose, molasses, salt, galactomannans, beta glucan, overheated proteins.

Leg and Bone disorders

1. Soft, easily bent bones and beak	Rickets, a deficiency or imbalance of vitamin D, calcium and phosphorus.
2. Hock enlargement and bowing of the legs in poult, chick, goosling, duckling (gastrocnemius or tendon of Achilles rarely slips from its condyles)	Niacin or Zinc deficiency
3. Enlarged tibiotarsal joint	Niacin deficiency
4. Perosis or slipped tendon in chicks, poults.	A deficiency cheifly of manganese, choline, folacin, biotin, Vitamin B_{12} or Zinc.
5. Bowed legs in ducks	Niacin deficiency
6. Shortening and thickening of leg bones in chicks	Zinc or manganese deficiency
7. Curled toe paralysis in chicks (Toes curled inwards)	Riboflavin deficiency
8. Extreme leg weakness and hens show a characteristic posture described as "penguin-like squat'	Vitamin D_3 deficiency

Blood and Vascular disorders

1. Macrocytic, hyperchromic anaemia	Folacin deficiency
2. Microcytic, hypochromic anaemia	Iron or copper deficiency
3. Internal haemorrhages from aortic rupture	Deficiency of Vitamin K
4. Exudative diathesis (a severe oedema produced by a marked increase in capillary permeability) in chicks, poults	Vitamin E or selenium deficiency

5. Enlarged heart in chicks
    and poults — Copper deficiency

Muscle disorders

1. Cardiac or gizzard myopathy
    in poults — Vitamin E or selenium
    deficiency

2. Muscular dystrophy with white
    areas of degeneration in skeletal
    muscle in chicks, ducks, poults — Vitamin E or selenium
    deficiency

Nervous disorders

1. Convulsions with head retraction/
    head drawn over back or
    polyneuritis in chicks, pigeons
    and quail — Thiamin deficiency

2. Convulsions and hyperexcitability
    in chicks, poults, duckling — Vitamin B_6 deficiency

3. Encephalomalacia (an ataxia resulting
    from haemorrhages and oedema within
    the cerebellum), tetanic spasm with
    head retraction, prostration with
    legs outstretched. — Vitamin E deficiency

4. Hyperirritability in chicks, poults,
    quail, ducklings — Magnesium deficiency

5. Fright reaction and tetanic spasms
    in chicks — Chloride deficiency

6. Cervical paralysis, neck extended
    in poults, quail — Folacin deficiency

7. 'Curled-toe' paralysis, gross enlargement
    of sciatic and brachial nerves with
    degeneration of myelin in chicks. — Riboflavin deficinecy

8. Ataxia characterised by a star-gazing
    posture (similar to that observed with
    thiamin deficiency) in young chicks. — Manganese deficiency

9. Ataxia in the young growing chick due
    to elevation in the cerebrospinal fluid
    pressure upon the brainstem — Vitamin A deficiency

Skin lesions

1. Dermatitis, scabs and crust around eyes,
    beaks and on the upper surface of the
    feet in chicks, poults; Crusty scabs
    around vents. — Pantothenic acid deficiency

2. Dermatitis, Incrustation in bottom of
    feet (ulcerated foot pad dermatitis)
    haemorrhagic cracks and necrotic
    toes in chicks and poults — Biotin deficiency

3.	Scaliness on feet in chicks	Zinc or niacin deficiency
4.	Lesions around eyes; eyelids stuck together in chicks and poults (cheesy exudate from eyes); salivary and tear glands may cease to function.	Vitamin A deficiency
5.	Inflammation of mouth cavity and tongue in chicks	Niacin deficiency
6.	Tongue deformity in chicks	Leucine, isoleucine or phenylalanine deficiency

Feather abnormalities

1.	Feather growth uneven, abnormally long feathers, feathers not lying smoothly in chicks and poults	Protein, amino acid imbalances
2.	Frizzled and rough feathers in chicks and poults	Calcium, niacin, zinc, or pantothenic acid deficiency
3.	Depigmentation in turkeys	Selenium deficiency

Information on Feed Ingredients

(a) Chemical composition and nutritive value of common poultry feed ingredients are presented in Table 16.

Table 16 Chemical Composition and Nutritive Value of Common Poultry Feed Ingredients.

Ingredients	DM %	ME Kcal/kg	CP	CF	EE	Ca	P %	Lysine	Methionine
Yellow Maize	89	3340	9	2.2	3.8	0.02	0.28	0.22	0.18
White Jowar	89	3200	10	2.3	2.8	0.03	0.28	0.21	0.16
Bajra*	91	2850	11.5	3.5	4.3	0.06	0.33	0.43	0.23
Broken Rice	89	2900	8.5	10.6	1.9	0.08	0.39	0.24	0.16
Wheat	89	3000	10	2.4	1.8	0.05	0.31	0.30	0.16
Ragi	92	2800	9	3.8	1.2	0.25	0.36	0.3	0.18
Oil or Fat	-	8000	-	-	-	-	-	-	-
DORB	91	2200	13.5	14.0	0.6	0.07	1.50	0.6	0.25
Rice Polish	90	3300	12	8	15.1	0.08	1.30	0.50	0.22
Wheat Bran	90	1300	15.7	11	3	0.14	1.15	0.59	0.23
Molasses	74	2300	3.0	-	-	1.10	0.12	-	-
Sunflower Cake	93	1900	27	28	1.1	0.37	1.0	1.13	0.58
SBM	89	2300	45	6.6	0.8	0.29	0.65	2.7	0.65
GNC-SE	92	2400	42	13	1.0	0.2	0.63	1.6	0.45
GNC-Exp.	90	2600	40	13	7.3	0.16	0.56	1.5	0.42
Rapeseed Cake	92	2300	35	11	1.4	0.72	1.12	1.7	0.65
Fish Meal	91	2400	42	1.0	5.0	3.73	2.43	3.2	1.1
Meat Meal	92	2400	45	8.7	7.1	8.27	4.1	2.5	0.65

*Bajra ME has been reported as 2675 or 2758 Kcal/kg (NRC, 1994; Sharma *et al.*, 1979) because of tough fibrous coat.

(b) **Maximum level of inclusion of feed ingredients:** Each ingredient has its maximum level of inclusion (Table 17) in the diet to obtain optimum performance. This is dictated by the presence of antinutritional/toxic factor(s), cost of the ingredient, difficulty in feed formulation, proper storage and shelf life of the feed, its capacity to induce imbalance of nutrients and reduce the performance of birds.

(c) **Availability and cost of feed ingredients:** In formulating balanced feeds, cost of feed ingredient is also taken into consideration in addition to the nutrients present so that least cost balanced feeds can be formulated.

Table 17 Maximum Level of Inclusion of some Common Poultry Feed Ingredients.

Feed ingredient	%
Maize	60
Sorghum white	30-40
Sorghum dark	10-20
Bajra	30-60
Ragi	30-60
Wheat	20-30
Rice bran	10-20
Deoiled rice bran	10-20
Rice polish	10-30
Wheat bran	5-10
Tapioca meal	5-15
Molasses	0-5
Maize gluten feed/meal	0-10
Groundnut cake	10-30
Sunflower cake	10-20
Safflower cake	5-15
Mustard cake	0-5
Soybean meal	40
Cottonseed cake (Decorticated)	0-10
Coconut cake	5-10
Fish meal	5-10
Meat meal	5-10
Blood meal	3
Silkworm-pupae meal	2-3
Rice broken	10-20
Fats and oils	5
Cottonseed meal	10
Sesame seed/tilseed meal	10-15

Examples of rations for broilers and layers are presented in Table 18, 19 and 20.

Energy feedstuffs are divided into high energy and low energy ones. Maize, wheat, broken rice, sorghum, fat and oils are high energy feedstuffs. Soya lecithin is a very good source of energy (5600 kcal ME/kg diet). Pearl millet, finger millet and other small millets, rice polish/bran, DORB, wheat bran, molasses, tapioca flour are examples of low energy feeds. Protein supplements are divided into vegetable and animal protein supplements. Roasted full-fat soybean meal is a good source of protein and fat, especially for broilers. Maize gluten, rice gluten, dried distillery grain with soluble (DDGS) are very good sources of protein.

TABLE 18. Corn Soya Based Broiler Rations

Ingredients	Pre-starter	Starter	Finisher
Maize	50	50.2	54.4
Soybean meal	41	39	33.8
Animal fat	4.8	6.5	7.5
Calcite	1.5	1.5	1.55
DCP	1.75	1.8	1.8
Salt	0.4	0.4	0.4
Lysine	0.07	0.03	0
Methionine	0.15	0.16	0.14
Choline chloride	0.1	0.1	0.1
Coccidiostat	0.05	0.05	0.05
Trace minerals and vitamins	0.2	0.2	0.2
Antibiotic supplement	0.1	0.1	0.1
	100	100	100

TABLE 19. Examples of some Broiler Rations

Ingredients	Pre-starter	Starter	Finisher
Maize	34	34.5	38.8
Wheat	10	10	10
Rice polish	5	5	5
Soybean meal	23.5	21.2	16
GNC-SE	10	10	10
Sunflower cake	5	5	5
Animal fat	4.9	6.6	7.6
Fish meal	5	5	5

Calcite	1.1	1.2	1.2
DCP	0.6	0.6	0.65
Salt	0.2	0.2	0.2
Lysine	0.16	0.13	0.04
Methionine	0.14	0.15	0.12
Choline chloride	0.1	0.1	0.1
Coccidiostat	0.05	0.05	0.05
Trace minerals and vitamins	0.2	0.2	0.2
Antibiotic supplement	0.1	0.1	0.1
	100	100	100

TABLE 20. Examples of some Layer Rations

Ingredients	Chick	Grower	Layer Phase-I	Layer Phase-II
Maize	35	20	24.5	25
Jowar	0	0	22	0
Broken rice	10	0	0	10
Bajra	0	25.7	0	10
Rice polish	15	0	4	0
DORB	8	25'	15	15.4
Wheat bran	0	5	0	6
Sunflower cake	0	10	0	10
GNC-SE	7	0	10	0
Soybean meal	17.5	7	11.3	9
Fish meal	5	5	5	5
Calcite	1.4	1.6	7.4	9
DCP	0.3	0	0.15	0
Salt	0.2	0.2	0.2	0.2
Lysine	0.08	0	0	0
Methionine	0.07	0.04	0.05	0
Choline chloride	0.1	0.1	0.1	0.1
Coccidiostat	0.05	0.05	0.05	0.05
Trace minerals and vitamins	0.2	0.2	0.2	0.2
Antibiotic supplement	0.1	0.1	0.1	0.1
	100	100	100	100

Feed formulation methods

(1) **By using Pearson square method or algebraic method:** It is possible to formulate simple diet by hand. Limited number of feedstuffs and fewer nutrients (CP, ME, Ca, P, etc) are taken into consideration. It is tedious

to formulate even a simple diet because substituting one feedstuff for another feed changes all the nutrients in the diet.

(2). Computerized feed formulations: In formulating commercial least cost diets with more feedstuffs and more nutrients to take into consideration, we need to use computers.

Trial and error formulation and linear programming (LP) are commonly used with computers for formulating the rations. Maximizing the net profit is the objective of the linear programming. Many software programmes are available for farmers and feed manufacturers; for example, simple excel based feed formulations from Central Avian Research Institute, Izatnagar, (UP) and from Dr. D.Chandrasekaran, Veterinary College and Research Institute, Namakkal (TN).

Steps in Feed Formulation: Example: Broiler Starter Feed

A 100 kg of least cost feed is formulated to provide the nutrients as per the specifications.

1. Fixed minor ingredients and slack space, 8.5 kg.
   These include nutrient and nonnutrient feed additives, and natural feed ingredients that are added at a later stage to balance the diet.

2. Levels of animal protein sources, 10 kg

	CP	ME
These (Fish meal, 7 kg and meat meal,	2.94	168 Kcal
3 kg) are added to diets since they	1.35	72 Kcal
are richer sources of limiting	4.29	240

   amino acids (lysine and methionine + cystine).

3. The level of cereal byproducts may be fixed. Deoiled rice bran, 3.0 kg (0.41% CP), (66 Kcal ME)

4. Vegetable protein sources and energy sources are added to provide the required amount of protein.

Amount of protein contributed by 21.5 kg of ingredients (Animal Proteins (fish meal and meat meal), DORB and the slack space) is 4.7 kg. That is the remaining 78.5 kg of ingredients are to provide 22–4.7 = 17.30 kg.

Groundnut cake (expeller) and maize are considered as vegetable protein source and energy source. The required protein level can be calculated by algebraic equation or by Pearson's formula.

Algebraic equation: Total of ingredients = 78.5 kg

Protein = 17.3 kg

Let X represents the soybean meal (SBM) & groundnut cake and Y represents maize. The average protein content of SBM & groundnut meal is 42.5% and of maize is 9%.

$$X + Y \quad = \quad 78.5 \text{ kg - I}$$
$$0.425\ X + 0.09\ Y \quad = \quad 17.30 \text{ kg - II}$$
$$0.09\ X + 0.09\ Y \quad = \quad 7.07 \text{ Multiply Eqa. I with } 0.09$$

-- -- --

$$0.335\ X \quad = \quad 10.23$$

SBM & GNC, $X = \dfrac{10.23}{0.335} \quad = \quad 30.50 \text{ kg}$

Maize $\quad Y = 78.5 - 30.5 = 48.0 \text{ kg}$

Pearson's formula: Total of ingredients = 78.5 kg
Protein = 17.30 kg

Protein as percent $\quad = \dfrac{17.30 \times 100}{78.5} = 22.00$

Protein in maize, $\quad 9\%$ _____ 20.5 kg maize

22.0

Protein in GNC, $\quad 42.5\%$ _____ 13.0 kg GNC & SBM

33.5 kg

Now maize and groundnut cake are proportioned for 78.5 kg.

$$\text{Maize} = \dfrac{20.5 \times 78.5}{33.5} = 48.0 \text{ kg} \quad 1603.20 \text{ Kcal}$$

$$\text{GNC} = \dfrac{13.0 \times 78.5}{33.5} = 30.5 \text{ kg} \quad \dfrac{747.25 \text{ Kcal}}{2350.45 \text{ Kcal}}$$

5. Balancing the ME content of the diet: The ingredients so far included, contributed 2656.45 kcal and the short fall (3100–2656.45) 443.55 Kcal can be met by supplementation of 5.6 kg animal fat/vegetable oil.

6. Balancing the P content of the diet: Available P has to be considered. P content of DORB, maize and SBM & GNC is 0.364 and only 30% of it is available; P content from animal proteins and inorganic sources is considered completely available. Thus the available P content is 0.40%. But the requirement is 0.5%.

7. Balancing the Ca content: The calcium content of the diet is 0.71%. The remaining calcium content to meet the requirement can be met by supplementation of 1.4 kg limestone and 0.4 kg bone meal.

8. The sodium content usually is not calculated and 0.5% addition of common salt meets the requirement. However, when feed ingredients from animal sources (e.g. fish meal and meat meal in this example) are included, it is necessary to calculate the sodium content and accordingly salt need to be supplemented. Calculations revealed that 0.2% common salt supplementation is required.

9. Balancing the limiting amino acid in the diet: Animal protein supplements are rich sources for lysine and methionine. Among the vegetable protein sources, soybean meal is a rich source for lysine. Further, lysine and methionine are available in synthetic form.

    The diet that is formulated here provide 1.06% lysine and 0.35% methionine. The remaining has to be met through supplementation of synthetic amino acids.

10. Balancing the crude fibre content of the diet: The diet that is formulated contain 4.8% crude fibre.

Finally, the diet has to be checked for the totals of the ingredients and for all the nutrients to ensure that it is well balanced.

Instead of a single cereal a combination of cereals or other energy sources may be used to reduce the cost of the diet. Similarly, instead of single

Feed Ingredients	% level	CP %	ME Kcal/kg	Ca %	P %	Lys %	Meth %	CF %
Fish meal	7	2.94	168	0.26	0.170	0.224	0.077	0.007
Meat meal	3	1.35	72	0.248	0.123	0.075	0.020	0.261
DORB	3	0.41	66	0.002	0.014	0.018	0.008	0.420
Maize	48	4.32	1603.2	0.010	0.134	0.106	0.086	0.056
GNC(Exp)	15.25	6.1	396.5	0.024	0.085	0.229	0.064	1.983
SBM	15.25	6.86	350.75	0.044	0.099	0.412	0.099	1.007
Animal fat	5.6	-	448	-	-	-	-	-
Limestone	1.4	-	-	0.54	-	-	-	-
Bone meal	0.4	-	-	0.116	0.050	-	-	-
Salt	0.2	-	-	-	-	-	-	-
Lysine	0.15	-	-	-	-	0.143	-	-
Methionine	0.15	-	-	-	-	-	0.15	-
Trace mineral mixture	0.40	-	-	-	-	-	-	-
Vitamin mixture	0.2	-	-	-	-	-	-	-
Total	100	21.98	3104	1.21	0.45	1.21	0.50	4.80

Note: A standardised mineral mixture may be added at 1.5 to 2% instead of limestone, bone meal, salt and trace mineral mixture.

vegetable protein supplement a combination of protein supplements may be used. Sterilized meat and bone meal (MBM) is a useful alternative to fishmeal and it is a source of protein and phosphorus. MBM is a useful alternative to fishmeal and dicalcium phosphate. However, the use of MBM is banned in cattle feed in India and other countries in view of its involvement in causing bovine spongiform encephalopathy and other zoonotic diseases.

Vitamins A, D_3, E, K, B_2, and choline chloride are necessarily added. Toxin binder, antibiotic additive, growth promoter and preservative are also added.

Formulating a ration - Balanced layer chick feed: Algebraic method

Steps in feed formulation

1. Write down the BIS (2007) Specifications for chick feed

Moisture, %, Max	CP, %, Min	ME, kcal/kg, Min	CF, %, Max	AIA, %, Max	Ca, %, Min	AP, %, Min	Lysine, %, Min	Methionine, %, Max	Salt, %,

2. Write down the nutritive value of the following feeds

Ingredients	DM, %	CP, %	ME, kcal/kg	CF, %	Ca, %	P, %	Lysine, %	Methionine, %
Maize								
Soybean meal								
DORB								
Rice polish								
Fish meal								

3. Fix the slack space at 5 per cent level. Slack space is reserved for
   - To add cereal grains and/or oil to balance ME level
   - To add calcium and phosphorus mineral source to balance their level in the ration
   - To add synthetic amino acids-lysine and methionine to balance
   - To add trace mineral and vitamin mixtures
   - To add necessary feed additives

4. Fix the level of animal protein   :   Fish meal-   8.0%
5. Fix the levels of cereal byproducts   :   DORB-   8.0%
                                         Rice polish-   7.0%

6. Calculate the total of these ingredients added so far and find out their CP contribution.

1	Slack space	5.0	0.0
2	DORB	8.0	1.08
3	Rice polish	7.0	0.84
4	Fish meal	8.0	3.36
	TOTAL	**28**	**5.28**

7. Choose the energy sources (cereals) and vegetable protein (oil cakes) sources and balance the CP level using Pearson square or algebraic method.

   • Total of ingredients other than maize and soybean meal = 28.0
   • Balance from maize and soybean meal = 100 - 28.0 = 72.0
   • Total protein requirement = 20 %
   • Protein already supplied = 5.28%
   • Balance protein required = 14.72%

   Adjustment of CP using Algebraic method:

   Let us consider, X = maize and Y = soybean meal

$$X + Y = 72.0 \qquad \text{Equation 1}$$
$$0.09 X + 0.45 Y = 14.72 \qquad \text{Equation 2}$$

   Multiplying Equation 1 with CP content of protein source (0.45)

$$0.45 X + 0.45 Y = 32.40 \qquad \text{Equation 3}$$

   Subtracting equation 2 from equation 3

$$0.45 X + 0.45 Y = 32.40$$
$$0.09 X + 0.45 Y = 14.72$$
$$0.36 X + 0 = 17.68$$
$$X = 17.68/0.36 = 49.11.$$

8. Level of maize in the ration is 49.0% (rounded)

   $Y = 72 - 49 = 23.0$. Level of SBM in the ration is 23.0%

9. Balancing the ME content of the diet

10. Balancing the available phosphorus content (thirty % of plant phosphorus is considered available)

11. Balancing the calcium content

Balancing of ME, Calcium and available phosphorus:

Ingredient	Inclusion level	CP,%	ME, kcal/Kg	AP, %	Ca, %
Maize (3340 kcal ME/Kg; 9% CP)	49.0	4.41	1637	0.041	0.001
Soybean meal (2300, 45.0)	23.0	10.35	529	0.045	0.067
DORB (2200; 13.5)	8.0	1.08	176	0.036	0.006
Rice polish (3300, 12.0)	7.0	0.84	231	0.027	0.006
Fish meal (2400, 42.0)	8.0	3.36	192	0.298	0.298
		20.04	2765	0.45	0.39
Balancing of ME: Include additional 1% of Maize				met the	
Maize	**1.0**	0.09	**33**	require	
		20.13	2798	-ment	
Balancing of Calcium: Include 1.70% of calcite (Ca-36%)					
Calcite	**1.7**	-	-	-	0.61
					1.0

12. Balancing the limiting amino acid content: Lysine and methionine
13. Balancing the crude fibre content
14. Balancing the sodium content

Balancing amino acids, crude fibre and sodium levels

Ingredient	Inclusion level	Lysine, %	Methionine, %	CF, %	Na, %
Maize	49+1	0.11	0.09	1.1	0.01
SBM	23	0.621	0.15	1.52	0.002
DORB	8	0.048	0.02	1.12	0.003
Rice polish	7	0.035	0.015	0.56	0.003
Fish meal	8	0.256	0.088	0.088	0.12
Calcite	1.7	-	-	-	-
		1.07	**0.36**	**4.4**	**0.14**
		met the require -ment		Within the limit	
Balancing of Methionine: include at 0.05%					
Methionine	**0.05**		**0.41**		

15. Feed additives:

Feed additives	Inclusion level
Trace mineral mixture	0.20
Vitamin AB_2D_3K	0.05
B complex vitamins	0.05
Choline chloride	0.10
Probiotic	0.05
Enzyme	0.05
Toxin binder	0.05
Coccidiostat	0.05
Total	**0.60**

Note: If fish meal is not included in poultry ration, addition of salt at 0.4% is necessary.

(Slack space adjustment: Slack space reserved: 5.0 minus (additional maize-1.0+ calcite-1.7+methionine-0.05+ feed additives-0.60) =1.65. DORB can be added to make up the ration 100.)

16. Final ration:

Maize	49.0 +1 = 50.0
SBM	23.0
DORB	8.0 +1.65 = 9.65
Rice polish	7.0
Fish meal	8.0
Calcite	1.70
Methionine	0.05
Feed additives	0.60 (listed above)
	100.00

Importance of Feeding During Different Physiological Stages

Feed requires special consideration since it represents nearly 65-70% of the cost of production of meat and eggs. The feed conversion efficiency in a bird is taken as an indicator of feed quality. The cost of producing a dozen eggs or a kg of meat is the true criterion for evaluating a diet.

During embryonic development, only - half of the ME present in the egg is utilized. The remaining half is adequate to meet the requirement of the hatched chick for 60-72 hours. However, it is recommended that chicks should be provided their first feed as soon as possible without waiting for the absorption of yolk.

In ovo feeding for better growth and stronger leg bones

There is high correlation between body weights in first 6 days and at 6 to 7 weeks of age in commercial broilers. Hence, early nutrition may play a significant role in poultry production and profitability. In ovo feeding refers to feeding embryonated eggs through administration of nutrients directly into the egg content (yolk sac or albumin). In ovo supplementation of amino acids (Bhanja and Mandal, 2005) and other micronutrients also provides scope for early post-hatch anatomical and functional growth of digestive system, post-hatch body weight and immunity.

Recent studies have showed that between El7 (embryo of 17 days old) and hatch the yolk contains low P, Cu, Mn and Zn reserves and respectively their uptake by the embryo is low. As the skeletal system is dependent upon such minerals for its proper development, this may be a nutritional limitation which could hinder bone development in broilers. Experimental in ovo feeding enrichment of eggs with a solution of PO_4, organic Cu, Mn and Zn, and vitamins A, E and D on El7 showed that the chicks had increased bone mineralization. This may suggest that elevating the mineral content of the egg either by in ovo feeding or by elevated organic mineral levels in breeder flocks' diet may improve bone development and reduce leg problems in broilers.

In ovo injection of 20 to 30 mg of threonine into yolk-sac of embryo modulated post-hatch growth and breast meat yield in broilers at marketable age; increased villi height (Kadam et al., 2008).

Physical form of the Diet

Feed may be in the form of mash or pellet. Mash feeding is the most common system practised. Pelleting and crumbling will result in less feed wastage. Nutrients are uniformly distributed without segregation as is observed in mash type of feed. Crumbled feeds are ideal for chicks and broilers. Feed consumption is increased and better growth rate and feed efficiency are achieved. The mash feed for poultry should have a gritty feeling and it should not be either too fine or too coarse.

Birds are given a chance to select their own feed, when feed ingredients are made available separately. This type of feeding is called Free choice (cafeteria) system. It is believed that a hen can balance her ration if given the opportunity.

Feeding of the Growers

Nutrition of growers (8 to 20 weeks) is critical as it influences their age at sexual maturity, size of the pullet eggs and overall performance of the bird in the layer house. Sometimes, it is desired to delay the sexual maturity of growing pullets to obtain uniform sized eggs and to avoid management problems incidental to laying. This is achieved by altering the lighting programme in the grower house and restricting the feed intake.

Restricted Feeding

Restricted feeding of birds during the growing period (particularly in the age group of 12 to 20 weeks) means an actual reduction of nutrient intake below minimum requirement of birds. Feed intake is reduced either by limiting the feed offered to 85-90% of normal feed intake or by diluting the conventional feed with fibrous material of low nutrient density or following a skip-a-day feeding. In the skip-a-day feeding, feed is provided on the first day at 85-90% level of the two days ration; on the second day the birds are not given any feed and some whole grain may be spread on the litter. Feed restriction is recommended until 21 to 22 weeks of age or up to 5% egg production level, whichever comes first. It is reported that low-protein or low-lysine diets are able to produce slightly more delay in sexual maturity than quantitative feed restriction. Pullet birds on restricted feeding require 5 to 10 days longer to reach sexual maturity. There is a reduction in the number of small eggs laid at the commencement of production.

Restricted feeding is also practised in broiler breeder farm to check the weight gain of breeders, since excess weight of breeders affect fertility and egg production.

Feeding During Hot Weather

Requirement of maintenance energy decreases 2.5-3.0 kcal ME/day/°C at environmental temperature above 21°C (example white leghorn layers); more energy is required for dissipation of heat (by panting). Therefore, the absolute energy requirement may not be less during hot weather. When the environmental temperature raises, birds of all types and ages consume 1 to 1.5% less feed per each 1°C raise in temperature between 20 and 30°C and 5% less feed in the temperature range of 32-38°C (more importantly less calcium and less electrolyte intake). This essentially means the birds receive less protein, vitamins and minerals and this have a disastrous effect on the bird performance. It is desirable, therefore, to increase the density of nutrients of the ration to compensate for reduction in intake.

Birds eat to satisfy their requirements of energy. The amount of feed needed per unit of production (eggs or meat) can be reduced by increasing the fat level of the diet or by increasing the cereals or starch content of the diet. The birds would eat less of a high energy ration and vice versa. The other nutrients, as well have to be adjusted to higher level.

Supplemental fat (5%) improves feed intake by about 15%. Fat improves palatability, reduce heat increment, decrease feed passage in the gut and increases nutrient absorption. Fats with more saturated fatty acids are preferred in hot humid climates.

Low protein diets increase the tolerance of birds to elevated environmental temperature because the heat production associated with the utilization of protein is greater than of carbohydrates and fats.

Feed formulation based on ideal protein concept economises nitrogen use, improves welfare of birds and minimizes feed cost and soil water pollution. Low-protein diets with balanced amino acids are preferred to high-protein diets with imbalanced amino acids.

High environmental temperature reduces egg shell quality. Hence, increase the calcium intake from 4g to 5g per bird per day to maintain egg shell quality. Provide shell grit as free choice feeding. Further, ground calcium source of about 1mm size is also provided for retaining in gizzard to meet the calcium needs for shell formation during the night times.

Heat stress causes alkalosis due to reduced electrolyte intake (and panting). Heat stress causes high potassium excretion through urine. Increase potassium allowance from 0.3 to 0.5%, increase dietary allowances for electrolytes (Na, K and Cl) by 1.5% per 1°C above 20°C.

High temperature may destroy vitamins present in feed. High moisture, rancid fats, trace minerals and choline enhance destruction of vitamins. High temperature decreases synthesis of vitamin C, absorption of vitamin A, reduces the immunity, reduces conversion of vitamin D_3 to its metabolically active form.

Metabolic heat production is about 20-70% less in starved-birds compared to that in fed-birds. Because of this, regular practice of feeding the birds at 9 AM during summer aggravates the ill-effects of heat stress. Therefore, the ideal feeding times are the early and late hours of the day during the hot weather.

Effect of heat stress on nutritional metabolism and egg productivity

Experimental findings obtained in heat-stressed ducks are explained here to make the readers aware on the impact of heat stress on poultry. Ducks exposed to heat stress decreased the feed intake, egg production and egg weight (Xianyong Ma et al., 2014). Similar to chickens, ducks also activate the thermolytic strategies to prevent illness and death. They show more hyperventilation or panting and wing-flapping. These adjustments to hyperthermia increase muscle activity and energy expenditure and are accompanied by some reduction in feed intake, egg production and egg weight, number of large follicles and ovarian weight. See the tables 21 and 22 for data on feed composition and nutritive value and performance of ducks.

Table 21 Basal dietary composition and nutrient level for egg-laying ducks

Diet ingredients	%	Metabolic energy (MJ/kg)	14.03[1]
Maize meal (7.8%)	57.5	Crude protein (%)	19.63[1]
Soybean meal (43.5%)	25.5	Calcium (%)	3.3
Wheat bran (15.7%)	4.8	Total phosphorus (%)	0.65
Fish meal (50%)	1.5	Available phosphorus (%)	0.42
Dicalcium phosphate	1.5	Methionine (%)	0.47
Limestone	7.4	Lysine (%)	0.95
L-Lysine HCl (78.8%)	0.06	Met + Cys (%)	0.74
Premix[2]	1.0	Thr (%)	0.66
Salt	0.3	Trp (%)	0.20
DL-Met (98.5%)	0.21	Arg (%)	1.16
Limestone	0.32	He (%)	0.70
		Leu (%)	1.49
Total	100.00	Dietary electrolyte balance (nmol/kg)	176

[1]Actually measured value; [2]Supplied the following per kilogram of diet: vitamin A, 9000 IU; vitamin D_3, 2500 IU; foilc acid, 0.6 mg; vitamin E, 22 mg; vitamin K_3, 2 mg; vitamin B_1, 1 mg; vitamin B_2, 3mg; vitamin B_5, 2 mg; vitamin B_{12}, 0.1 mg; nicotinamide, 38 mg; biotin, 10 μg; manganese, 85 mg; zinc, 80 mg; iron, 30 mg; copper, 15 mg, the carrier is zeolite.

Table 22 Effect of high temperature on production performance of laying ducks

Variable	N[1]	Control	Heat stress	P-value[2]
Body weight (kg/duck)	60	1.21	1.18	0.084
Feed intake (g/pen/day[3])	30	140.14	123.48	0.039
Egg production (%[4])	30	87.54	81.16	0.045
Egg weight (g)	60	66.84	65.44	0.049
Feed/egg conversion ratio (g/g)	30	2.39	2.32	0.120
Energy content in eggs (MJ/g)	12	7.02	6.83	0.158
Protein content in eggs (%)	12	11.86	11.34	0.078

[1]Number of observations in each mean; [2]from ANOVA for P value; [3]calculated from per pen data for 28-days; [4]eggs per bird per day over 28-days; source (Xianyong Ma et al., 2014).

Respiratory alkalosis: Hyperventilation or panting in birds exposed to greater ambient temperature resulted in reduced HCO_3^- and partial pressures of CO_2 in blood, consequently respiratory alkalosis. Alkalosis reduces blood ionized Ca (the form utilized by the shell gland) and blood HCO_3^- also has an important role in $CaCO_3$ formation in the eggshell.

Carbonic anhydrase stimulates HCO_3^- generation in the shell gland and contributes to deposition of $CaCO_3$ in the shell. The other important ones in egg shell calcification are osteopontin (a component of the organic matrix of the chicken egg shell) and calcium binding protein.

The adverse effect of heat stress on eggshell quality has been well documented. Heat stress in ducks decreases eggshell strength and thickness, egg yolk colour and Haugh unit of eggs. Heat stress, further, decreases the expression of the carbonic anhydrase and calcium binding protein genes in the shell gland (Xianyong Ma et al., 2014). The decrease in quality of eggshell is related to increased respiratory alkalosis, reduced blood flow through the shell gland, reduced carbonic anhydrase in the shell gland and kidneys, and reduced calcium turnover. Reduction of feed intake is an important factor that leads to the deterioration of egg quality during heat stress.

Endocrine disturbance from the heat stress: As a signature element of the stress response, cortisol concentrations were more than doubled in the heat-exposed ducks while thyroxine decreased to about 75% that of the control ducks. There were striking decreases in the activities of glutamic-pyruvic transaminase and glutamic-oxaloacetic transaminase and there were increased activities of lactate dehydrogenase and alkaline phosphatase. These changes suggest that protein metabolism or turnover was affected by the heat stress, which was reflected in the reduced protein laid (see Table 22) in the ducks after 28-day of heat exposure (Xianyong Ma et al., 2014).

Antioxidant status: Lin et al. (2006) considered that oxidative stress is part of the stress response of broiler chickens to heat exposure and Whitehead and Keller (2003) found diminished antioxidant status in heat deprived chickens. Heat-exposed ducks showed decreased antioxidant capacity.

Liver tissue is one of the most sensitive organs synthesizing HSP 70 in response to hyperthermia and does so in a temperature-dependent fashion. It has been described in a variety of species that up-regulation of the HSP 70 gene enhances resistance to heat and other stresses. The expression of HSP 70 gene in the liver was noticeably increased in heat-stressed ducks (Xianyong Ma et al., 2014). Enhanced expression of the HSP 70 gene in the liver of the heat-stressed ducks suggests a protective role.

It may be concluded that heat stress decreased the productivity of the ducks, which was related to a reduced feed intake, protein synthesis, endocrine dysfunction, low antioxidant capacity, and derangement of calcium and phosphorus balance. A strategy for promoting feed consumption or nutrient availability may partially overcome (the reduced feed intake due to heat stress) the unfavourable influence of heat stress on productivity because the decreased ovarian and oviductal weights might be pivotal in the reduction of egg production.

Voluntary Feed Intake

Voluntary feed intake is the amount of feed that a bird consumes when it has unlimited access to a diet. Voluntary feed intake of birds reflect the quality of feed, health of the flock and management of the farm. If a flock consumes less than the predicted level of intake it tells that feed quality is poor and has nutritional deficiencies; it can be a useful warning of errors in management or indicative of an outbreak of disease.

The mechanisms controlling appetite are complex-overall control of feed intake is influenced by the hypothalamus in the base of the brain, but the pathways that transmit instructions are still incompletely understood. Current hypotheses assume that the hypothalamus responds to physical and chemical changes in the circulating fluids of the body.

1. *Thermostatic theory:* It has been suggested that the heat produced after food is consumed raises the temperature of blood and hypothalamus, so that the desire to eat is lessened. This theory would explain why birds eat less at high ambient temperatures and why feed with a low heat increment such as fats can cause obesity.

2. *Glucostatic theory:* This proposes that there are glucose receptors in the hypothalamus which are sensitive to the rate at which glucose is being utilised by them. Low utilisation rates lead to hunger sensation.

   The above theories can possibly explain short-term regulation of feed intake; long-term regulation is probably concerned with the prevention of excess fat deposition.

3. *Lipostatic theory:* According to this theory the hypothalamus is sensitive to concentrations of circulating metabolites mobilized from endogenous fat stores. Since the amount of fat mobilized is proportional to the size of fat deposits, a lipostatic mechanism keeping the fat content constant, could control body weight.

No one hypothesis alone describes adequately the observed feed intake behaviour. Therefore it is likely that multiple factors are responsible.

Factors that Influence Voluntary Intake

The most important factors that affect feed intake are the characteristics of the bird, quality of feed, and the environment.

Attributes of the bird: The characteristics of the bird that influence feed intake are body weight, rate of live weight gain, output of eggs. Heavy birds consume more feed than light birds. Birds that grow faster than the average normally consume more feed than the average. At a given weight, immature birds of broiler strains consume more feed than birds of an egg laying strain. The intake of dietary energy by laying hens is related to their rate of egg production. A 1% increase in egg production is associated with a 2% increase in feed intake. Laying birds have been shown to consume 20% more feed on egg forming days than days when eggs are not formed. Feed intake increases markedly when birds go through the hormonal change two weeks prior to the onset of egg production.

Dietary factors: An increase in dietary energy results in a decrease in intake. If the diet is deficient in one or more essential nutrients, appetite is depressed and this is associated with a decline in growth or reproductive performance. The intake of pelleted feed can be up to 8% greater than the intake of the same feed presented as a meal. This may be due to partly an effect of partial cooking of the feed.

Environment factors: Light intensity and day-length have some effect on voluntary feed intake. Longer days stimulate egg production and therefore encourage hens to consume more feed. In case of chicks, maximum feed intake and growth rate are obtained when they are reared in continuous light. With broilers too much light may increase activity and therefore reduce efficiency of feed utilization. Ambient temperature has a major effect on feed intake.

Calcium for growing pullets: Additional calcium may be given when 5 per cent of the pullets come to lay. By keeping the dietary calcium level low during the growing period, the efficiency of calcium utilization is kept high and this will help the birds to absorb more calcium on a high calcium diet at the onset of lay. Feeding high calcium diet just before the onset of laying help the birds to store calcium in the medullary bones which can be used for the subsequent eggshell formation.

Most of the calcium in the diet of growing bird is used for bone formation, whereas in the mature laying bird most dietary calcium is used for eggshell formation. An excess of dietary calcium interferes with the availability of other minerals, such as P, Mg, Mn and Zn. A ratio of approximately 2 calcium to 1 nonphytate P is appropriate for most poultry diets, except for layer birds where it is as high as 6:1.

Calcium for Layers

Layer rations should be adequate in calcium and the recommended level of inclusion is 3.0%-3.5%. A part of the dietary calcium may be fed as oyster shell or limestone chips for better shell quality. The requirement for calcium is more in the afternoon since this is the time of the day that the egg would be in the shell gland. The feeding of limestone or oyster shell on a continuous free choice basis is not recommended by some researchers. Since the birds' capacity to retain calcium is limited, there is nothing to be gained by feeding high levels of calcium in a ration or feeding large quantities of oyster shell or limestone at free choice.

Check the following if any eggshell problem (shellless eggs or thin shelled eggs) is noticed in the layer farm.

1. Check the calcium content of the diet.
2. Check the layer shed temperature - Higher than normal temperature reduce the shell thickness.
3. Check vitamin D_3 level - a deficiency causes thin and rough shell with reduced egg production.
4. Check the health status - respiratory diseases may affect shell quality.
5. Check the age of the birds - shell quality declines during the end of the production cycle.

Retention of calcium during the first 40 weeks is about 55% and decreases thereafter with age. Thus, requirement of calcium increases with age. Heavy birds consume more feed, hence dietary concentration of calcium should be less.

Calcium for eggshell formation: It has been shown to retain only about 50% of the ingested calcium in hens receiving 3.5 to 4% calcium in all mash layer diet. So a hen taking in 3.6 g of calcium per day retains about 1.8 g of calcium during the approximately 18 hr time when feed is available. Thus the hen retains about 100 mg of calcium per hour.

Since average egg contains about 2.0 to 2.2 g of calcium, the hen receiving her total calcium from an all mash ration must withdraw approximately 0.2 to 0.4 g of calcium from her bones during the night when the egg is still being calcified but no calcium is available from the feed. Eggshell quality may be improved by supplying the hen with dietary calcium 24 hours per day. The dietary supply of calcium is met in the form of calcium carbonate in the all mash ration and the remaining in the form of oyster shell (large particles) at free choice. Absorbing calcium at the rate of 100 mg per hour for 24 hours, the hen should be able to retain 2.4 g of calcium, slightly more than the 2.0 to 2.2 g needed to make a good eggshell. Hence free choice calcium source is advocated.

High producing hens may hold the egg in the uterus for a much shorter time than hens laying at lower rates. Oyster shell or calcite grit is needed much more in diets for high producing hens than for those which retain the egg in the shell gland over a longer period of time.

A level of 4% oyster shell together with 3.5% pulverized limestone (total dietary calcium of about 3.5%) should insure maximum calcium absorption throughout 24 hrs each day. Shell grit dissolves slowly in the acidic medium of the proventriculus and ventriculus so that a continuous supply of calcium is provided to the intestine.

Shell grit feeding

In deep litter layers, shell grit is made available as free choice feed by filling it in few feeders during the period of peak egg production (25-45 weeks). The calcium deficiency is commonly seen in caged layers (cage layer fatigue) due to reduced activity within the cage. Many hens show spontaneous recovery if removed from the cages and allowed to walk normally on the floor. This indicates that a lack of exercise may be a partial cause. Cage layer fatigue is more prevalent in single-hen cages than in multiple-hen cages. When two or more hens are caged together, they get more exercise because of competition for feed and water. A high incidence of cage layer fatigue can be prevented by ensuring the normal weight-for-age of pullets at sexual maturity and by giving pullets a high calcium diet (minimum 3.5 % Ca) for at least 7 days prior to first oviposition.

About 2.5 g calcium per day is needed for normal metabolic process in laying chicken. To ensure this, a layer ration should contain minimum of 3.5 % calcium; so that by consuming 115-120 g feed, the bird will get 4.0 to 4.2 g calcium, out of which about 2.5 g will be available to the birds. Diets must provide adequate quantities of calcium and phosphorus to prevent deficiencies. Adding calcium to young birds by top-dressing the feed with 10 kg of oyster shell or limestone in per 1000 layers will often help the condition. In older hens, calcium deficiency is less likely than phosphorus or vitamin D_3 deficiencies, so top-dress feed with equivalent level of dicalcium phosphate.

Diet and Egg Size

Egg size is largely dependent upon the level of dietary protein and level of linoleic acid. Higher intake of balanced protein produce larger eggs. So feeding higher levels of proteins at the onset of production will help to increase egg size more rapidly. A level of 1% linoleic acid in the diet is considered adequate for maximum egg size.

Phase Feeding During Laying Phase

Egg type layers are maintained even up to 80 weeks of age. The production cycle of layers may be divided into 3 phases. It is reported that the requirement of protein and amino acids are reduced particularly in phase 3. It is known that the requirement of calcium increases while that of phosphorus decreases with each succeeding phase.

Phase (Age)	Egg production	Egg weight	Body weight
Phase I (up to 36 weeks age)	Rises and reaches the maximum	Gradually increases	Gradually increases
Phase II (37 to 56 weeks age)	Production maintained	Gradually increases	Gradually increases
Phase III (from 57 weeks age)	Production declines	Gradually increases	Slightly increases

Feeding for Broiler Skin Colour and Egg Yolk Colour

The colour of yellow skin in chickens is due to a group of chemicals known as xanthophylls, substances closely related to the carotenoids. Carotenoid pigments impart yellow pigment to the fat deposits of chicken and to egg yolk. Not only are xanthophylls easily oxidized from natural feed ingredients but the fat and skin of the chicken also lose their yellow colour in this manner. To maintain yellow skin colour and yellow yolk colour, the birds are to regularly consume the xanthophylls.

There are many xanthophylls capable of imparting a yellow-orange colour-hydroxy carotenoid pigmenting compounds. Alfalfa leaf meal has lutein, yellow maize has cryptoxanthine, zeaxanthin. Similarly petals of a marigold species (*Tagetes erecta*) and algae (*Spongiococum excentricum*) are rich source of xanthophylls.

Xanthophylls differ in colour transmission. It takes about 3 weeks to produce the desired colour in a broiler. The older the broiler, the higher the percentage of xanthophylls transferred from the feed to the skin, but the oxidation of xanthophylls is also greater in older birds. Zeaxanthin is far superior in producing a darker pigment (than lutein). Approximate xanthophyll quantity necessary is 11 to 66 mg/kg feed.

Forced Moulting

Moulting is a normal process of chickens and other feathered species. It occurs in both sexes. Decrease in day length is normal trigger for moulting. Minor stresses such as temporary feed or water shortage and diseases, can also initiate a partial or premature moulting. Moulting supposedly gives a hen a period of rest during which she rejuvenates her bodily processes, preparing herself for the next laying cycle.

Forced moulting of flock is suggested whenever the egg production is less and egg prices are less.

Effect of Diet on Egg Hatchability

A marked deficiency of any one or more of the nutrients such as calcium, manganese, protein, vitamin A, vitamin D, riboflavin and choline in practical diets causes a reduction or even a cessation of egg production.

Low or reduced hatchability causes heavy loss to the poultry breeder. Hatchability is markedly influenced by the composition of diet. It is a much more sensitive indicator of the adequacy of a given diet than is the egg production. Dietary factors that affect the hatchability of eggs are the quantity and quality of protein, the amounts of several essential minerals and vitamins. It is necessary that a fertile egg contains all the nutrients in the requisite amounts for successful development of the embryo as the avian embryos have (unlike mammalian foetuses) no other source for nutrients. Nutrition of the breeding hen determines to a large extent the hatchability of fertile eggs.

* Higher energy intake (in the breeding hen) is reported to cause a slight increase in the yolk weight. If other nutrient concentration is not increased, a general or specific deficiency may develop and affect the hatchability.

* Marginal deficiency of protein causes a reduction in the egg size though the amino acid composition of egg protein remains unaltered. Diets should contain 12 to 15% protein to obtain optimum hatchability. Excess dietary protein increases the requirement of birds for vitamin A, biotin, vitamin B_{12} and Ca and thereby influences the hatchability of eggs.

* The essential fatty acid linoleic acid is essential in the diet of breeder hens for the normal hatchability of eggs.

* Vitamins A, D, E and K, riboflavin, thiamin, pantothenic acid, nicotinic acid, pyridoxine, folic acid, biotin and vitamin B_{12} are essential in the diet of breeding hen. Vitamin content of the diet is reflected upon their concentration in the eggs. All these vitamins influence the hatchability of eggs and viability of the hatched chickens.

* Riboflavin deficiency results in poor hatchability and is reflected in clubbed down embryos. Biotin deficiency is reflected in parrot beaks (crooked beaks) in embryo. Pantothenic acid deficiency shows unhatched embroys suffering from subcutaneons haemorrhages. Thiamin deficiency may result in early embryo mortality. High incidence of embryonic deformities and death occurs in eggs produced by hens fed a folic acid-deficient diet. This is preventable by folic acid injection into the eggs prior to incubation and by feeding of folic acid rich diets. Similarly vitamin A, vitamin E, vitamin B_{12} are needed in proper amounts to avoid early embryo mortality around 2,1 to 3 and 8 to 14 days, respectively.

* Mineral elements are essential for the development of embryo. Hence deficiency of the minerals like Ca, P, Mn, Zn, Mg, Fe, Cu, I, Md and Se causes embryonic mortality and abnormalities. Similarly excess of Ca, P, Se, etc. are also undesirable and depress hatchability.

* Manganese deficiency in the diet of the breeding hen causes a condition in embryonic chicks known as nutritional chondrodystrophy. "Parrot" beak resulting from a disproportionate shortening of the lower mandible is also seen. This deficiency causes mortality of the embryo around 18 to 21 days. In case of deficiency of zinc, absence of legs and wings are noticed in the embryo and feather down may appear "tufted".

Importance of Vitamin E in Poultry Feeding

Commercial broilers are subjected to stress and this stress decreases lymphocyte numbers and increases the susceptibility to viral diseases.

Reactive oxygen metabolites are produced endogenously by normal metabolic processes. Exogenous contributors to oxidative stress include dietary imbalances, disease and environmental pollutants.

The mechanism of action of vitamin E involves (1) a general antioxidant effect, preventing peroxidation and free radical damage to sensitive lymphoreticular cells, (2) a specific antioxidant effect in suppressing prostaglandin biosynthesis by inhibiting the oxidation of L-arachidonic acid, by affecting key enzymes of the oxidative phosphorylation (e.g. interfering with coenzyme Q and cytochrome biosynthesis), and by altering the receptor function of the cell membrane of lymphocytes.

It has been reported that broilers subjected to environmental and immune stress need higher vitamin E supplementation. Vitamin E levels of 100-300 IU/kg have been demonstrated to be effective against E. coli, Ranikhet, coccidiosis and a combination of bird density, litter quality, E. coli, coccidiosis and fat rancidity.

Cannibalism and Feather Picking

It occurs in flocks fed fibre-free diets. It is considered that chicken diets should contain 3-4% crude fibre. This problem is more likely with pelleted or crumbled diet. A methionine deficiency may lead to feather picking apart from limiting weight gain.

Fatty Liver and Kidney Syndrome (FLKS)

Diets dificient or marginal in biotin can lead to FLKS in young broilers. This condition is most commonly seen in 2-4 week old birds fed wheat-based diets (wheat contain little available biotin). Pyruvate carboxylase enzyme is biotin-dependent. Death is caused by hypoglycemia due to failure of hepatic gluconeogenesis which in turn is triggered by inadequate levels of pyruvate carboxylase. Stress is a major contributor to the severity of FLKS. Stress likely induces an epinephrine-induced catabolism of the already low glycogen reserves.

Fatty Liver Haemorrhagic Syndrome (FLHS)

It is a condition where there is increased accumulation of fat in the liver. It is a common occurrence in laying hens and breeders. Pullets carrying an excess of body fat are more prone for this condition. Causes are:

1. Low protein, high energy rations
2. Rations with amino acid imbalance or deficiency

3. Diets low in lipotropic factors such as choline, methionine and vitamin B_{12}
4. Certain moulds or mould toxins may also cause this condition
5. Liver haemorrhages occur in laying hens fed rapeseed meal that contains high levels of glucosinolates.

Solution: Increase the level of dietary protein by 1 to 2% or supplementation of 50 g of copper sulfate, 500 g of choline, 3 mg of vitamin B_{12}, 5000 IU of vitamin E and 500 g of DL–methionine per 1000 kg of feed may help.

Cage Layer Fatigue and Bone Breakage in Layers

High producing laying hens maintained in cages sometimes show paralysis around the time of peak egg production. The condition is caused by a fracture of the vertebrae that subsequently affects the spinal cord. The fracture is due to an impaired calcium flux related to the high output of calcium in the eggshell. Because of depletion of medullary bone reserves, the bird utilizes cortical bone as a source of calcium for the eggshell. The condition is rarely seen in deep litter system, suggesting that reduced activity/exercise is a predisposing factor.

A high incidence of cage layer fatigue (CLF) can be prevented by ensuring the normal weight-for-age of pullets at sexual maturity, and such pullets receive a high-calcium diet (minimum 3.5% Ca) at least 14 d prior to first oviposition. Older caged layers are also very susceptible to bone breakage, especially during their removal from the cage and during transport to processing. It is not known if CLF and bone breakage are related.

Tibial dyschondroplasia (TD)–Role of 1,25 [OH]$_2$D$_3$ and vitamin C

Tibial dyschondroplasia (TD) is a significant cause of lameness and economic loss in young, fast-growing broiler chickens. The actual lesion, an avascular, cartilaginous mass, is seen in the growth plate of the tibiotarsus. Microscopic examination of the growth plate from a normal chick reveals that it consists of layers of chondrocytes, surrounded by collagenous extracellular matrix. Proximally, the cells are arranged in ordered columns, but the arrangement becomes more random further down the growth plate. The top-most layer of the growth plate consists of small, disc-shaped proliferating chondrocytes. Next layer, the cells develop into a thin, 3-4 cell thick layer of pre-hypertrophic chondrocytes, which are more larger and more spherical. Finally, the cells fully differentiate to form hypertrophic chondrocytes and the processes which result in mineralization of matrix can commence.

Microscopic examination of the growth plate of a chick affected by TD reveals an accumulation of cells at the pre-hypertrophic stage, which is indicative of a failure of the differentiation process.

It has been reported that vitamin C and vitamin D reduce the incidence of tibial dyschondroplasia. 1, 25-dihydroxycholecalciferol (1, 25[OH]$_2$D$_3$) is the metabolically active form of cholecalciferol (vitamin D$_3$). It is synthesized by the animals and birds in two stages in the liver and kidney and the synthesis is closely regulated with several feedback loops. 1, 25[OH]$_2$D$_3$ acts to increase plasma calcium by increasing absorption of dietary calcium via synthesis of a specific duodenal calcium binding protein. It also reduces calcium excretion by the kidneys and stimulates osteoclastic bone resorption. It has also been shown to have a role in cell differentiation. Low dietary calcium and thus hypocalcaemia trigger the release of parathyroid hormone, which in turn produce the metabolically active form of vitamin D$_3$, under normal conditions, to have normal blood calcium. Putting 1, 25[OH]$_2$D$_3$ in the feed seems to override the control mechanisms, resulting in increased absorption of dietary calcium.

A potential role exists for ascorbic acid in reducing the incidence of tibial dyschondroplasia. Ascorbic acid is a cofactor for metalloenzymes such as the cytochromes and lysyl oxidase and proplyl oxidase, the latter two being important in collagen synthesis.

Ascites

Metabolic diseases such as ascites in broiler chickens result in significant economic losses to the poultry industry. The syndrome is multifactorial and mainly caused by exogenous (e.g.environmental factors) and/or endogenous factors (e.g.faster growth rates, reactive oxygen species). Ascites syndrome or pulmonary hypertension syndrome is also known as pulmonary arterial hypertension syndrome. Ascites can be attributed to imbalances between cardiac output and the anatomical capacity of the pulmonary vasculature to accommodate ever-increasing rates of blood flow.

Watery Whites

"Watery" whites (albumen) generally suggest that the eggs were not cooled properly or became overheated before gathering from the shed. Old and stored eggs may have "watery" whites. It is possible to have a strain of bird which lays a very high percentage of eggs with firm whites by breeding. The watery white contains the same amount of water and protein as the thick white. The difference lies in the colloidal structure of the water protein micelle. Albumen quality is important in preparation of egg products such as egg albumen powder, egg yolk powder, etc.

Dietary Fatty Acids and Body Fat

The composition of body fats can be influenced by dietary fatty acids in monogastrics and birds (see page no. 393). Cottonseed oil, rapeseed oil and fish oils can impart undesirable colour/flavour to meat and eggs.

Cottonseed oil has two cyclopropenoid fatty acids (sterculic acid and malvalic acid) which are incorporated into the yolk membrane. On storage, the yolk membrane becomes permeable to albumen. This causes a salmon colouration of the yolk. Some iron also diffuses out of the yolk to give pink albumen. Cyclopropeniods increases the deposition of stearic acid and palmitic acid in fat depots as the desaturase enzymes are inhibited. The amount of stearic acid also increases in egg yolks and, on refrigeration, yolks become rubbery-like balls. Residual gossypol may also be present in some oils and can give an olive colour to the yolks.

Off flavour in eggs from birds that ate flaxseed is due to trimethyl amine. Rapeseed oil and mustard oil may contain from 20 to 40% erucic acid which causes an accumulation of fats in the heart muscle of rats, monkeys and ducks. Rapeseed (*Brassica napus*), Crambe (*Crambe abyssinica*) belong to crucifera family. These high erucic acid oilseed plants have glucosinolates. Refer Chapter 19 of *Principles of Animal Nutrition and Feed Technology* for more information.

Fish oils present in poultry diets tend to impart a fishy flavour to meat and eggs because they are rich in polyunsaturated fatty acids.

Salt Poisoning

Water containing 1.5% NaCl is toxic for laying hens, but a lower level of 0.1% salt may delay the onset of egg production. The safe upper limit for salts in drinking water is less than 3000 ppm. The measurement of the concentration of all constituents dissolved in water is referred to as "total dissolved solids" (TDS). Water containing 1000 ppm TDS is good for poultry.

Salt in the drinking water is much more toxic than in the feed. Turkeys and ducks are more susceptible to salt poisoning than chickens. As per the BIS specifications a maximum level of 0.6% salt in the diet is optimum. Depending on the salt content of feed ingredients (e.g. fish meal), the level of added salt is adjusted. The symptoms of salt poisoning are watery droppings, inability to stand, increased water intake, muscular weakness, convulsions and death. Severe congestion and haemorrhages are observed upon postmortem in the alimentary canal, liver, lungs, kidneys and muscles.

Essentiality of use of NCFR in animal feeding

There is a stiff competition for food between humans and animals. Only 2% of rice and wheat, 5% of sorghum, 10% of barley and maize and 50% of bajra and ragi are diverted to livestock and poultry feeding. There is great demand for animal products as animal products support physical and intellectual development of young people and pregnant mothers. Hence more animal products (milk, meat and eggs) are to be produced economically.

The use of NCFR has become essential in animal feeding due to limited availability of conventional feed ingredients to minimize the competition of animals with human beings. Now more and more NCFR are finding place in today's compound animal feeds. Because of this, the prices of compound feeds never directly or proportionally increase when the prices of conventional raw materials go up.

Non-starch polysaccharides (NSP): However, these NCFR (sunflower meal, rapeseed meal, copra meal, palm kernel meal, etc) have higher concentrations of NSP such as β-mannans (mainly glucomannans and galactomannans) and arbinoxylans, which depress the utilization of metabolizable energy in monogastric animals. Soluble NSP (Table 23) are non-digestible. They increase viscosity of digesta and reduce digestion of nutrients. Hence they are called anti-nutrients. High levels of NSP may reduce the absorption of glucose and decrease the production of glucose dependent insulinotrophic polypeptide and insulin (Nunes and Malmlof, 1992). It is possible that this problem can be reduced by supplementation of diets with exogenous enzymes. These include mannanase, xylanase, amylase, proteinase, phytase.

Table 23 Non-starch polysaccharide (NSP) content of feeds

| Groups | Feeds | Non-starch polysaccharide, % | | | NSP, % | |
		Soluble	Insoluble	Total	Neutral	Acidic
Cereal and millets	Maize	1.83	3.23	5.06	4.64	0.42
	Sorghum	1.53	2.51	4.04	3.59	0.45
	Peral millet	2.67	6.32	9.00	8.51	0.48
Vegetable protein supplements	Groundnut meal, expeller	3.67	12.24	15.91	13.60	2.31
	Sunflower meal	3.67	18.31	21.98	17.63	4.34
	Soybean meal	2.22	14.15	16.37	14.31	2.05
Cereal byproducts	Deoiled rice bran	3.40	27.39	30.79	28.49	2.31
	Rice polish	2.54	17.98	20.52	19.12	1.39

Source: R.P.Senthilkumar and V.Balakrishnan (2013) IJAN, 30, 2, 221-223; enzymatic colorimetric method of Englyst and Hudson (1987)

Table 24 Composition (% DM) of the NSP in maize grain and soybean meal

NSP component	Maize	Soybean meal
Arabinose	1.9	2.0
Xylose	2.4	1.8
Mannose	0.2	0.6
Galactose	0.4	2.9
Glucose	2.6	6.7
Uronic acid	0.6	2.5
Total NSP	8.1	17.2

Level of Uncoventional Feeds

Level of inclusion of certain unconventional feeds in poultry diets and antinutrients present in feedstuffs are given in Table 25 and Table 26, respectively.

Table 25 Level of inclusion of certain Less commonly used feeds and Unconventional feeds in poultry Diets*

S. No	Feedstuff	Chicks and Broilers	Growers and Layers	Reasons
1	Ambadi cake	10	20	High in fibre
2	Cane molasses	2	5	Higher levels cause wet litter
3	Cottonseed meal	10	10	Iron supplementation is required to bind gossypol
4	Deoiled mango seed kernel meal	3	5	Contains tannins
5	Deoiled salseed meal	3	6	Contains tannins
6	Dried poultry manure	0	5	Problem of pathogens
7	Feather meal	2	2	Low in lysine, methionine and tryptophan; poorly digestible
8	Fish meal	10	10	Poor quality, pathogenic microbial contamination
9	Guar meal	3	5	Proper heat treatment is required
10	Hatchery byproduct meal	2	3	Rancidity; Pathogenic microbial contamination
11	Karanja cake	5	10	Contains karanjine; only solvent extracted cake should be used
12	Linseed meal	3	5	Linatin, linamarine and indigestible mucilage
13	Maize gluten meal	10	20	Prone to contamination with mycotoxins

14	Maize gluten feed	10	20	High in fibre and prone to mycotoxin contamination
15	Meat meal; meat and bone meal	5	5	Pathogenic microbial contamination
16	Niger cake	5	10	High in fibre
17	Palm kernel meal	10	20	High in fibre
18	Peanut /Groundnut leaf meal	3	5	As a source of carotenes
19	Poultry byproduct meal	5	5	Pathogenic microbial contamination; low in methionine
20	Poultry offal meal	3	3	Pathogenic microbial contamination; low in methionine, low in digestibility
21	Rapeseed /Mustard seed meal	3	5	Due to presence of erucic acid, tannins and glucosinolates
22	Rubber seed meal	5	10	May contain HCN; not suitable for breeders
23	Safflower seed meal	5	10	High in fibre
24	Sesame seed / til seed meal	10	15	High in phytates and oxalates
25	Silkworm pupae meal	2	3	Low in threonine
26	Subabul leaf meal	5	10	Contains mimosine
27	Sunflower meal	10	20	High in fibre
28	Squilla meal	5	5	Low in lysine, methionine, threonine, tryptophan and arginine
29	Tapioca tuber meal	20	30	Contains HCN

*Source: Handbook of Poultry Nutrition by V.R.REDDY and D.T. Bhosale 2004, IBD Co (Publishing Division), Lucknow, India.

Table 26 Important anti-nutrients present in feedstuffs*

S. No	Feedstuff	Anti-nutrient substances
1	Soybean seeds	Protease inhibitors (trypsin inhibitors), haemagglutinins, saponins, estrogens, lipoxygenase (antivitamin A), antivitamin D, non-starch polysaccharides
2	Castor bean meal	Ricin, Haemagglutinins (lectins)
3	Lucerne leaf meal	Saponins, tannins,
4	Cassava (tapioca)	Cyanogenetic glycoside
5	Linseed meal	Cyanogenetic glycoside, linatine (antivitamin E)
6	Rape seeds and mustard seeds	Glucosinolates , tannins, erucic acid

7	Cottonseed meal	Gossypol
8	Sorghum	Tannins
9	Sal seed meal	Tannins
10	Mango seed kernel	Tannins
11	Tamarind seed meal	Tannins
12	All plant feedstuffs	Phytates
13	Subabul (*Leucaena leucocephala*)	Mimosine
14	Neem seed meal	Nimbidins (nimbine, nimbinin and nimbidine)
15	Kidney bean	Haemagglutinins (lectins), antivitamin E
16	Sweet clover	Dicumarol (antivitamin K)
17	Wheat	Arabinoxylans (non-starch polysaccharides)
18	Barley, oats	(1-3,1-4)- β-glucans (non-starch polysaccharides)
19	Guar meal	Trysin inhibitor and gum

*Source: Handbook of Poultry Nutrition by V.R. REDDY and D.T. Bhosale 2004, IBD Co (Publishing Division), Lucknow, India.

Improved Native Chickens

Small-scale backyard poultry production has remained an important source of food and income for a majority of rural poor families. Based on the research findings at Project Directorate on Poultry, Hyderabad the requirements of Vanaraja (Table 27) and Gramapriya (Table 28) are furnished in the latest ICAR requirements (ICAR, 2013).

Table 27 Nutrient requirements (as fed basis) of Vanaraja (egg and meat type) breeders*

Nutrients	Chicks (0-6 wk)	Growers (7-16 wk)	Pre-breeder (17-23 wk)	Breeder (>23 wk)	Male breeders (>23 wk)
ME (kcal/kg)	2800	2700	2700	2700	2750
Crude protein (%)	21	18	16.5	16	14
Calcium (%)	1.1	1.0	1.5	3.0	0.8
Available phosphorus (%)	0.45	0.45	0.38	0.30	0.30
Lysine (%)	1.10	0.85	0.80	0.75	0.68
Methionine (%)	0.46	0.40	0.36	0.35	0.33
Arginine (%)	1.11	0.85	0.87	0.91	0.83
Tryptophan (%)	0.20	0.16	0.1.5	0.16	0.14
Threonine (%)	0.70	0.61	0.52 '	0.52	0.48
Vitamin A (IU/kg)	15,000	22,500	18,000	15,000	10,000
Vitamin D_3 (IU/kg)	4,000	6,000	4,800	4,000	2,000

Vitamin E (IU/kg)	100	150	120	100	200
Vitamin K (mg/kg)	4	6	4.8	4	4
Pyridoxine (mg/kg)	6	9	7.2	6	6
Thiamin (mg/kg)	4.4	6.6	5.28	4.4	4.4
Riboflavin (mg/kg)	20	30	24	20	20
Pantothenic acid (mg/kg)	30	45	36	30	30
Niacin (mg/kg)	66	99	79.2	66	66
Choline (mg/kg)	1,200	1,800	1,440	1,200	1,500
Folic acid (mg/kg)	4	6	4.8	4	4
Biotin (mg/kg)	0.25	0.375	0.3	0.25	0.25
Vitamin B_{12} (mg/kg)	0.03	0.045	0.036	0.03	0.03
Manganese (mg/kg)	100	150	120	100	120
Zinc (mg/kg)	100	150	120	100	100
Iron (mg/kg)	80	120	96	80	80
Copper (mg/kg)	20	30	24	20	20
Iodine (mg/kg)	2.5	3.75	3	2.5	2.5
Selenium (mg/kg)	0.25	0.375	0.3	0.25	0.35

* Source: ICAR (2013)

Table 28 Nutrient requirements of Gramapriya (as fed basis) breeders at different ages*

Nutrients	Chicks (1-6 wk)	Growers (7-16 wk)	Pre-breeder (17-23 wk)	Breeder (>23 wk)	Males (>23 wk)
ME (kcal/kg)	2800	2700	2700	2700	2750
Crude protein (%)	21	18	16.5	16	14
Calcium (%)	1.1	1.0	1.5	3.0	0.8
Available phosphorus (%)	0.45	0.45	0.38	0.30	0.30
Lysine (%)	1.10	0.85	0.80	0.75	0.68
Methionine (%)	0.46	0.40	0.36	0.35	0.33
Arginine (%)	1.11	0.85	0.87	0.91	0.83
Tryptophan (%)	0.20	0.16	0.15	0.16	0.14
Threonine (%)	0.70	0.61	0.52	0.52	0.48
Vitamin A (IU/kg)	15,000	22,500	18,000	15,000	10,000
Vitamin D_3 (IU/kg)	4,000	6,000	4,800	4,000	2,000
Vitamin E (IU/kg)	100	150	120	100	200
Vitamin K (mg/kg)	4	6	4.8	4	4
Pyridoxine (mg/kg)	6	9	7.2	6	6
Thiamin (mg/kg)	4.4	6.6	5.28	4.4	4.4

Riboflavin (mg/kg)	20	30	24	20	20
Pantothenic acid (mg/kg)	30	45	36	30	30
Niacin (mg/kg)	66	99	79.2	66	66
Choline (mg/kg)	1,200	1,800	1,440	1,200	1,500
Folic acid (mg/kg)	4	6	4.8	4	4
Biotin (mg/kg)	0.25	0.375	0.3	0.25	0.25
Vitamin B_{12} (mg/kg)	0.03	0.045	0.036	0.03	0.03
Manganese (mg/kg)	100	150	120	100	120
Zinc (mg/kg)	100	150	120	100	100
Iron (mg/kg)	80	120	96	80	80
Copper (mg/kg)	20	30	24	20	20
Iodine (mg/kg)	2.5	3.75	3	2.5	2.5
Selenium (mg/kg)	0.25	0.375	0.3	0.25	0.35

* **Source:** ICAR (2013)

FEEDING OF DUCKS

General Information on Production Traits

Ducks occupy an important position next to chicken farming in India. Feeding of ducks in rural India is mostly done under range system. Duck keepers move from village to village with their flocks. Ducks mostly feed on grains, insects, forage, etc. that are available in different fields after harvesting the crop. They also get fish, etc. from the local streams, canals. Farmers may hire the duck keeper to keep the ducks on their farm lands in order to get the manure during the nights. Eggs are collected the next day morning.

Khaki Campbells are noted for their egg production potential and yield 250-300 eggs per year. Khaki Campbell duck originated by crossing a Malaysian Indian Runner female with a Rouen male. A strain of Khaki Campbell ducks developed in Holland produced between 335 and 340 eggs per duck per 365 days, an average for several years from a flock size of 50,000 ducks. The egg size was 73.4 g. This indicates their potential.

In China Peking Duck is a famous food and the roasted ducks have been the most relished dish of Emperors and high officials in Peking since 1368 AD. They were taken to New York in 1873 after one hundred and twenty four day voyage and there became Pekin Ducks. Of several breeds of meaty ducks, the Pekin duck has been by far the most popular meat duck in the world. White Pekin ducks are broiler type. They attain a body weight of 3.3

Table 29 Approximate Body Weights and Feed Consumption of White Pekin Ducks to 8 Weeks of Age.

Age (Weeks)	BW (kg)		Weekly Feed consumption (kg)		Cumulative Feed consumption (kg)	
	Male	Female	Male	Female	Male	Female
0	0.06	0.06	-	-	-	-
1	0.27	0.27	0.22	0.22	0.22	0.22
2	0.78	0.74	0.77	0.73	0.99	0.95
3	1.38	1.28	1.12	1.11	2.11	2.05
4	1.96	1.82	1.28	1.28	3.40	3.33
5	2.49	2.30	1.48	1.43	4.87	4.76
6	2.96	2.73	1.63	1.59	6.50	6.35
7	3.34	3.06	1.68	1.63	8.18	7.98
8	3.61	3.29	1.68	1.63	9.86	9.61

kg to 3.6 kg by 8 weeks of age and cumulative feed consumption is about 10 kg (9.6 to 9.9 kg) (Table 29). Central Duck Breeding Farm (CDBF), Hessarghatta, Bangalore imported Vigova-Super M broiler ducks from Vietnam. Vigova would weigh 3 kg at 49 days of age.

Digestive System and Feeding Habit

Ducks do not have a crop and their proventriculus is cylindrical. The absence of a crop is probably responsible for the faster rate of passage of ingesta in ducks than in broilers.

Ducks are voracious eaters and foragers too. Apart from compound feeds, snails, fingerlings, earthworms, and insects, vegetation also form a part of their diet when reared in ponds which reduce the feed cost. Ducks have difficulty in swallowing dry mash. When fed dry mash, they will take mouthful and swill it down at the nearest water source, thus wasting a great amount of nutrients in the water. This kind of feeding behaviour is related to the structure of the bill.

The structures of the duck's bill which allow efficient straining of submerged food materials as well as the consumption of the most dry food particles of appropriate size, are not well designed for the consumption of mixed feeds in the dry mash form. Most mashes form a sticky paste when mixed with saliva and adhere to the papillae and other structures bordering the outer margin of the tongue and upper and lower bill. This caking interferes with the movement of the food mass to the tongue where it is normally rotated and coated with saliva and then propelled back to the esophagus for swallowing. This interference results in a reduction in feed intake and an increase in feed wastage which occurs when the duck attempts to shake or wash off the mash adhering to its mouthparts.

Pellet feeding has become popular and is practiced in all the commercial farms of the developed countries because of wastage and labour intensive nature of wet mash feeding. Ducks prefer pellets to mash when given a choice. The acceptable pellet size for a newly hatched pekin duckling is 3.97 mm pellet diameter. During the first two weeks for starter duck rations, the pellet diameter is 3.18 mm to 3.97 mm with length not more than 8 mm. Excessively long pellets are also difficult for the duckling to swallow. After about two weeks of age, Pekin duckling can consume pellets of 4.76 mm in diameter and about 13 mm in length without difficulty.

Nutrient Requirement of White Pekin Ducks

NRC (1994) gave two-feed programme (Table 30). A diet containing 22% protein for the period of 0 to 2 weeks and a 16% protein diet for the period from 2 to 7 weeks. These requirement data are presented on the basis of 90% dietary DM, which approximates most feeding conditions. Nutritional requirements of ducks differ considerably from those of chickens, and ducks are less affected by dietary bulk than chickens; hence some lower cost feed ingredients can be used at fairly high levels in duck feeds. It was reported that the ME_n values of several feedstuffs were very similar for ducks and broiler chickens.

The studies carried out by different workers in India at College of Veterinary Science, Hyderabad and NRC (1994) have been utilized for finalizing the requirements of ducks [ICAR, (2013); Table 31]. Ducks are comparatively sensitive to deficiency of vitamin E and selenium. Niacin requirement of 45 mg/kg diet has to be ensured to prevent leg weakness in ducks. Choline supplementation improves growth of ducklings.

Aflatoxin poisoning in ducks: Ducks are very much susceptible to aflatoxin while guinea fowls and chickens are the most tolerant. Ducks can tolerate only to the extent of 0.03 ppm as against 0.2 ppm in case of chickens. Muller *et al.* (1970) fed graded levels of aflatoxin to a variety of birds and found that the order of toxicity ranged from greatest for ducklings through turkey poults, goslings, pheasants to the lowest level of toxicity in chicks. Fernando *et al.* (1977, 1984) reported that aflatoxin B_1 is more toxic to ducks than is aflatoxin M_1. Aflatoxin metabolism is 90 times faster in the duck liver than in rat liver. A number of studies have indicated

Table 30 Nutrient Requirements of White Pekin Ducks as Percentages or Units per kg of Diet (90% DM) (NRC, 1994).

Nutrient	Unit	0 to 2 weeks 2900	2 to 7 weeks 3000	Breeding ducks 2900
		←———————— Kcal ME/kg diet ————————→		
Protein and amino acids				
Protein	%	22	16	15
Arginine	%	1.1	1.0	
Isoleucine	%	0.63	0.46	0.38
Leucine	%	1.26	0.91	0.76
Lysine	%	0.90	0.65	0.60
Methionine	%	0.4	0.3	0.27
Methionine + Cystine	%	0.7	0.55	0.50
Tryptophan	%	0.23	0.17	0.14
Valine	%	0.78	0.56	0.47
Macro-minerals				
Calcium	%	0.65	0.60	2.75
Chloride	%	0.12	0.12	0.12
Nonphytate P	%	0.40	0.30	
Sodium	%	0.15	0.15	0.15
Magnesium	mg	500	500	500
Trace minerals				
Manganese	mg	50	-	-
Selenium	mg	0.20	-	-
Zinc	mg	60	-	-
Water soluble vitamins				
Niacin	mg	55	55	55
Pantothenic acid	mg	11	11	11
Pyridoxine	mg	2.5	2.5	3.0
Riboflavin	mg	4	4	4

Dash marks indicate that no estimates are available.
In such cases, requirements of broiler chickens may be seen as a guide.

that the reason for the exceptional toxicity of aflatoxin B_1 for ducks is that this species contain a very high level of enzyme in the liver to convert aflatoxin B_1 to 'aflatoxicol' ($B_2 \rightarrow B_1 \rightarrow$ aflatoxicol).

Even though aflatoxin cause serious damage to both growing ducklings and laying ducks, no aflatoxins have been found to be carried over into eggs; nor have they been shown to cause any testicular damage in drakes. Hafez *et al.* (1979) could find no aflatoxins in eggs of ducks fed 8.1 mg of aflatoxin B_1 per kg of diet over a 3 week period. The hens soon stopped laying and showed follicular atresia of the ovaries (Look for more information on aflatoxin production and control in Chapter 17 of *Principles of Animal*

Table 31 Nutrient requirements (as fed basis) of Ducks*

Nutrients	Starter	Grower	Rearer	Layer
Age, weeks	0-8	8-16	16-20	>20
Crude protein (%)	20.5	. 16.5	15	16.5
ME (kcal/kg)	2,800	2,650	2,500	2,650
Linoleic acid (%)	1.0	1.0	0.8	1.0
Lysine (%)	1.0	0.75	0.60	0.75
Methionine (%)	0.45	0.35	0.30	0.3
Methionine + Cysteine (%)	0.85	0.65	0.60	0.75
Calcium (%)	1	1	1	3
Available phosphorus (%)	0.42	0.35	0.35	0.35
Manganese (mg/kg)	60	50	40	50
Sodium (%)	0.17	0.15	0.15	0.17
Chlorine (%)	0.12	0.12	0.12	0.12
Vitamin A (IU/kg)	3,200	2,250	2,250	4,000
Vitamin D3 (IU/kg)	400	350	350	650
Vitamin E (IU/kg)	20	20	15	20
Vitamin K (mg/kg)	2.5	2	2	2.5
Riboflavin (mg/kg)	5	4	4	6
Niacin (mg/kg)	60	55	50	50
Pantothenic acid (mg/kg)	10	8	8	12
Pyridoxin (mg/kg)	3	2.5	2.5	3
Choline (mg/kg)	1,000	750	500	750
Biotin (mg/kg)	0.10	0.10	0.10	0.10
Folic acid (mg/kg)	0.60	0.40	0.40	0.60

* Source: ICAR (2013)

Nutrition and Feed Technology).

Accumulation of Methylmercury

In a few instances, mercury has been known to contaminate lakes or ponds via spills from factories. Methylmercury is produced in large part by microorganisms in the bottom of lakes and ponds where natural deposits of mercury compounds are found in the soil of the lake bed. These microorganisms methylate the inorganic mercury, thus producing a fat-soluble form of mercury that can be taken up by the algae or other plant life in the lake. Small fishes consume the algae while larger fishes and diving ducks consume the small fishes, thereby accumulating methylmercury in their fatty tissues particularly in the liver. Dabbling ducks may also accumulate methylmercury from the water plants that they consume.

Nutrient Requirements for Japanese Quail

Japanese quails reach adult body weight in about 5-6 weeks and start laying eggs for the next 12 to 18 months. Japanese quails are prolific breeders and have the ability to produce four generations in a year. Their meat and eggs contain less fat and cholesterol and thus are more healthy. Hence Quails are becoming popular as an alternate meat bird to the broiler chicken. Since feed consumption is low, broiler quails require high levels of protein and critical amino acids in the diet. The egg weight of egg line quails is about 10 g. Quails require more choline than chickens. Work on nutrient requirements had been done at Central Avian Research Institute (CARI), Izatnagar. ICAR (2013) requirements are furnished in Table 32.

Body Weight, Feed Consumption and Feed Efficiency of Japanese Quail*

Age, weeks	Body weight, (g)		Av. feed consumption g/bird/day	Cumulative feed efficiency
	Male	Female		
0	7.4	7.4	-	-
1	22.8	23.4	3	1.33
2	46.3	48.0	8	1.93
3	73.3	77.4	11	2.26
4	90.5	100.6	15	2.93
5	111.9	122.3	17	3.44
6	124.5	151.7	21	4.01
Adult (10-12 weeks)	139.8	170.6	23.8	3.00

* *Source:* Page No. 58 of Feeding of Poultry by B. Panda, V.R. Reddy, V.R. Sadagopan and A.K. Shrivastav. ICAR, 1984.

Table 32 Nutrient requirements (as fed basis) of Japanese quails (ICAR, 2013)

Nutrients	Growing		Breeder/layer (5-30 wk)	
	0-3 wk	3-5 wk	Meat line	Egg line
ME (kcal/kg)	2,900 o	2,950	2,950	2,850
Crude protein (%)	25.0	21.5	20.0	18.6
Lysine (%)	1.45	1.20	1.10	1.00
Methionine (%)	0.55	0.50	0.45	0.40
Methionine + Cysteine (%)	0.90	0.80	0.80	0.70
Arginine (%)	1.80	1.50	1.25	1.15
Threonine (%)	1.12	0.92	0.80	0.70
Linoleic acid (%)	1.00	1.00	1.00	0.90
Calcium (%)	0.85	0.85	3.00	3.00
Available phosphorus (%)	0.45	0.35	0.35	0.32

Sodium (%)	0.15	0.15 o	0.15	0.14
Copper (mg/kg)	5.0	5.0	5.0	4.5
Iron (mg/kg)	80	60	60	55
Manganese (mg/kg)	50	60	60	54
Zinc (mg/kg)	60	50	50	45
Vitamin A (IU/kg)	2,500	2,500	3,300	2,970
Vitamin D3 (ICU)	400	400	900	810
Vitamin E (IU)	10	10	25	22.5
Thiamin (mg/kg)	2.0	2.0	2.0	1.8
Riboflavin (mg/kg)	4.0	4.0	4.0	3.6
Pyridoxine (mg/kg)	2.5	2.5	3.0	2.7
Vitamin B)2 (mg/kg)	0.003	0.003	0.003	0.003
Folic acid (mg/kg)	1.0	1.0	1.0	0.9
Niacin (mg/kg)	55	55	20	18
Pantothenic (mg/kg)	11.0	11.0	15	13.5
Choline (mg/kg)	2,000	1,500	1,500	1,350

Feeding of Turkey

Turkey birds are mainly reared for meat purpose in India since turkey provides excellent meat. Turkey birds are reared in Central Poultry Breeding Farm (CPBF), Hessarghatta near Bangalore. They are as efficient as chicken in the utilization of feed for growth. The breeds reared in CPBF are Broad Breasted Bronze turkey and Broad Breasted Large White turkey. The data on average body weight and feed efficiency as published by CPBF, Hessarghatta is presented hereunder.

Age, weeks	Average body weight, g
Day old	43
4th	568
8th	1615
12th	2989
16th	4137
20th	4787
24th	6175

Age, weeks	Feed consumption/bird kg	Feed/gain
0-4	0.606	1.067
0-8	2.600	1.610
0-12	6.114	2.046
0-16	11.123	2.689
0-20	16.350	3.416
0-24	22.291	3.610

Nutrient requirements of Turkeys are higher because of their faster growth. The protein requirement of poults is 28% during 0 to 4 weeks and the energy requirement for the corresponding period is 2800 Kcal ME_n per kg diet. The energy and protein requirement of turkey (20 to 24 weeks for males and 17 to 20 weeks for females) are 3300 Kcal ME_n/kg diet and 14% (NRC, 1994). Female birds grow at a slower rate than males. However, the feeding standards suggested are common for both female and male birds. Turkey's requirement particularly for vitamins A, D, B_{12}, niacin and choline is substantially higher than for chick.

Turkey birds have special requirements for lysine and methionine. Lysine has special role in feathering, as lysine-deficient Bronze poults show a characteristic white barring of the primary and secondary feathers of the wings. The requirement of protein can be brought down to 24% (ICAR, 2013; Table 33) during 0-4 weeks age with appropriate supplementation of lysine and methionine.

Table 33 Nutrient requirements (as fed basis) of Turkey (ICAR, 2013)

Nutrients	0-6 wk	6-12 wk	12-18 wk	18 wk pre-laying	Breeder
ME (kcal/kg)	2,800	2,800	2,650	2,600	2,650
Crude protein (%)	24.0	22.0	18.0	15.0	15.0
Arginine (%)	1.5	1.4	0.90	0.65	0.6
Lysine (%)	1.5	1.2	1.05	0.72	0.6
Methionine (%)	0.55	0.45	0.35	0.25	0.2
Threonine (%)	0.95	0.85	0.70	0.55	0.45
Linoleic acid (%)	1.0	1.0	0.80	0.8	1.10
Calcium (%)	1.2	1.0	0.80	0.6	2.25
Phosphorus (%)	0.55	0.5	0.38	0.3	0.35
Sodium (%)	0.17	0.15	0.12	0.12	0.12
Chloride (%)	0.15	0.14	0.13	0.12	0.12
Copper (mg/kg)	10.0	8.0	6.0	6.0	8.0
Iodine (mg/kg)	0.4	0.4	0.4	0.4	0.4
Iron (mg/kg)	80	60	55	50	80
Manganese (mg/kg)	60	60	60	60	60
Selenium (mg/kg)	0.2	0.2	0.2	0.2	0.2
Zinc (mg/kg)	70	65	40	22	65
Vitamin A (IU/kg)	5,000	5,000	5,000	5,000	5,000
D_3 (IU/kg)	1,100	1,100	1,100	1,100	1,100
E (IU/kg)	12	12	10	10	25
K (mg/kg)	1.75	1.5	0.85	0.625	1.0

Thiamin (mg/kg)	2.0	2.0	2.0	2.0	2.0
Riboflavin (mg/kg)	4.0	3.6	3.0	2.5	4.0
Pyridoxine (mg/kg)	4.5	4.5	3.5	3	4.0
Vitamin B_{12} (mg/kg)	0.003	0.003	0.003	0.003	0.003
Biotin (mg/kg)	0.25	.0.2	0.12	0.1	0.2
Folic acid (mg/kg)	1.0	1.0	0.8	0.7	1.0
Niacin (mg/kg)	60.0	60.0	45.0	40.0	40.0
Pantothenic acid (mg/kg)	10.0	9.0	9.0	9.0	16.0
Choline (mg)	1,600	1,400	1,050	875	1,000

Feeding of Geese

Geese are largely herbivorous. Geese are reared under three different systems: (i) the goslings are fed starter diets for 2 weeks in confinement and thereafter allowed for foraging; (ii) the goslings are fed limited amounts of feed throughout the growing period and allowed for foraging; (iii) the goslings are provided feed for *ad libitum* consumption in confinement. The energy and protein requirement of geese during 0 to 4 weeks is 2900 Kcal ME_n/ kg diet and 20% while the requirement of energy and protein after 4 weeks is 3000 Kcal and 15%. (NRC 1994). Please see appendix to find the rations for ducks, turkeys and Japanese quails P. 456.

Approximate Body Weights and Feed Consumption of Commercially Reared Male and Female Geese.*

Age, weeks	Av. BW, (kg)	Feed Consumption, (kg)	Cumulative Feed Consumption (kg)
0	0.11	0.00	0.00
2	0.82	0.96	0.96
4	2.05	2.93	3.89
6	3.05	3.20	7.09
8	4.05	4.34	11.43
10	4.85	4.68	16.11

* *Source:* Page no. 41 of Nutrient Requirements of Poultry, NRC publication, 1994.

Nutrient Requirements for Guinea Fowl

Guinea fowl meat is attractive in appearance, although darker than chicken. Their FCR for meat production at 12-14 weeks of age is 3.5:1. Live weight and dressed weights are 1400 and 1000 g, respectively (Table 34). Egg production starts at 18 weeks of age. They may lay as few as 60 eggs to as many as 200 eggs in a year with about 40 g in weight. Guinea fowl (pearl, lavender and white colour) is superior as free range bird. They are reared primarily for meat purpose. They are resistant to common diseases of chicken, are more tolerant to mycotoxins and have excellent foraging capabilities.

Table 34 Growth performance of Guinea fowl (0-18 weeks of age)*

Age in weeks	Body weight, g	Feed intake/ Bird,g	FCR
2	39	119	6.2
4	81	182	4.3
5	191	378	3.4
6	353	609	3.7
10	597	714	2.9
12	860	819	3.1
14	1063	959	4.7
16	1193	1120	8.6
18	1220	1204	44.5

* Day old chick weighs 20 g; average feed intake/bird during 18 weeks was 6.1 kg and FCR was 5.0; based on three year data. Source: B.K.Shingari, K.L.Sapra and R.K.Mehta (1994) Poultry International, July 1994, pp 54.

Guinea fowl are considered to be bad parents (jack is male and jenny is female). Therefore, the young or keets should not be brooded under the hens, rather they should be artificially brooded like commercial chicks. Guinea chicks or keets are not able to learn to feed and drink water quickly and many die of starvation. It has been found beneficial to place one or two day-old chickens in the flock so that keets follow them to feeders and drinkers and start to eat and drink as quick as possible.

ICAR (2013) provided the nutrient needs of guinea keets (Table 35 and 36) and guinea fowl (Table 37) based on the work carried out at CARI, Izatnagar (India).

Table 35 Recommended dietary density of nutrients in the diets of guinea keets for hot seasons in tropics (ICAR, 2013)

Nutrients	Starter (0-4 wk)	Grower (5-8 wk)	Finisher (9-12 wk)
Crude Protein (%)	22	20	18
ME (kcal/kg)	2,700	2,900	2,900
ME (kcal/g CP)	123	145	161
Lysine (%)	1.11	0.80	0.80
Methionine (%)	0.43	0.40	0.35
Cysteine (%)	0.28	0.25	0.22
Calcium (%)	1.00	0.90	0.80
Phosphorus (%)	0.65	0.60	0.55

Table 36 Recommended dietary density of nutrients in the diets of guinea keets for cold seasons in tropics (ICAR, 2013)

Nutrients	Starter (0-4 wk)	Grower (5-8 wk)	Finisher (9-12 wk)
Crude Protein (%)	24	20	18
ME (kcal/kg)	2,900	3,000	3,000
ME (kcal/g CP)	121	150	167
Lysine (%)	1.11	0.93	0.82
Methionine (%)	0.45	0.40	0.35
Cysteine (%)	0.28	0.25	0.22
Calcium (%)	1.00	0.90	0.80
Phosphorus (%)	0.65	0.60	0.55

Table 37 Recommended dietary concentration of nutrients in the diets of breeder guinea fowl (ICAR, 2013)

Nutrients	AMEn (kcal/k DM)		
	2,800	2,900	3,000
Crude Protein (%)	13-14	14-15	14-16
Lysine (%)	0.75	0.80	0.85
Methionine + Cysteine (%)	0.50	0.55	0.57
Calcium (%)	3.70	3.90	4.00
Phosphorus (%)	0.67	0.69	0.70

Nutrient Requirements for Emu

Emu is the second largest flightless bird in ratites group. Emu is popular for low fat red meat. The department of poultry science, CVSc, Hyderabad (Sri Venkateswara Veterinary University, Tirupati) has been doing pioneering research work on emu since the year 2000. ICAR (2013) requirements (Table 38) are based upon these reports.

Chicks weigh about 370 to 450 g while adults weigh 35 to 45 kg. Emus attain sexual maturity at 18 to 24 months and breeding occurs during winter season. Each adult female (after 3 years of age) lays on an average 30 eggs during a breeding season and the male sits on the brooding eggs for 52 days without feed and water. Emu has the ability to utilize dietary forage.

Table 38 Nutrient requirements (as fed basis) of Emus (ICAR, 2013)

	Starter (0-14 wk age / up to 10 kg body wt.)	Grower (15-34 wk age / 10-25 kg body wt.)	Finisher (35 wk age to slaughter/ 25-40 kg body wt.)	Breeder (4-5 wk before breeding)	Maintenance (non-breeding)
ME (kcal/kg)	2,700	2,600	2,600	2,600	2,400
Crude protein (%)	20	18	16	20	15
Lysine (%)	1.0	0.8	0.7	0.9	0.63
Methionine (%)	0.45	0.4	0.35	0.40	0.25
Methionine + Cysteine (%)	0.75	0.7	0.60	0.76	0.47
Tryptophan (%)	0.17	0.15	0.13	0.18	0.12
Threonine (%)	0.50	0.48	0.42	0.60	0.38
Calcium (%)	1.5	1.5	1.5	2.50	1.6
Available phosphorus (%)	0.55	0.5	0.40	0.4	0.4
Sodium chloride (%)	0.40	0.3	0.30	0.4	0.3
Crude fibre (max) (%)	9	10	10	10	10
Vitamin A (IU/kg)	15,000	8.800	8,800	15,000	8,800
Vitamin D3 (ICU/kg)	4,500	3,300	3.300	4,500	3,300
Vitamin E (IU/kg)	100	44	44	100	44
Vitamin B12 (mg/kg)	45	22	22	45	22
Choline (mg/kg)	2,200	2,200	2,200	2,200	2,200
Copper (mg/kg)	30	33-	33	30	33
Zinc (mg/kg)	110	110	110	110	110
Manganese (mg/kg)	150	154	154	150	154
Iodine (mg/kg)	1.1	1.1	1.1	1.1	1.1

Precision Feeding

One of the main objectives of raising poultry is to produce unadulterated wholesome food in the form of chicken meat and eggs to the consumers as a profitable enterprise with least contribution to climate change. Precision animal nutrition (PAN) is defined as providing the animal with the feed that precisely meet its nutritional requirements for optimum productive efficiency to produce better quality animal products and to contribute cleaner environment and thereby ensure profitability (Reddy and Krishna, 2009). Simply put, the provision of nutrients required for optimum production with no wastage is the precision feeding. The driving force behind PAN is economics and environment compatibility.

The tools to achieve PAN include more precise ration formulation based on nutritive value of each batch of ingredients, proper weighing and mixing of ingredients, improved ingredient and feed processing techniques, use of feed additives and implementing phase feeding.

Contribution of nutrients to the cost of feed

"All nutrients are essential, but no ingredient is indispensable". The cost of ingredients based on nutrient density (energy and protein) should get priority over mere cost of feed ingredients when formulating feeds. Herein an illustrated example (Table 39) is presented on the contribution of nutrients to the cost of feed (V.Ramasubba Reddy. 2014).

Use of feed additives

Feed additives play pivotal role in the present scenario of intensive production and in the competitive environment. Many feed additives offer flexible and cost-effective solutions. Their benefits include increased feed quality and palatability, improved nutrient availability, digestibility and animal performance, improved final product, economization of cost of animal protein and reduce environmental pollution associated with the poultry industry.

Feed additives may be nutritional additives and zootechnial additives. Nutritional additives provide nutrients to animals to achieve optimal growth e.g. amino acids. Zootechnical additives enable more effective use of nutrients in the feed e.g. enzymes. Higher levels of trace minerals such as copper, zinc, selenium and chromium are added since they enhance performance and immunity and reduce stress. Feed additives are generally used in concentrated forms.

Table 39 Approximate contribution of nutrients to the cost of feed

Sl. No.	Nutrient component	% cost	Remarks
A	Energy, protein and amino acids		
1	Energy	50	
2	Protein (amino acids)	40	
B	Minerals		
1	Phosphorus	2.6	
2	Calcium	0.1-0.6	0.1% in growing and 0.6% in layers
3	Sodium and chloride	0.2	
4	Potassium, magnesium and sulphur	—	Not supplemented in commercial diets
5	Trace minerals	0.6	Added in higher quantities than the requirement
C	Vitamins	1.0	Added in higher quantities than the requirement
D	Feed additives		

Source: Ramasubba Reddy, V. Precision Feeding - Poultry IN: Samanta, A.K., Bhatta, R., Sejian, V., Kolte, A.P.Malik, P., Sirohi, S.K. and Prasad, C.S. (2014). Invited Lectures: Climate Resilient Livestock Feeding Systems for Global Food Security. Global Animal Nutrition Conference, April 20-22, 2014, Bangalore, India, 286pp

Antibiotics are classified as feed antibiotics and therapeutic antibiotics to curb the use of therapeutic antibiotics at sub-therapeutic levels for animal production (since antibiotics favour proliferation of antibiotic resistant microorganisms, which have serious consequences for disease control in humans and animals).

One of the keys to maximizing the genetic potential of the birds is to maintain a healthy gut. **Eubiotics** are defined as non-antibiotic products maintaining the desired balance of the good bacteria and pathogens or eubiosis in the digestive tract. The products that maintain health and performance by modulating the gut flora are (1) direct-acting gut flora modulators (organic acids and essential oil components) reduces colonization of pathogens on the intestinal wall, (2) probiotics (3) prebiotics and (4) immune modulators (nucleotides and immunoglobulins).

The **probiotics** are not substitute of antibiotics in birds with serious infections, but are useful in restoring the normal bacterial population that was otherwise altered due to administration of antibiotics. Probiotics are active against a wider range of conditions when multiple-strain preparations are used.

The most striking feature of modern broilers is their maximum growth potential in the first week. Maximum growth is possible with dietary incorporation of functional ingredients such as nucleotides, glutamic acid, inositol, etc through enhancing nutrient utilization, growth, immunity and disease prevention.

The other additives include toxin binders and mould inhibitors, coccidiostats, acidifiers, antioxidants, appropriate non-therapeutic antibiotics.

Multiple benefits of feed additives by phytase superdosing with a high-efficacy single-enzyme xylanase

Enzymes are a group of feed additives that is used on a large scale, everywhere in the world. Their known effects include unlocking certain undigestible ingredients or breaking down long protein or sugar chains in raw materials. The substantial anti-nutrient effect of phytate is now becoming more widely recognized. The use of high phytase doses capable of degrading the vast majority of dietary phytate, known as superdosing (AB Vista designed the latest generation phytase, Quantum Blue), showed additional beneficial effects in terms of animal health, and is already been put into practice at some farms. Xylanase degrades the NSP arabinoxylan; arabinoxylan oligosaccharide is a degradation product. This has a prebiotic effect for poultry to prevent colonization of Salmonella in the gut. This is a 'hidden' beneficial effect of the enzyme xylanase.

Nowadays nutritionists are looking for more technically advanced feed additives that have proven benefits and are more focused on gut health and immunity enhancing effects. Further, it is also looked for additives that can enhance the end-product quality from the animal. When the target is phytate elimination, improving the availability of that phytate through the action of a well-targeted xylanase should be an advantage. When both the enzymes are optimized for efficacy, that advantage translates into a genuine performance gain.

Sodium metabisulphite addition to sorghum-based diets

Reducing agent sodium metabisulphite caused oxidative-reductive depolymerisation of starch polysaccharides in sorghum grain. Inclusion of reducing agent enhanced the apparent ME and N-corrected AME and feed conversion efficiency in broiler chickens (Selle et al., 2014).

Dimethylglycine and betaine

Sarcosine, dimethylglycine (DMG) and trimethylglycine (betaine) are N-methylated analogues of glycine. DMG is a more potent enhancer of emulsification than glycine, sarcosine and betaine. These are the intermediate metabolites in the choline pathway (Figure 3).

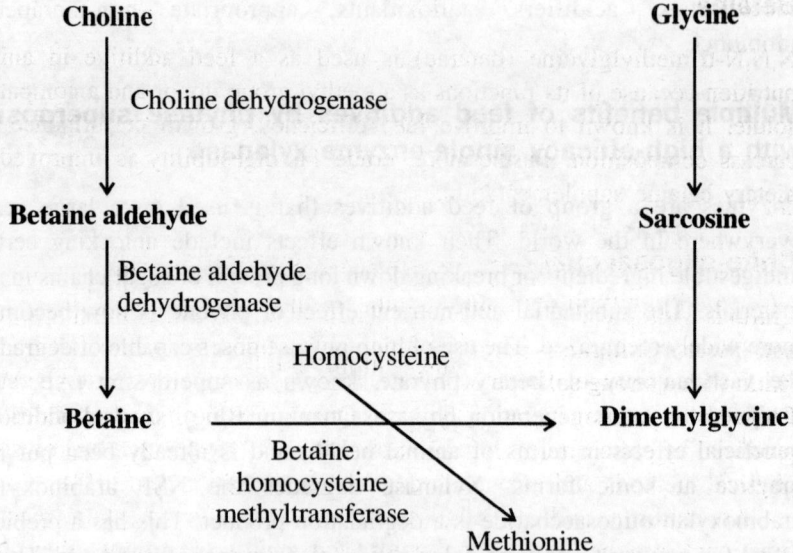

Figure 3   Overview of the choline pathway in which dimethylglycine (DMG) is an intermediate metabolite (Cools, A., et al., 2010. Animal 4:12, 2004-2011)

N,N-dimethylglycine (DMG) is a naturally occurring glycine derivative, which is useful as additive to broiler diets as it improves nutrient digestibility and reduces the development of broiler ascites syndrome.

Enhanced emulsification of dietary fat by use of additives with surfactant properties (N,N-dimethylglycine [DMG] and betaine) is suggested to facilitate liberation of non-fat nutrients from a fatty insulation, rendering them available for enzymatic digestion and absorption (Kalmar et al. 2011). Dietary DMG has also shown to improve carcass characteristics by decreasing fat deposition and increasing meat yield. DMG not only reduces feed costs, but also has potential environmental benefits because of improved protein utilisation, which has been demonstrated by reduced N excretion into urine (Kalmar et al., 2010).

It does not accumulate in edible parts of broiler chickens when supplemented at a dosage of 1 g Na DMG/kg and, therefore, does not pose a consumer risk of involuntary intake of DMG intended as a broiler feed additive (Kalmar et al., 2012). As methyl donation capacity and anti-oxidative action are both associated with increased insulin sensitivity, DMG can possibly influence insulin sensitivity; reduced blood lactate level and improved athletic performance in men, horses and dogs are also reported.

Betaine

N,N,N-trimethylglycine (betaine) is used as a feed additive in animal nutrition because of its functions as a methyl group donor and a compatible solute. It is known to improve feed efficiency, growth performance and carcass composition. Furthermore, crude fat digestibility is improved by dietary betaine supplementation.

Chito-oligosaccharides as feed supplements

Chitin is widespread in nature as component of exoskeleton of shrimps, crabs and insects. Chitosan is commercially manufactured from chitin by treating chitin with a strong solution of sodium hydroxide at an elevated temperature. Chitosan is a non-toxic polyglucosamine. Chito-oligosaccharides are produced by chitosan depolymerization using acid hydrolysis, hydrolysis by physical methods and enzymatic degradation (Lodhi et al., 2014).

As chitosan and its oligosaccharide derivatives contain reactive, functional groups like amino acids and hydroxyl groups, they have antimicrobial, anti-inflammatory, anti-oxidative, antitumor, immunostimulatory and hypocholesterolemic properties when fed as dietary additive for farm animals. Due to these properties, chitosan can be effective as a pro-health feed supplement for farm animals, as well as an alternative to feed antibiotics. The health promoting properties of chitosan are reflected in improved growth performance (body weight gain and/or feed conversion ratio) and digestibility of nutrients in young animals, that is, broiler chickens and weaned pigs (Swiatkiewicz et al., 2014).

Foot pad dermatitis (FPD)

Foot pad dermatitis (FPD) is a widespread problem in poultry production and constitutes a welfare issue, especially when exposed to higher litter moisture content. Foot pad becomes necrotic. Experimental results suggest that it is advisable to combine the Zn-methionine at 150mg/kg diet and biotin at 2000 ug/kg diet to improve the health of foot pads in chickens exposed to litter with critical moisture content of 35%.

9

Swine Nutrition

General Information on Growth Potential

Pigs are highly prolific among meat producing livestock, having a gestation period of 114 days. The pigs excel all other type of farm animals in the efficiency of converting feed into high quality pork. Feed alone accounts for 80% of cost of production. If adequately fed, a young pig (of breeds like Large White Yorkshire, Landrace, etc.) can reach 5 times its birth weight at the end of 3 weeks and 10 times its birth weight in 5 weeks. It is well acknowledged that LWY pigs are acclimatized to the tropical climatic conditions of India. However, the growth rates differ from that of their counterparts in their home tract. A growth rate of this magnitude requires a skillfully formulated feeding programme and good management. It has been reported that an average gain of 700 g per day from birth to slaughter is possible with the latest production systems, which means we can look for producing a 100 kg pig in 143 days of age.

Nutrient Requirements and Modeling for Pigs

Nutrient requirements are expressed for the monogastric animals like poultry and pigs as per cent of the diet or the amount per kg of the ration since they are generally fed in groups rather than individual feeding practised in case of cattle and buffaloes (where absolute requirements are given). The latest requirements available are NRC Nutrient requirements of swine, 2012 (11th revised edition); ICAR (2013), and BIS specifications for pig feeds, 1986. Similarly ARC requirements are also available. NRC requirements are on 90% DM basis and are for Large White Yorkshire, Landrace, Berkshire, etc. breeds (Tables 1 and 2), while BIS specifications are on 100% DM basis for indigenous and improved pigs and crossbred pigs, as well probably (Tables 3, 4 and 5).

Table 1 Nutrient Requirements of Swine Allowed Feed *Ad libitum* (90% DM) (Adapted from NRC 1988).

Intake and performance levels	Swine Live weight (kg)				
	1-5	5-10	10-20	20-50	50-110
Expected wt. gain g/day	200	250	450	700	820
Expected feed intake, g/day	250	460	950	1900	3110
Expected efficiency, feed/gain	1.25	1.84	2.11	2.71	3.79
Metabolizable energy, Kcal/kg	3220	3240	3250	3260	3275
Protein %	24	20	18	15	13
Indispensable amino acids (important only)					
Lysine %	1.40	1.15	0.95	0.75	0.60
Methionine + cystine %	0.68	0.58	0.48	0.41	0.34
Threonine %	0.80	0.68	0.56	0.48	0.40
Tryptophan %	0.20	0.17	0.14	0.12	0.10
Linoleic acid (%)	0.1	0.1	0.1	0.1	0.1

Requirement (% or amount/kg diet)[a]

Mineral elements					
Calcium %	0.90	0.80	0.70	0.60	0.50
Phosphorus, total %	0.70	0.65	0.60	0.50	0.40
Available P %	0.55	0.40	0.32	0.23	0.15
Iron, mg	100	100	80	60	40
Copper, mg	6	6	5	4	3
Manganese, mg	4	4	3	2	2
Zinc, mg	100	100	80	60	50
Selenium, mg	0.3	0.3	0.25	0.15	0.10
Vitamins					
Vitamin A, IU	2200	2200	1750	1300	1300
Vitamin D, IU	220	220	220	150	150
Vitamin E, IU	16	16	11	11	11
Vitamin K, mg	0.5	0.5	0.5	0.5	0.5
Niacin, available, mg	20	15	12.5	10	7
Pantothenic acid, mg	12	10	9	8	7
Riboflavin, mg	4	3.5	3	2.5	2
Vitamin B_{12}, µg	20	17.5	15	10	5

[a]The amino acids, minerals and vitamins requirements are based upon the types of ingredients.
  1 to 5 kg pigs, diet has 25 to 75% milk products
  5 to 10 kg pigs, diet has 5 to 25% milk products
  10 to 110 kg, a corn-soybean meal diet

NRC requirements are minimum standards without any safety allowances. Therefore, they should not be considered as recommendations. National Research Council reports provides updated advice on the energy and nutrient requirements of swine to help maintain an efficient, profitable, and environmentally conscious swine industry. The 11th revised edition of Nutrient Requirements of Swine (NRC, 2012) evaluates the most recent scientific literature to provide updated information, including a review of the value of corn and soybean-based byproducts from the biofuel industry as food for swine, and revised and revamped nutrient tables. The report also includes updated and expanded computer models to estimate energy, amino acid, calcium and phosphorus requirements for swine at different life stages.

NRC (2012) developed a computer model to calculate the requirements of nutrients and energy for growing-finishing pigs (gilts, barrows and intact males), gestating sows, and lactating sows. These computerized models take

Table 2 Nutrient Requirements of Breeding Swine (Adapted from NRC 1988).

Intake levels	Bred gilts, sows and adult boars	Lactating gilts and sows
DE, Kcal/kg diet	3,340	3,340
ME, Kcal/kg diet	3,210	3,210
CP %	12	13

Table 3 Requirements for Pig Feeds [IS 7472:1986 (Clause 3.3)]. reaffirmed in 2001

Sl. No.	Characteristic	Requirement		
		Pig Starter/ Creep Feed	Pig Growth Meal	Pig Finishing/ Breeding Meal
1.	Moisture content, percent by mass, Max	11.0	11.0	11.0
2.	Crude protein (N2 × 6.25), percent by mass, Min	20.0	18.0	16.0
3.	Crude fat or ether extract, percent by mass, Min	2.0	2.0	2.0
4.	Crude fibre, percent by mass, Max	5.0	6.0	8.0
5.	Total ash, percent by mass, Max	8.0	8.0	8.0
6.	Acid insoluble ash, percent by mass, Max	4.0	4.0	4.0
7.	Metabolizable energy (Kcal/kg), Min	3360	3170	3170

Note: The values specified for requirements (2) to (6) are on moisture free basis.

Table 4 Requirements for Pig Feeds to be Declared (Clause 3.4).

Sl. No.	Characteristic	Requirement		
		Pig Starter/ Creep Feed	Pig Growth Meal	Pig Finishing/ Breeding Meal
1.	Calcium (as Ca), percent by mass, Min	0.6	0.6	0.6
2.	Available phosphorus, percent by mass, Min	0.6	0.4	0.5
3.	Iron (as Fe), mg/kg, Min	100	90	80
4.	Copper, mg/kg, Min	8	6	6
5.	Manganese, mg/kg, Min	30	30	20
6.	Zinc, mg/kg, Min	50	50	50
7.	Common salt (as NaCl), percent by mass, Max	0.5	0.5	0.5

Note: The values specified for requirements (1) to (7) are on moisture free basis.

Table 5 Requirements for Pig Feeds (Clause 3.5).

Sl. No.	Characteristic	Requirement		
		Pig Starter/ Creep Feed	Pig Growth Meal	Pig Finishing/ Breeding Meal
1.	Niacin, mg/kg	17	14	10
2.	Pantothenic acid, mg/kg	11	10	10
3.	Riboflavin, mg/kg	3	2.4	2.2
4.	Vitamin B_{12} activity, µg/kg	15	11	11
5.	Vitamin A, IU/kg	1700	1300	1300
6.	Vitamin D, IU/kg	190	180	130

into account lean growth rate, gender, environmental temperature, pen space, energy density of the diet and other variables. Distinct models are used for growing pigs, gestating sows, lactating sows, etc. The model uses values for metabolizable energy, standardized ileal digestible (SID) amino acids, and standardized total tract digestibility (STTD) of phosphorus as the basis for all calculations.

Diets are most correctly formulated using values for SID of amino acids because values for SID amino acids in different feed ingredients are additive in mixed diets, which is not always the case for apparent ileal digestibility. Values for SID of amino acids are determined by correcting values for apparent ileal digestibility of amino acids for basal endogenous losses. However, the basal endogenous losses of amino acids are relatively variable among the experiments. Hence. SID of amino acids are calculated by using the equation of Stein et al. (2007). Feed composition tables in NRC (2012), therefore, contain values for the SID of amino acids, and requirements are also expressed as SID amino acids.

Total tract digestibility versus ileal digestibility

For lipids, values of total tract digestibility are influenced by microbial synthesis of lipids, and it is. therefore, more accurate to use values for ileal digestibility. Total ileal endogenous losses of lipids are used to determine the true ileal digestibility of lipids. It is recommended (NRC, 2012) that where values for lipid digestibility are used, true ileal digestibility values should be determined.

In case of carbohydrates, the apparent ileal digestibility is used to determine digestibility of monosaccharides, disaccharides, and starch, because monosaccharides are absorbed only in the small intestine. However, for oligosaccharides and non-starch polysaccharides, fermentation takes place in the large intestine, and therefore, values for apparent total tract digestibility of these nutrients are calculated. No endogenous losses of carbohydrates have been demonstrated (contrary to amino acids, lipids and phosphorus) and it is, therefore, not necessary to correct values for carbohydrate digestibility for endogenous losses. As a consequence, values for apparent digestibility can be used to characterize the digestibility of carbohydrates.

In case of phosphorus, values for standardized total tract digestibility (STTD) are used and these values are obtained by correcting values for apparent total tract digestibility for basal total tract endogenous loss of phosphorus. Since the endogenous losses of phosphorus from pigs are relatively constant, a value of 190 mg /kg DMI can be used to correct values of apparent total tract phosphorus digestibility while calculating values for STTD.

Evolution of Energy and Protein Requirements for Indian Pigs

Energy requirements are expressed as the amount of metabolizable energy (ME) per kg diet. ME consists of 94 to 97% DE (Average 96%). The loss of energy as gas produced in the digestive tract of swine is usually between 0.5 and 1% DE. The quality and quantity of protein in the diet affect the relationship between ME and DE. ME decreases if protein is of poor quality. ME also decreases with excess protein because the amino acids not used for protein synthesis are catabolized and used as source of energy and the N is excreted as urea. Therefore, as the N content of the urine increases,

ME of the diet decreases. A correction is sometimes made to ME values for N gained or lost from the body (ME_n). This correction of N equilibrium may be valid for mature animals. N retention is usual in growing animals. Therefore, the correction probably is not necessary.

Energy metabolism is influenced by the physiological state of the animal, ambient temperature, and physical activity.

Paul et al. (2007) compiled data from 27 feeding trials conducted on growing pigs from different research institutions across India. The estimated maintenance requirement of DE is in the range of 123.3 kcal to 167.8 kcal per kg $W^{0.75}$ for different body weights. The corresponding value for NRC (1998) and ARC (1981), respectively, are 110 kcal and 109.46 kcal per kg $W^{0.75}$. ICAR (2013) preferred the NRC & ARC values as they are mostly based on calorimetric studies along with comparative slaughter studies. Thus, the value of 110 kcal DE (106 kcal ME) /kg$W^{0.75}$/day is adopted as maintenance energy requirement and a value of 8.97g /kg$W^{0.75}$/day is used for protein (CP) calculation (Paul et al., 2007).

As growth pattern, body composition and carcass traits of Indian crossbred and indigenous pigs are different from those of elite exotic pigs, eventually their requirements will also vary. Thus, for the calculation of DE, CP and amino acid requirements for daily gain, values suggested by Paul et al. (2007) at respective phases of growth have been taken into consideration.

Nutrient Requirements (NRC, 2012) of growing-finishing pigs

Requirements of all nutrients for weanling, growing, and finishing pigs are calculated for 7 separate weight groups, i.e., 5-7 kg, 7-11 kg, 11-25 kg, 25-50 kg, 50-75 kg, 75-100 kg, and 100-135 kg.

Requirements of all nutrients are provided for mixed sex groups. For pigs greater than 50 kg, requirements for calcium, phosphorus, and amino acids are also calculated separately for gilts, barrows, and entire males. For pigs of 50 to 105 kg weight range, requirements for calcium, phosphorus, and amino acids are also provided separately for pigs based on the rate of deposition of protein (115, 135, or 155 g/day) to illustrate the influence of protein deposition on nutrient requirements. For finishing pigs (i.e., pigs greater than 105 kg) the requirements for calcium, phosphorus and amino acids are provided for male pigs that are immunized against gonadotropin hormone. Similarly, requirements for calcium, phosphorus, and amino acids for entire male pigs or barrows and gilts fed diets containing 5 or 10 ppm ractopamine from 115 to 135 kg are also provided because inclusion of ractopamine in the diets increases the requirements for nutrients.

ME for maintenance of pigs in different physiological states (NRC, 2012)

ME for maintenance (ME_m) can be predicted in growing-finishing pigs, gestating sows and lactating sows using the following equations (maintenance energy in growing-finishing pigs are better predicted from $BW^{0.60}$ than from $BW^{0.75}$):

ME_m growing-finishing pigs = 197 kcal/kg $BW^{0.60}$

ME_m gestating sows $\quad$ = 100 kcal/kg $BW^{0.75}$

ME_m lactating sows $\quad$ = 110 kcal/kg $BW^{0.75}$

Ratios Among Amino Acids (Ideal Protein)

In determining amino acid requirements, a fundamental concept of this publication is that there is an optimal dietary pattern among essential amino acids that corresponds to the needs of the animal. This optimal dietary pattern is often called "ideal protein." The basis for ideal protein has been discussed by several authors, including the Agricultural Research Council (1981), Fuller and Wang (1990), Baker and Chung (1992), Cole and Van Lunen (1994), and Baker (1997).

NRC 10th revised edition (1998) gave the estimated requirements of young weanling pigs from 3 to 20 kg, and of growing-finishing pigs from 20 to 120 kg body weight (Table 6). The amino acid requirements are generated (by the model) for pigs (equal ratio of barrows and gilts) of a high-medium lean growth rate (325 g of carcass fat-free gain/day) from 20 to 120 kg and housed under ideal temperature and space conditions. Separate requirements for barrows and gilts of three lean growth rates from 50 to 120 kg are also furnished. Requirements for minerals, vitamins and linoleic acid are also given.

Amino acid requirements (estimated by the sow models) for gestating sows of 125 kg to 200 kg body weight with gestation weight gain of 30 to 55 kg and anticipated litter size of 11 to 14 and lactating sows (175 kg) with daily weight gain of 150 to 250 g are given (Table 7). Dietary minerals, vitamin and fatty acid requirements of gestating and lactating sows are also furnished.

Amino acid, mineral, vitamin and fatty acid requirements of sexually active boars are also given separately.

Table 6 Nutrient requirements of swine (10th revised edition, 1998) of growing - finishing animals when allowed feed *ad libitum* on 90% DMB[a]

	Growing-finishing Swine					
Live weight, kg	3–5	5–10	10–20	20–50	50–80*	80–120**
ME, Kcal/kg diet	3265	3265	3265	3265	3265	3265
CP, %	26.0	23.7	20.9	18.0	15.5	13.2

[a] Mixed gender of pigs with high-medium lean growth rate of 325 g per day
* Barrows require 14.9% CP while boars need 16.3%
** Barrows require 12.7% CP while boars need 13.8%

Table 7 Nutrient requirements of swine (10th revised edition, 1998) of gestating and lactating sows and boars when allowed feed *ad libitum* on 90% DMB

	Gestating sows		**Lactating sows**	**Sexually active boars**	
Live weight	**125 kg to 200 kg**		**175 kg***		
ME, Kcal/kg diet	3265	3265	3265	3265	3265
CP, %	12.9	12.4	16.3-18.4**	17.2- 19.2[b]	13.0

* Assumes 10 pigs per litter and a 21-day lactation period; daily weight gain of pigs is from 150 to 250 g; anticipated lactational weight change from nil to 10kg weight loss.
** Anticipated lactational weight change 'nil'; b Anticipated lactational weight loss '10 kg'

Efficiencies of utilization of dietary amino acids for maintenance and protein synthesis in growing-finishing pigs: Efficiency of utilization (above maintenance) of standardized ileal digestible lysine for protein deposition decreases from 0.682% in pigs at 20 kg BW to 0.568% in pigs at 120 kg BW (NRC, 2012).

Energy Requirements of the Sow

A factorial approach was used to arrive at daily energy and feed intakes recommended for pregnancy and lactation. The long-term reproductive efficiency of the sow is promoted by minimizing weight loss during lactation.

Pregnancy: It was suggested that sows should be fed and managed to gain a net of 25 kg throughout pregnancy for at least the first 3 or 4 parities. The increase in weight of the placenta and other products of conception should be approximately 20 kg, for total of 45 kg gestation weight gain of the sow. If pregnant sows are offered feed *ad libitum*, they will consume more energy than they require for maintenance and the development of the products of conception. Such sows deposit more body fat and protein. Hence it is necessary to limit the energy intake of gestating sows.

The energy restriction during gestation has little effect on either litter size or birth weight. It was reported that the feed intake between 1.7 and 2.3 kg/day during pregnancy (maintained for five parities) had no significant effect on the total number of pigs born. The majority of experiments on this topic have demonstrated that birth weights of piglets progressively increase when sow feed or energy intake increase during pregnancy up to 6.0 Mcal of DE/day.

If the feed intake is restricted, as it is for gilts and boars used for breeding, the daily nutrient intake (but not energy) must be maintained at the level recommended for market pigs. Therefore, the nutrient-to-energy ratio (See Poultry Nutrition) of the diet must be increased.

Lactation: Energy requirements during lactation include a require-ment for maintenance and a requirement for milk production. ME_m for lactating sow is 110 Kcal/kg $W^{0.75}$/day, while it is 100 kcal for the gestating sow (NRC, 2012). Please see Table 7 for NRC (1998) requirements.

Energy requirement for milk production is 2 Mcal of DE/kg milk. It is calculated by assuming that the gross energy of milk is 1.3 Mcal DE/kg of milk and a 65% efficiency of utilization. The contribution from body weight loss of sows fed at the recommended levels may be determined on the assumption that weight is 30% fat and 13% protein. This weight loss would then contain about 4.5 Mcal/kg, which is converted into milk energy with an efficiency of 85% (NRC, 1998).

Requirement for Protein and Amino Acids

Dietary protein has been supplied mainly for the lean growth of animals. To enhance lean growth and to spare costly protein with the advent of ideal amino acid profile, researchers have focussed on the relationship between lean growth and amino acids rather than protein.

Gilts and boars require higher percentages of amino acids (and therefore CP; Table 6) than barrows do, since gilts and boars consume less feed and are naturally leaner. It was reported that maximal carcass leanness requires a greater intake of amino acids than does maximal rate of weight gain.

The availability of amino acids in the protein of dietary ingredients has been determined for a limited number of protein sources fed to swine. The primary method to determine availability has been to measure the proportion of a dietary amino acid that has disappeared from the gut when digesta reach the terminal ileum. These values are more appropriately termed "*ileal digestibilities*" Refer Chapter 15 of *Principles of Animal Nutrition and Feed Technology* for more information.

The three amino acids of greater practical importance are lysine, tryptophan and threonine. Cereal grains and vegetable protein supplements are likely to be deficient in lysine, methionine + cystine and tryptophan, soybean meal being an exception. Animal protein sources are rich in lysine, tryptophan and methionine. Fish meal should not be fed at levels higher than 10% as otherwise objectionable fishy flavour may develop in the pork.

Valine is the 5th or 6th limiting amino acid in nursery diets for piglets, while it could be second or even first limiting amino acid in sows.

Water requirement in pigs

Pigs contain between 48 and 82% water, depending on size, and water is needed for most biochemical reactions in the body. *Readers may refer chapter 3 'Composition of animal body' - in Principles of Animal Nutrition and Feed Technology textbook.* Requirement for water is between 80 and 120 mL per kg BW in growing-finishing pigs and non-lactating sows. Many factors influence the intake of water by pigs, which include level of feed intake, dietary ingredients, ambient temperature and humidity, and health status of the animal. That is why, it is recommended that water is freely available to pigs. Specific considerations should be given to lactating sows because of their high water requirement for milk synthesis. Lactating sows may drink up to 40 L of water per day and sow feed intake may be improved if they are offered feed mixed with water prior to consumption.

Clinical Signs of Amino Acid Deficiencies or Imbalances in Swine

The primary sign is usually a reduction in feed intake that is accompanied by increased feed wastage, impaired growth and general unthriftiness. Swine can tolerate high intakes of protein with no ill effects, except occasional mild diarrhoea. But large intakes of individual amino acids can lead to a variety of negative syndromes that have been classified as toxicity, antagonism and imbalance, depending on the nature of the effect.

Antagonism commonly occur among amino acids that are structurally related and this prejudice their utilization. An example is the lysine-arginine antagonism, in which excessive dietary lysine increases the requirement for arginine. Similarly the addition of as little as 20 g of leucine to a 1 kg diet deficient in isoleucine may have deleterious effects on performance. A reduction in feed intake is common in most of the amino acid imbalance situations.

Minerals and Vitamins

Deviating from NRC (1998), values for the standardized total tract digestibility (STTD) of phosphorus are used as the basis for estimating requirements of phosphorus by pigs in NRC (2012). It is concluded that phosphorus requirements of growing-finishing pigs may be calculated from nitrogen retention because a straight line relationship has been observed between body contents of nitrogen and phosphorus. It is also concluded that the requirement for phosphorus to maximize body weight gain and feed efficiency is only 85% of the phosphorus needed to maximize bone mineralization.

New knowledge about the need for vitamin D showed that its requirement is greatly increased because results of recent research indicated that sow and litter performance is improved if greater levels of vitamin D are included in the diets.

A common problem of calcium- or phosphorus-deficient sows is a paralysis of the hind legs known as posterior paralysis. It occurs most frequently in high milk producing sows towards the end or just after the end of lactation.

There is no evidence that pigs have an absolute requirement for cobalt, other than its role in vitamin B_{12}. Cobalt can substitute for zinc in the enzyme carboxipeptidase and for part of the zinc in the enzyme alkaline phosphatase. It has been shown that supplemental cobalt prevents lesions associated a zinc deficiency.

Parakeratosis, piglet anaemia, goose stepping are described elsewhere (Chapter 10 of *Principles of Animal Nutrition and Feed Technology*).

Osteochondrosis: It signifies a fault in the load-bearing joints which is non-inflammatory and involves the cartilage tissue around the end of the bone. It seems to be more common now in Western countries. There is a strong genetic component and the rate of heritability is between 20% and 60%. There is also conjecture that it is related to selection for heavier hams, since this change in conformation brings more weight to bear on the rear legs with proportionately less on front limbs.

Pigs with high porcine somatotropin (PST) levels seem more predisposed to osteochondrosis than with low levels.

Feeding of Pigs

Feeding systems

Pig farming is an effective enterprise for improving the socio-economic status of resource-poor farmers. Pigs are reared under scavenging, semi-scavenging and intensive systems of production. In India majority of pigs are indigenous and are reared under free-range scavenging system with little or no input. Indigenous and crossbred pigs are also reared under semi-intensive system wherein they are allowed to scavenge for the whole day and are.supplemented with household kitchen or hotel waste, rice bran, wheat bran, pressmud, etc. Pigs of exotic and crossbred are reared under intensive system in the sheds on scientific lines. Body weights of indigenous pigs maintained in AICRP units under intensive system of production are presented in Table 8.

Table 8 Body weight changes (kg) of indigenous pigs

Age (week)	Jabalpur	Tirupati	Izatnagar	Khanapara	Average
Birth	0.7	0.78	0.68	0.83	0.75
4	3.61	4.07	3.95	3.96	3.90
8	7.59	8.12	7.32	8.01	7.76
12	9.3	11.47	10.75	10.98	10.63
16	13.16	15.83	14.7	17.39	15.27
20	16.27	22.47	20.81	22.59	20.54
24	21.99	30.82	25.5	28.36	26.67
28	24.72	35.24	31.35	32.56	30.97

Source: S.S.Bhatia (1996)

Pigs have a large intestine constituting 35 to 45% of the volume of gastrointestinal tract. Fermentative digestion occur in caecum and colon. It has been estimated that fermentation products chiefly VFA may meet 25 to 30% of the maintenance requirements of pigs. An adult pig can conveniently handle 3-5 kg of leafy succulent green feeds (10-15% DM). Source of fibre, levels of fibre and other nutrients are the factors that decide the maximum level of crude fibre the pigs can handle. In growing-fattening pigs 6-8% CF may be used while the adult's ration may contain 10-12%. It has been reported that an increase in dietary fibre by 1% (beyond the specified) depressed the digestibility of gross energy by about 3.5%.

Pigs less than 2 to 3 weeks old have insufficient pancreatic amylase and intestinal disaccharidases. Hence after 2 weeks of age only, pigs are to be fed starch-or cereal-based diets. Glucose and lactose are effectively used by pigs less than 7 days old. Afterwards only, pigs can utilize fructose and sucrose. The amount of antibiotics added ranges from 0.4 to 2 g per 100 kg of feed depending upon the type of antibiotic feed supplement.

Feeding of Piglets

Creep feed is the feed given to suckling pigs behind a barrier (or creep) which allows only piglets to have access to the feed. This kind of arrangement avoids the risk of injury to piglets from overlaying by sows. The creep feeding is essential for piglets suckling their mothers for the faster growth. The sow's milk (which is at peak at 3 weeks of age) is unable to support the growth of piglets exclusively on milk. Hence creep feeding is introduced at 7-10 days of age and continued up to 56 days of age at which piglets are weaned from the mother. If weaning is practiced at an early age of 3 weeks (Segregated early weaning, SEW) a special pre-starter ration should be used.

Iron dextran injection (i/m) is to be given on 4th and 14th day of age to prevent piglet anaemia.

NRC (1988) suggested three levels of protein, viz. 24%, 20% and 18% during 1-5 kg, 5-10 kg and 10-20 kg body weight, respectively (Table 1, see also Table 6 for NRC 1998) while BIS (1986) suggested one level of protein (20%) only (Table 3). Phase feeding, as suggested by NRC, helps the piglets to make rapid gains during early age. All boars are castrated at weaning age except some boars needed for breeding purpose.

Feeding of Growing-Finishing Pigs

Pigs are fed starter, grower and finisher diets as per the requirement. Dividing postweaning phase into starter, grower and finishing is arbitrary and differs with the breed and growth pattern. NRC (1979) has these phases as up to 20 kg, 20-35 kg, and 35-65 and 65-110 kg respectively, while NRC (1988) stated them up to 20 kg, 20-50 kg and 50-110 kg body weight (Table 1, see also Table 6 for NRC 1998). The CP (%) and ME (Kcal/kg diet) requirements are 18 and 3250, 15 and 3260 and 13 and 3275, respectively (NRC 1988). BIS (1986) specified only three types of feeds for pigs and these are creep/starter diet (rations to be fed up to weaning), pig growth meal (rations to be fed from weaning to 35 kg live weight) and pig finisher/ breeding meal (rations to be fed from 35 kg live weight) (Table 3).

The average birth weight of a LWY piglet is 1.2 kg while a *desi* piglet may weigh 0.7 kg. By 8 weeks of age yorkshire pig weighs about 12 kg and it attains a weight of 65 to 70 kg by 6 months of age. It has been found that 65-70 kg is the optimum weight for slaughter for economic pork production in India while in the US and Europe, yorkshire and landrace pigs are slaughtered at 90-100 kg body weight.

Split-sex feeding and Multiphase feeding in swine

In precision animal nutrition it becomes important to feed "the animal with diets that are formulated to match its nutrient requirement, as .an animal's nutrient requirement changes with age, sex, and growth potential. Examples of this are split-sex feeding and phase feedi ig.

Pigs are fed as per different growth phases depending upon age and body weight. This phase feeding is followed mainly due to differences in the performance under different agro-climatic conditions and genetic makeup. Nutrient requirements of swine (NRC, 1998; Table 6) of growing-finishing animals from 3 - 120 kg body weight are stated, in six growing stages (3-5, 5-10, 10-20, 20-50, 50-80, and 80-120 kg), as 3265 kcal ME/kg diet and variable content of CP from 26% decreased to 13.2% as they advance in age. For Indian conditions, Ranjhan (1981) and BIS (1986) recommended only three stages viz. weaning, growing and finishing.

Barrows require feeds with lower protein content compared to boars in the weight groups of 50-80 kg and 80-120 kg; similarly gestating and lactating sows require variable nutrients. As laying down of lean muscle mass gives way to fat cells and thus growth potential of pigs change over time during growing-finishing stage, feed composition has important effect on animals' performance and manure composition. Non-retained dietary nutrients are excreted. This is a great economic loss to the farmer and contributes environmental pollution in terms of nitrogen and phosphorus.

Given that the optimal concentration of nutrients in the diet progressively decreases during the growth period, phase feeding has to be practiced concomitantly adjusting the dietary nutrient concentrations to match the animals' requirements. This kind of multiphase feeding can be an efficient approach to significantly reduce feeding costs and N and P excretions in pig production systems.

Influence of Nutrition on Nutrient Excretion: To reduce nutrient excretion, it is recommended that diets be frequently adjusted to match the requirements of the animals. Split-sex feeding will also allow for more accurate nutrient provision and, therefore, reduce nutrient excretion. Exogenous enzymes may sometimes be used to improve the digestibility of nutrients with low digestibility such as phosphorus in plant based feed ingredients. Proper balancing of dietary digestible amino acids and use of correct calcium to phosphorus ratio are also necessary to reduce nutrient excretion. Strategies that may be used to reduce nutrient excretion include use of synthetic amino acids, formulation of diets based on ideal protein, use of microbial phytase and possibly other exogenous enzymes.

Importance of proper feeding of sows during gestation

Several studies indicated that both feed composition and the amount of feed offered during late gestation are of major importance in preventing reproductive problems in the peripartal period and the first few days of lactation. The peripartal period is a critical period in commercial pig production. During the last third of gestation, the sow's metabolic and hormonal state dramatically changes. Sows can become catabolic during the last month of gestation, which was evidenced by increased concentrations of non-esterified fatty acids (NEFA) and glycerol in plasma. This is due to increased fetal demand and can lead to reduced appetite and, in very rare cases, even to porcine ketosis. After day 85 of gestation, insulin sensitivity decreases. Poor glucose tolerance has also been reported and related to an increased number of stillborn piglets, post-partum hypophagia, hypogalactia and subsequently to increased pre-weaning piglet mortality.

Overfeeding sows during late gestation and high back fat thickness at parturition predispose to several problems in the first few days post partum: low voluntary feed intake, higher catabolic rate, increased NEFA mobilization and decreased insulin secretion.

In this regard, it is important to consider not only the amount of energy but also the source from which the energy is derived. For instance, when sows were fed extra energy from fat, a decreased glucose tolerance and an increased number of stillborn piglets were observed in comparison to starch as source of energy. Further, feed additives can have an influence on production results.

Choline has beneficial effect on sow and piglet performance. Betaine, a metabolite of choline, significantly improved total tract digestibility of crude fat, crude ash and crude fibre (CF) in weaned piglets without affecting digestibility of crude protein (CP) and nitrogen-free extract (NFE) (Eklund et al., 2006). The supplementation of N, N-dimethylglycine (DMG) in parturition feed of sows has an emulsifying effect. This resulted in improvements in not only fat digestibility, but also the digestibility of the protein and the nitrogen-free dietary fraction. DMG can act as a methyl donor and, additionally, has anti-oxidative properties.

Feeding of Breeding and Lactating Pigs

Breeding gilts/sows and boars and lactating sows need to be fed on restricted quantity of feed. Green leaves may be included in their feeding. NRC (1988) suggested 12% CP and 3210 Kcal/kg diet ME for breeding animals and 13% CP and 3210 Kcal/kg diet ME for lactating sows (Table 2, see also Table 7 for NRC 1998).

After weaning the piglets at 8 weeks of age, the sow should be flushed, i.e. put on a more nutritious ration and then mated during the first heat period. A well balanced comparatively high protein ration a couple of weeks before breeding is required for 'flushing' to obtain greater litter size and weight.

During gestation period, gilts and sows are fed on restricted feeding (2.0 to 3 kg) without getting them over-fat. A daily gain in weight of 0.25-0.3 kg throughout the gestation period is satisfactory. Three or four days before farrowing, the ration should be made more laxative through the introduction of more wheat bran. Bran may be substituted for about half of the regular ration. On the day it farrows, gilt/sow should be given plenty of slightly warm water but no feed. On the next day, it can be given 1 to 1.5 kg laxative ration. On the succeeding days, the amount fed can be increased through gradual introduction of the regular lactation ration so that sow is on full feed in about 7 days after farrowing.

The requirements of the lactating sow are greater than those during the gestation period. A rule of thumb method is to provide daily 2 to 3 kg ration for maintenance plus 0.2 to 0.5 kg for each piglet the sow is nursing. In case of indigenous pigs, an adult pig is offered 2 kg feed per day. During gestation it is increased to 2.5 kg by 70th day and continued till parturition. The lactating sow is offered 2.5 kg plus 0.25 kg per piglet till the piglets are weaned. Examples of some diets for pigs are presented in Table 9.

Climatic Environment and Nutrition

The high environmental temperature and high relative humidity of tropical climates can greatly affect the nutrient requirements of pigs. High ambient temperatures decrease the appetite of the pig as a sort of physiological adaptation. A poor appetite decreases the feed intake resulting in poor growth performance of the animal. As the pig tends to eat to satisfy its energy requirements, its diet in tropics should not contain the same energy levels

Table 9 Examples of Starter, Grower and Finisher Diets for Pigs (% Composition) (to meet the Nutrient Requirements as Specified by BIS, 1986).

Feedstuff	Creep/Starter diets CP 20% ME 3370 Kcal/kg on DMB CP 17.8% ME 3000 Kcal/kg on 89% DM				Grower diets CP 18% ME 3170 Kcal/kg on DMB CP 16.2% ME 2850 Kcal/kg on 89% DM				Finisher diets CP 16% ME 3170 Kcal/kg on DMB CP 14.4% ME 2850 Kcal/kg on 89% DM		
Maize	70	60	-	-	52	55	-	-	57	-	-
Jowar	-	-	60	-	-	-	55	-	-	57	-
Bajra	-	-	-	60	-	-	-	55	-	-	57
GNC (exp)	20	20	16	18	15	13	13	11	8	8	6
DORB	-	8	9	5	25	23	21.5	20	28	26.5	25
Fish meal	7.5	10	10	10	6	7	7	7	5	5	5
Mineral mixture with salt	2.5	2.0	2.0	2.0	2	2	2	2	2	2	2
Vegetable oil/ Animal fat	-	-	3.0	5.0	-	-	1.5	5	-	1.5	5
Vitamins A, B₂, D₃	←				25 g / 100 kg						→
Vitamin 'B' complex	←				25 g / 100 kg						→

recommended for temperate regions because these high energy diets can result in protein deficiency. Experiments conducted by the author at AICRP on pigs, Tirupati with LWY pigs showed that pigs fed on low-energy diets (10% less than that of NRC, 1979) increased their feed intake to satisfy their energy needs which resulted in sufficient intake of other nutrients to support maximum gains.

Experimental Data on LWY Pigs from Birth to 66 kg BW

(The Author's MVSc Thesis Work).

1. Creep feed and starter feed

Composition				Feed consumed/ piglet
Maize	70	Up to 8 weeks	:	8.5 kg
Groundnut cake (exp)	20	From 8 weeks to a body		
Fish meal	7.5	weight of 20.9 kg	:	37.0 kg
Mineral mixture	2.0			
Salt	0.5			
fortified with AB₂D₃	100			
25 g and Vitamin B complex 25 g				

2. Grower diets: At about 20 kg BW barrows were assigned to 4 grower diets. Composition is presented here

Ingredients %	G1	G2	G3	G4
Maize	35.0	58.0	28.0	52.0
Groundnut cake (exp)	12.5	15.0	18.5	21.0
Wheat bran	44.0	18.5	45.0	18.5
Fish meal	6.0	6.0	6.0	6.0
Mineral mixture	2.0	2.0	2.0	2.0
Salt	0.5	0.5	0.5	0.5
fortified with AB_2D_3				
	100	100	100	100

3. Finisher diets: At 35 kg BW the barrows were shifted to the respective finisher diets

Ingredient (%)	F1	F2	F3	F4
Maize	38.0	64.5	35.0	58.0
Groundnut cake (exp)	7.0	10.0	13.5	16.0
Wheat bran	47.5	18.0	44.0	18.5
Fish meal	5.0	5.0	5.0	5.0
Mineral mixture	2.0	2.0	2.0	2.0
Salt	0.5	0.5	0.5	0.5
fortified with AB_2D_3				
	100	100	100	100

4. Performance Characteristics of Pigs Fed Diets Containing different Levels of Protein and Energy.

Parameter	D1 G1-F1	D2 G2-F2	D3 G3-F3	D4 G4-F4
Initial weight, kg	21.13	20.83	20.53	21.22
Age of pigs, days	95.8	92.5	88.3	96.0
Final weight, kg	67.88	64.65	65.88	65.0
Age of pigs, days	179.6	178.0	168.8	181.3
Amount of feed consumed /pig, kg	175.8	170.8	173.1	155.2
Feed/gain, kg	3.75	3.90	3.82	3.54

From the data furnished here (p. 292 and 293), the amount of feed consumed by one pig from birth to slaughter can be calculated and total cost of feed can be derived. Diets with varying energy protein ratios can be used accordingly for economic swine production.

Efficiency of Feed Conversion in Swine

The amount of feed required for an animal to make a unit gain in weight is called feed efficiency. Pig is superior to beef cattle, goats or sheep in converting animal feed to human food.

Factors that Affect the Feed Efficiency

1. Diet should have optimum energy protein ratio. It should be balanced with vitamins and minerals.
2. Diets with low quality protein and diets with higher levels of fibre increase the amount of feed nutrients, especially nitrogen, lost in excreta.
3. At low environmental temperatures, the animal's maintenance energy requirement is increased and there is a reduction in the supply of energy available for growth and hence feed efficiency decreased.
4. Data from many experiments show that feed efficiency in swine is 30 to 40% heritable.
5. Young animals require less feed per unit of gain than older and more mature ones. In baby pigs, growth rate is rapid and body cells multiply fastly. Baby pigs are most efficient in utilizing feed nutrients. In growing pigs (20-35 kg) and finishing pigs (35-65 kg) the cells still continue to multiply, but multiplication is not as rapid as in the baby pig phase. The feed efficiencies are 3.13 to 3.35 and 3.82 to 4.13 for growing and finishing LWY pigs.
6. Usually as pigs grow older and become heavier the percentage and amount of fat increases. Decreasing excess fat will increase feed efficiency since fat has about 90% DM whereas lean tissue has about 30% DM.
7. Faster gaining animals usually make more efficient gains than slower growing animals.

Cost per kg gain decreases as litter size is increased, death loss is curtailed, rate of gain and feed efficiency are increased, leaner pig is produced and efficiency of other production practices are increased.

Development of economic rations

Conventional feedstuffs like maize, groundnut cake, soybean meal and fishmeal are given top priority in formulating pig diets. A key task for nutritionists is to achieve cost optimization of feed formulation. The ever-increasing cost of these ingredients coupled with short supply has necessitated the search for utilization of alternative unconventional low cost feed ingredients. There is a global boom in the use of byproducts from non-food crop production as well as human food processing in animal feeding. Towards this several experiments have been conducted by replacing maize with rice polish and molasses (Krishna Rao and Prasad 1980), tamarind seed and molasses (Thomas and Prasad 1983; Reddy et al. 1986 b), *variga grain* (*Panicum milaceum*) (Seshi Reddy et al. 1984), bagasse and molasses in 9:1 ratio (Reddy et al. 1985), tamarind seed or rice polish (Reddy et al. 1986 b).

Krishna Rao and Prasad (1980) reported that partial replacement of maize with zinc-supplemented rice polish diet was superior to the maize diet. Molasses could safely be added at 10% level. Maize could not be completely replaced with variga, although 50% replacement could be beneficial (Seshi Reddy et al. 1984). Twenty parts of maize could be replaced with bagasse and molasses mixture without any adverse effect on economy of feed conversion (Reddy et al. 1985). Maize could be completely replaced with 30% tamarind seed and 10% molasses for economic pig rearing (Thomas and Prasad 1983; Reddy et al. 1986 b). Replacing maize partially with 20% rice polish and 10% molasses appeared to be better than complete replacement of maize with 30% rice polish and 15% molasses (Thomas and Prasad 1983).

Efforts of complete replacement of maize with bajra, groundnut cake with deoiled sunflower cake; wheat bran with deoiled rice bran; fishmeal with synthetic amino acids-lysine and methionine did not yield favourable results (Srinivasa Rao et al. 1992). Studies of Karunakar Rao et al. (2005) indicated that replacement of bajra with tamarind seed kernel in grower diets or along with tapioca waste in finisher diets resulted in poor performance in pigs.

Effect of feed processing on energy and nutrient digestibility

Feed processing such as grinding, extrusion, expander processing, pelleting, gelatinization, micronization and hydrothermal treatment may improve the digestibility and fermentability of nonstarch polysaccharides and other nutrients and thereby increase energy utilization of feed ingredients. Heat treatment may also inactivate antinutritional factors in the feed. However, extrusion, expander processing and pelleting of feeds usually results in improved feed conversion rates. Lesser particle size of feed has been emphasized (because of greater exposure for enzymatic action) since it could significantly improve feed efficiency and reduce the N level in the faeces. Particle size of 700 microns is recommended for swine feeds. However, a feed using finely ground wheat may give rise to stomach ulcers.

Supplementation of enzymes

Commercial application of enzymes focused on removing the antinutritional effects of NSPs present primarily in viscous grains (wheat, rye, barley or triticale), nonviscous cereal grains (sorghum, maize) and other feedstuffs, increasing utilization of phytate P and also to alleviate environmental pollution; and improving the digestibility of vegetable proteins. The NSPs, proteins, phytic acid and various minerals are present as complex compounds in the cell walls of plants. Nutrients bound to NSP or phytate are released by NSP degrading enzymes or phytases so that the digestibility of the protein and of various minerals (Ca, Mg, Zn, etc.) can be improved as a concomitant effect.

In monogastric animals, enzymes such as proteases, amylases, lipases are produced and there is a need to supplement them in young animals (newly weaned piglets may produce inadequate amounts of certain enzymes) and in adults (when fed on certain feeds) to further their digestive capacity. Bedford and Schulze (1998) reviewed the currently available enzymes used as feed supplements and prospects for further developments of enzymes such as glycanases (carbohydrate degrading enzymes) as alternatives to in-feed, antibiotics for the improved production performance.

Non-nutritive feed additives

Non-nutritive feed additives that may be included in diets fed to pigs are antibiotic growth promoters, anthelmintics, acidifiers, direct-fed microbials, non-digestible oligosaccharides, plant extracts, exogenous enzymes (i.e., carbohydrases and phytase), feed flavours, mycotoxin binders, antioxidants, pellet binders, flow agents, and ractopamine. US FDA regulates the use of antibiotic growth promoters, anthelmitics and ractopamine. Readers may refer chapter on 'Feed Additives' in textbook "Principles of Animal Nutrition and Feed Technology" for their description.

Harmful contaminants that may be present in feed ingredients or diets

The contaminants that may be present in feed ingredients or diets include chemical, biological, and physical contaminants. Potential chemical contaminants include pesticides, mycotoxins, heavy metals, melamine, and dioxins. Biological contaminants include bovine spongiform encephalopathy (BSE), chronic wasting disease. *Bacillus spp., Clostridium spp., Escherichia coli, Mycobacterium spp., Pseudomonas spp., Salmonella enterica*, and

Staphylococcus spp., while physical contaminants include plastic, glass, metal, and vermin carcasses that accidentally may end up in the feed supply.

Porcine epidemic diarrheoa

Porcine epidemic diarrheoa (PEDv) killed around seven million young pigs in the US since it was first identified there in 2013. The causative virus is spread in faecal matter. Animal feed is the suspected source the disease got into the US. The disease is believed to have its origins in China, according to the World Organization for Animal Health (office international des epizootis OIE).

Feed containing pork products are widely used in European Union (EU) countries. Due to concerns of the spread of PED virus in North America and Asia, European Union officials have proposed new rules for the treatment of imported pig blood for use in animal feed. Porcine blood products like plasma are commonly used in the diets of weaned piglets. Any blood products to be imported to the EU for use in pig feed must have been treated at 80° F, followed by storage for six weeks at room temperature. This would ensure any 'corona virus' present in such blood products is inactivated.

10

Horse Nutrition

The members of Equidae family *viz* horses, donkeys, mules and ponies played an important role, since time immemorial, in the service of mankind.

Horses are used for riding, racing, pleasure, recreation, exercise, work, polo, etc. commercial and recreation activities. Light horses are horses used primarily for riding, driving, showing, racing, or utility on a farm. A light horse is capable of more action and greater speed than a draft horse, which is a large breed of horse used for work. In many countries of the world, especially in Europe, horses are also used as a source of meat for human consumption. In some countries, horsemeat sells for more than beef and amounts to 4-6% of total meat consumption. A number of breeders have used small ponies to breed miniature horses. Many are used as pets, in parades, shows, circuses, and other activities. Ponies are very popular, especially with children. Ponies are used in many research studies on feeding and nutrition. The pony is defined as being under 14 hands, 2 inches by the American Horse Show Association (Table 1).

Table 1 Approximate Body Weights of Ponies and Horses.

Height (hh)	Type	Weight (kg)
10	Pony	200
12.2	Pony	300
13	Pony	350
14.2	Pony	450
13	Foal/ weanling	200
14.2	Cob horse	500
15	Hack horse	450
16	Thoroughbred horse	550
16	Hunter horse	600
16.2	Hunter horse	650
17	Shire horse	1000

Breeds of Horses

India possesses nine horse breeds, out of which six breeds are well recognized. These are Marwari (from Rajasthan), Kathiawari (from Gujarat), Spiti (from Himachal Pradesh), Zanskari (from Ladakh), Manipuri (from Manipur) and Bhutia (from Sikkim, Darjeeling, Arunachal Pradesh and Bhutan). Exotic horse breeds introduced in India are English Thoroughbred, Connemara, Haflinger, Water, Arab and Polish.

Andhiyur (Erode, TN) 'annual shandy' attracts good horses for sale (apart from other breeds of livestock); one Marwari horse of pedigree breed of 6.5 feet tall was stated to cost Rs 25 lakhs in the year 2014.

Strategies in Different Herbivorous Animals

Horses are specialised herbivores adapted to life on open grasslands. A herbivore is confronted with a food which consists of between 20 and 50% dry matter of a refractory material which its own digestive enzymes cannot handle. Though the horse is a herbivorous animal, it differs greatly from the ruminants in the anatomy and physiology of its digestive tract.

The horse has evolved over millions of years to become a fleet-footed herbivore. Different herbivore species have developed different strategies. For example, let us compare geese, ruminants and horses. Geese manage to extract enough nutrients from the vegetative parts of plants merely by eating very large quantities of plant material, since the efficiency of digestion of the food as a whole is very low. Their gizzards squeeze the cell contents out of the cell walls. The time required for the meal to pass through a goose is six to eight hours only.

Ruminant animals developed a complex stomach of rumen, reticulum, omasum and abomasum. The weight of the digestive tract and its contents represents approximately 37.5% and 45% of the ruminant animal's total weight (in sheep and cattle, respectively) as opposed to 3.7% in dogs, 8% in humans and 14% in pigs, all simple stomached animals, while in horses it is approximately 20% of total weight. Reticulo-rumen provides conducive environment to rumen microorganisms to attack the feed where it stays for up to 5 to 7 days. The ruminant can derive a higher proportion of energy from a given weight of fibrous feed than can any other animal.

The digestive system, or the alimentary canal, in the horse is about 100 ft long from the mouth to the anus. It takes about 65 to 75 h for feed to proceed from the mouth to the anus. Feed passage time in equines is quicker than in ruminants, 36-48 h compared with 72-96 h, on a similar diet. The entire tract can be divided into two functional parts: the foregut and the hindgut. The foregut functions similar to pig, which is also a simple stomached animal. The function of hindgut is qualitatively similar to ruminant animal, though efficiency wise it is incomparable. That's why, the horse is somewhere between the pig and the ruminant in its utilization of feeds. Ruminants are foregut fermentors while horses are hindgut fermentors.

Horses have mobile nostrils and flexible upper lip to assist in the selection and gathering of food. The grass is cropped close to the ground using the incisor teeth. Horses have to process the fibrous feeds that contain a very hard, sand-like substance called silica before swallowing. To overcome the quick wear and tear to the teeth, cement like substance forms a layer resembling bone over the dentine of the tooth. Further, horse has high crowned teeth, which grow continuously throughout its life to compensate for wear. Anatomical structure of skull and teeth exert substantial crushing force and a side-to-side shearing action, which effectively grind fibrous herbage into a pulp.

Microbiota in the Gastrointestinal Tract of Equines

- *Streptococcus equi* isolated from the cheek and tongue epithelium cells of ponies has been associated with strangles, a mouth and nose disease. The oesophagus is colonized by obligately and facultatively anaerobic bacteria (Meyer et al., 2010). Yeasts are present, but in low numbers.
- Lactobacillus and Streptococcus spp. isolated from the fundic section of the stomach ($10^8 - 10^9$ CFU/mL) represent almost the entire population of anaerobic bacteria. Lactobacilli are the most prevalent.
- The mucosae and lumen of the duodenum, jejunum and ileum contain between 10^6 and 10^7 viable bacteria per mL, of which most have proteolytic activity.
- Glands in the large intestine secrete mucus, but no digestive enzymes.
- The caecum contains mainly amylolytic, cellulolytic, glucolytic, hemicellulolytic, lactate fermenting and proteolytic bacteria. It is, however, important to note that only 20% of the total number of bacteria in the large intestine is proteolytic and that most of the protein digestion takes place in the small intestine. Cellulolytic bacteria inhabit the caecum more often than the colon.
- Anaerobic fungi have also been isolated from the caecum and are between 10^1 and 10^4 zoospores per mL content.
- The Archaea present in horses constitute approximately 3.5% of the total microbial cell numbers. The methanogen population in the caecum is approximately 10^5/mL.

- Methanogens remove excess hydrogen via anaerobic metabolism and, by doing that, favour the growth of fermentative bacteria. Acetogenic bacteria convert H_2 and CO_2 to acetate.
- Protozoa of 10^3 and 10^5 per mL have been isolated from the caecum and colon of ponies. Protozoa assist in the degradation of hemicellulose and pectins and upon removal, dry matter (DM) digestion decreases.
- Prebiotics (short chain fructooligosaccharides) could be effective in keeping a balanced microbial population in the hindgut, especially under stressful situations such as those experienced with a starch overload in the diet.

Digestive System-digestion and Absorption

Digestive system

Horse (*Equus caballus*) is a monogastric, hindgut fermenting animal, i.e. most of the feed is degraded in the caecum and colon (Figure 1). Production of large quantities of saliva (10–12 L/day) helps to transport the feed through a 1.2–1.5 m long oesophagus and buffers the digesta (Cunha, 1991). The oesophagus enters the stomach at the oesophageal section (Figure 2). This part of the stomach is non-glandular, but pepsin and other proteolytic enzymes are secreted by glands in the pyloric section (Pillineer, 1993). Transition of digesta through the stomach is relatively rapid, although a large portion remains for 2–6 h in the anaerobic fundic (lower) section of the stomach.

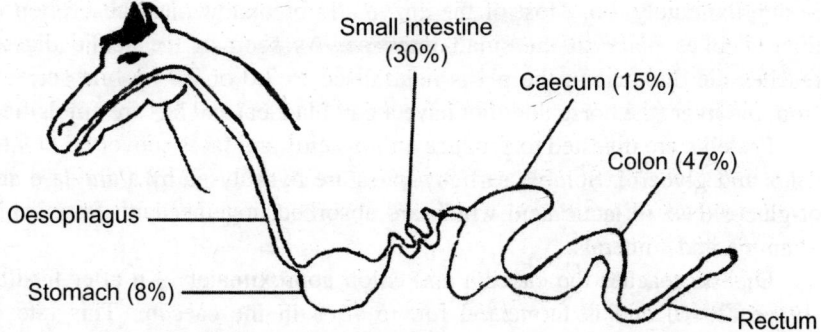

Figure 1   Schematic presentation of the equine gastro-intestinal tract (adapted from Cunha, 1991)

The foregut consists of mouth, pharynx, esophagus (4-5 ft), stomach (8-10% of the total digestive tract) and small intestine (30% of the digestive

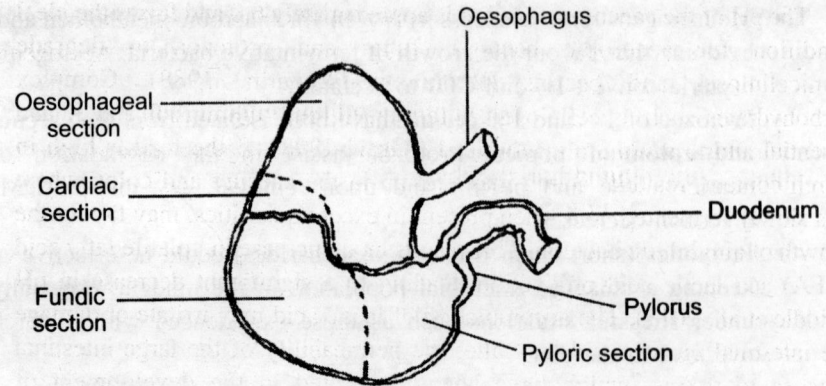

Figure 2 Anatomy of the stomach (adapted from Pilliner, 1993)

tract; about 70 ft long). The capacity of a mature cow's stomach is over 10 times that of a mature horse. Hence, the stomach of the horse requires frequent consumption of small quantities of feed and are evolved to feed for prolonged periods rather than to take large, spaced meals. The hindgut is the large intestine (some mention it as caecum and large intestine). The large intestine (60-62% of the digestive tract) consists of the caecum (15%; 4 ft long), large colon (38-40%; 10-12 ft long), small colon (9%; 10-12 ft long), rectum (1 ft long) and anus.

Dynamics of pH through the gastrointestinal tract of the horse

Carbohydrates are fermented to lactic acid and the pH of the digesta decreases to approximately 2.6. Most of the enzymatic breakdown and absorption of digesta takes place in the small intestine. As soon as the acidic digesta reaches the duodenum, the pH is neutralised to 7.0 or 7.4 by bile secreted from the liver (the horse does not have a gall bladder) and fats are emulsified.

Proteins are digested to produce amino acids and fat is converted to fatty acids and glycerol. Soluble carbohydrates are hydrolysed by a-amylase and ot-glucosidase to lactic acid which are absorbed, together with fatty acids, vitamins and minerals.

Digesta reaches the caecum and colon approximately 3 h after feeding (Frape, 2010) and is fermented for 36-48 h in the caecum. This rate of transition is only possible if the roughage component of the feed is kept optimal. The caecum of 25-35 L has two valves situated relatively close to each other. The ileum enters at the position of the first valve and further passage to the colon is through the second valve. The motility and capacity of the caecum increase during feeding to optimise interaction between the bacteria and digesta.

The pH of the caecum and colon is approximately 6.0 and forms the ideal condition for anaerobic bacteria, fungi and protozoa to degrade hemicelluloses and pectins (Bonhomme-Florentin, 1988). Complex carbohydrates such as cellulose are fermented, and vitamins B and K and essential amino acids are synthesised (Pagan, 1998). If the feed is high in starch content, residual starch may end up in the caecum and colon where it is slowly fermented, and when present in excess quantities, may favour the growth of amylolytic bacteria. This results in an increase in volatile fatty acid (VFA) and lactic acid production, leading to a significant decrease in pH (Biddle et al., 2013). The accumulation of lactic acid may irritate or damage the intestinal mucosa and may alter the permeability of the large intestinal mucosa to toxins, which have been implicated in the development of laminitis.

When the pH drops below 6.0, the growth of many fibre-fermenting microorganisms, such as *Ruminococcus albus* and *Fibrobacter succinogenes*, is suppressed, whilst the number of acidophiles, such as *Streptococcus bovis* (renamed *Streptococcus lutetiensis*), Lactobacillus spp and Mitzuokella spp. increases. This leads to more lactic acid production in the hindgut and a further drop in pH. A decrease in pH may lead to hindgut acidosis and the developing of colic and anorexia. If the pH remains below 5.8 over an extended period, the epithelial lining may be damaged and nutrients are not optimally absorbed. On the other hand, if the carbohydrate level in the feed is too low, non-lactic acid bacteria dominate, the pH increases, and CO_2 and VFA are produced (Frape, 2010). It is thus important to ensure that the microbiota in the gastrointestinal tract is always in a well-balanced state.

Carbohydrate Digestion

The foal has a small digestive tract and the caecum does not become fully functional until it is about 15-24 months old. So foals and young horses are limited in their ability to use much forage.

Starch is fermented to lactic acid by lactobacilli and streptococci in the fundic section of the stomach and further enzymatically degraded in the small intestine to glucose, which is transported across the gastrointestinal wall. Residual carbohydrates are fermented in the hindgut, i.e. the caecum and colon. Lactic acid produced in the small intestine is not well absorbed and is transported to the caecum and colon where it is fermented to propionate (Frape, 2010). The intake of starch has to be carefully controlled, as excessive quantities may increase blood-glucose levels from the normal 4.4-4.7 mmol/L to more than 6.5 mmol/L after 2 h of feeding. The critical capacity for hydrolysable carbohydrate overload in horse ranges from 0.2%

to 0.4% of body weight (BW) per meal. It was suggested that starch intake has to be limited to 1-1.5 g/kg BW/day.

Horses with blood glucose concentrations of greater than 200 mg/dL usually have serious underlying causes of colic. Celluloses are fermented by bacteria in the caecum and colon to acetate, butyrate and propionate. As much as 1.0 g of VFA are produced per kg BW. The fatty acids are rapidly absorbed into the bloodstream. Excessive, unabsorbed levels of VFA decrease the pH, especially in the lower intestine, and may depress the growth of fibrolytic microorganisms, Salmonella spp. and *Escherichia coli*.

Lactose can be digested by young horses, but horses older than 3 years appear to have limited lactase activity. As a consequence, sudden introduction of lactose-containing feedstuffs to mature horses may induce digestive disturbances.

Horse is only two-thirds as efficient as the ruminant in the digestion of hay

Feed and nutrients not digested in the stomach and small intestine flow to the large intestine, where they are digested by anaerobic microbial fermentation. However, the horse is only about two-thirds as efficient as the ruminant in the digestion of average-quality grass hay. The higher the quality of the forage, the better it is digested by the horse. The horse comes closer to the ruminant in the digestion of a high-quality lucerne hay. Microbial action in the caecum produces volatile fatty acids, vitamins, and amino acids. The volatile fatty acids produced may supply about one-fourth of the horse's energy needs. The volatile fatty acid concentration in the caecum and colon will vary with the kind of diet fed and with the ratio of grain to roughage used. With high-grain diets the total concentration of volatile fatty acids and the percentage of acetic acid decreases, the levels of propionic, isovaleric, and valeric acids increase.

Glucose derived from digestion of nonstructural dietary carbohydrates enters the portal vein. VFA available from fermentation of structural carbohydrates are absorbed in the caecum and colon and constitute important sources of energy. As a consequence of this digestive and metabolic strategy, the horse has plasma glucose concentrations intermediate between those of ruminants and simple stomached omnivores.

Protein Digestion - Need for dietary supply of indispensable amino acids

Protein digestion starts in the small intestine, which is the main site for conversion to amino acids and absorption of majority of amino acids. But the amino acids synthesized by the bacteria in the caecum and large intestine are not too efficiently utilized by the horse. Only 1-12% of the amino acids are of microbial origin. Most of the essential amino acids are thus obtained from plant material. Amino acids in the large intestine are decarboxylated to amines and excess amino acids are deaminated to urea in the liver. Urea is secreted into the ileum and transported to the caecum where bacteria hydrolyse it to ammonia. The levels of ammonia are carefully controlled in the liver by converting it to urea. Excessive levels can lead to ammonia toxicity. Ammonia is used for protein synthesis by bacteria containing glutamate dehydrogenase (e.g. *Bacteroides thetaiotaomicron, R. albus, R. flavefaciens* and *Megasphaera elsdenii*) or bacteria possessing the dual enzyme system glutamine synthetase and glutamate synthase (e.g. *Selenomonas ruminantium*). Some lactic acid bacteria, specifically Lactobacillus spp. and *S. lutetiensis*, produce decarboxylases that convert free amino acids into monoamines. An imbalance of monoamines may mimic naturally occurring amines such as serotonin, epinephrine and dopamine in the blood, resulting in excessive vasoconstriction, especially in the digits. Young horses, therefore, cannot depend on amino acid synthesis in the caecum to supply their indispensable amino acid needs. Hence, the diet fed must supply the indispensable amino acids, especially lysine.

Fat Digestion

A well-balanced equine diet consists of only 4% (w/w) fat. If effectively digested, fat is an excellent source of energy, provided that the fat is highly digestible and is fed at sensible levels, i.e. 250-500 mL/day for well-exercised horses. A high-fat ration (8%) had no effect on the pancreatic lipase activity and concentrations as high as 15% had no effect on digestion in the small intestine. It has been reported that the balance of the microbial flora in the large intestine is disturbed when the fat content in feed is raised to higher than 75-100 g fat/100 kg bodyweight per meal. Fat is enzymatically degraded to fatty acids and glycerol in the small intestine and then absorbed. Fatty acids are converted to ATP and acetate in the mitochondria by enzymes of the β-oxidation pathway.

There are many conflicting reports on the effect fat on crude fibre digestibility. Several researchers reported that the addition of fat to the diet does not affect the apparent digestibility of cell wall contents, neutral detergent fibre or acid detergent fibre. Other reports showed an increase in apparent digestibility of either neutral detergent fibre or acid detergent fibre with fat-supplemented diets. A change in fibre digestion will have an effect on the flow rate of the digesta, and thus an effect on the microbial composition in the caecum and colon.

A high fat intake may decrease precaecal starch digestion, leading to increased fermentation in the caecum. Excess levels of fat in the diet may thus reduce microbial fermentation of fibre digestibility. To maintain a balanced energy state, the intake of other nutrients has to be lowered with an intake of additional fat.

The composition of body fat in the horse is similar to that of dietary fat since the fatty acids are absorbed from the small intestine before they can be altered by microorganisms in the large intestine.

Vitamins

Fat soluble vitamins, i.e. A (retinol), D (calciferol), K and E (tocopherol) need to be supplied in the diet. Vitamin A is produced from beta-carotene. Changes in diet intake or metabolism will thus affect the absorption of these vitamins. Most water-soluble vitamins, i.e. vitamins B_1 (thiamine), B_2 (riboflavin), B_3 (niacin), B_5 (pantothenic acid), B_6 (pyridoxine), B_{12} (cyanocobalamin), B_{15} (pangamic acid), folic acid, biotin, choline and vitamin C (ascorbic acid) are produced by gastrointestinal microbiota (Cunha, 1991; Frape, 2010; Pilliner, 1993).

Vitamins play an important role in carbohydrate, fat and protein metabolism and vitamin requirement is directly linked to the fitness level and physiological conditions of the horse, such as lactation, pregnancy and growth. During exercise, gastrointestinal blood flow decreases as muscular blood flow increases. This causes a decrease in dry matter digestibility and an increase in passage rate. Fit horses consume less forage and the capacity of the hind gut shrinks, thus less microbiota are available to produce the vitamins required. An active horse on a high energy diet requires more vitamins. During intense exercise, increased oxygen consumption may damage the cell membranes in muscles, the lungs and other tissues, increasing the requirement for vitamin E and vitamin C (NRC, 2007). Horses that are fed hay and grain usually have a higher requirement for vitamin E compared to horses consuming good pasture. Vitamin E supplements are not always the answer. Horses that were fed hay and oats did not maintain their vitamin E levels despite receiving a supplement of 80 IU vitamin E/kg DM. No negative side effects were observed when additional vitamin E was added to the feed, suggesting that it may be prudent to provide vitamin E in excess of the current recommendations if horses are intensely exercised.

Minerals

Calcium and phosphorus are of special importance in horses in the development of quality bone simply because some athletic activity may put more stress on bones. Calcium is absorbed from the small intestine, while phosphorus is absorbed from the small and large intestine. Secretion of phosphate into the caecum and ventral colon, and reabsorption in the dorsal and small colon, seems to have a VFA buffer purpose. The calcium and phosphorus requirements of two-year old horses weighing 500 kg are 36.7 g/d and 20.4 g/d, respectively (NRC, 2007). This is much higher than the previous recommendations of 24 g of calcium and 13 g of phosphorus for two-year old horses not-in-training, and 34 g calcium and 19 g of phosphorus for two-year old horses in-training. Availability of Ca, P and vitamin D in sufficient amounts are important for bone formation.

Magnesium plays a role in calcium and phosphorus metabolism, and serves as an enzyme activator and co-factor in the metabolism of carbohydrates, fats and proteins. Magnesium is absorbed in the lower part of the small intestine and to a lesser extent in the large intestine.

Potassium is absorbed just before it reaches the caecum and is associated with acid-base balance, regulation of fluids and carbohydrate metabolism. Potassium and sodium are important in sugar and amino acid absorption, functioning of the nervous system and transport of substrates across the cell membrane. Reabsorption of sodium takes place within the large intestine. Sodium deficiency leads to dehydration and the insufficient utilisation of digested protein. Chloride is an important component in bile and hydrochloric acid. A chloride deficiency is highly unlikely if the sodium requirements are met.

Sulphur in the body is estimated to be 1.5 g/kg BW and is present in the form of amino acids and water-soluble vitamins containing sulphur and heparin. Organic sulphur is present in plant protein amino acids, whereas inorganic sulphur makes up about 10-15% of plant sulphur, and is used for protein synthesis by the gut microbiota. Trace minerals such as iodine, copper, zinc and selenium need much care while supplementation.

Carbohydrates

Carbohydrates form the largest part of the energy supply. There are two types of carbohydrate: soluble and insoluble. Primarily the soluble carbohydrates (starches and sugars) are digested in the small intestine and are absorbed as simple sugars. High starch feeds such as oats and barley are rapidly digested in the small intestine and provide the horse with 'instant energy'. This burst of energy may be one of the reasons why cereal grains can have a 'heating' effect on a horse's temperament. However, if soluble sugar content is high (as is found in lush, well fertilized grasses), all that is ingested is not digested in the small intestine but passes into the hindgut, upsetting the pH of the contents and cause digestive upset. In severe cases the horse or pony will suffer from laminitis. Some horses become 'hot' (excited) when fed soluble carbohydrate feeds such as oats or barley and alternative way of providing energy (e.g. sunflower oil) is better.

Most of the complex or insoluble carbohydrates (cellulose and fibre) are digested by microorganisms in the caecum and colon, and volatile fatty acids, vitamins, and amino acids are produced. The release of energy is slow and such feeds are considered as 'non-heating'. Horses digest crude fibre about two-thirds as efficiently as do ruminants. Digestion coefficients are similar for ponies and horses. Legume forages are better for horses over grasses because of their higher content of soluble carbohydrates. Horses need quality forage at a minimum of 0.5% body weight.

Fats and Energy

Although carbohydrates form the bulk of energy supply, fats and fatty acids are important in horse nutrition. Adding fat to their diet increases energy density and decreases diet volume, total feed intake, and digestive tract volume which should be helpful for horses. Fat provides energy in a '**non-heating**' form and is unlikely to cause temperament upsets. Adding fat also increases the level of protein required and may increase the level of certain vitamins and minerals needed for utilization of the extra calories provided. Normally 5-10% fat may be added in the diet of high-level performing horses, though levels of up to 20% fat can be added to diets with good results. Extra fat in the diet demands the addition of vitamin E. Linoleic acid is the primary source of essential fatty acids, and it is assumed that well-balanced diets supply the horse's requirements for it. Rancidity in feeds, however, may destroy unsaturated fatty acids (linoleic acid is one of them) and so rancidity should be guarded against since it destroys other nutrients as well.

Protein and Amino Acids

Protein in the diet is not required as such. It is needed as a source of indispensable amino acids and of nitrogen for synthesis of dispensable amino acids. However, protein level is still used and is a good guide for meeting amino acid needs. Lysine is an indispensable amino acid for the young horse. Methionine and threonine may also be indispensable amino acids for the horse under certain conditions. High energy diets increase protein needs since protein requirements are directly related to calorie level. Adding urea to horse diets is not recommended, although the horse may make use of it when low-protein diets are fed.

The horse can tolerate some excess protein in the diet. The extra protein is broken down by the body and is used as a source of energy, just like carbohydrates or fats. However, since protein is a more expensive source of energy, it should be fed in excess only as insurance against a possible need for more protein or amino acids in the diet for valuable horses.

The utilization of protein for energy produces three to six times more heat than the utilization of carbohydrates or fat. This may be beneficial in a cold environment, but contributes to excessive sweating and heat exhaustion during physical activity, particularly in a warm environment. Occasionally, allergies to a specific protein in certain feedstuffs occur. This results in **urticaria** or **hives** or frequently called '**protein bumps**' overall or small portions of the animal's body; sometimes diarhoea or respiratory problems may be seen.

Water Needs

An adequate intake of clean, fresh water at all times is very important. A horse, or any other animal, will survive longer without feed than without water. A loss of 10% of a horse's body water can lead to disorders (digestive disturbances such as colic and founder), and a 20% water loss results in death. A horse needs 2-4 kg water per kg of feed. The water needs of the animal may be increased considerably by the duration and degree of physical activity, temperature, humidity, the stage of its life cycle, the kind and level of diet fed, etc.

Working / exercising horses need about 20 to 30 % more water and it is higher in lactating mares (Table 2).

Table 2 Daily water consumption by different classes of horses*

Class of horse	Minimum (litre)	Maximum (litre)
Maintenance, 500 kg (thermo-neutral)	27	36
Maintenance, 500 kg (warm environment)	36	68
Lactating mare, 500 kg	45	68
Working (moderate), 500 kg	45	54
Working (moderate), 500 kg (warm environment)	54	81
Weanling, 300 kg (thermo-neutral)	27	36

* Source: NRC, (2007)

A number of mineral elements, such as sodium, chloride, potassium, calcium, etc. are lost in the sweat and urine during physical activity. Electrolyte loss increases as per the duration and degree of physical activity and with increasing temperature and humidity. The loss of these minerals causes depressed feed intake, fatigue, muscle weakness, and decreased performance. Hence such losses need to be replenished. The estimated sweat losses of horses on light, moderate, heavy and very heavy exercising programmes are 0.25%, 0.5%, 1.0% and 2.0% of body weight/day, respectively. Based on these estimates, the feed of an exercised horse has to be supplemented with 3.1 g sodium, 5.3 g chlorine and 1.4 g potassium to replace the minerals lost in 1 L of sweat (NRC, 2007). This could, however, be less in cool environments. The use of electrolytes and frequent watering is helpful, especially in endurance races or prolonged exercise or activity. However the horse should be cooled before being allowed to drink all the water it wants, after strenuous activity.

Nutrient Requirements of Horses

The National Research Council (NRC), USA Sub-committee on Horse Nutrition published the requirements in 1966 and later revised them in 1973 and 1989 (Nutrient requirements of horses, 5th revised edition) based on the work done in temperate regions.

Proper formulation of diets for horses depends on adequate knowledge of their nutrient requirements. These requirements depend on the breed and age of the horse and whether he or she is exercising, pregnant, or lactating. A great deal of new information bas been accumulated since the publication 17 years ago of the last edition of Nutrient Requirements of Horses (1989). The latest edition (NRC, 2007 sixth revised edition) provides a new set of requirements based on revised data. Nutrient requirements for all classes of horses and ponies during various physiological life phases are established. The effects of physiological factors (such as exercise) and environmental factors (temperature and humidity) are also covered. Nutrient Requirements of Horses is intended to ensure that the diets of horses and other equids contain adequate amounts of nutrients and that the intakes of certain nutrients are not so excessive that they inhibit performance or impair health.

The nutrient requirements for equine have been less studied in India (ICAR, 2013). Some studies have been carried out at Military Equine Stud farm at Babugarh in collaboration with the Indian Veterinary Research Institute, Izatnagar and at Veterinary College, Rajasthan Agricultural University, Bikaner. ICAR (2013) requirements are developed with due consideration on the findings of Indian research workers; NRC (2007) requirements have been used majorly to arrive at recommendations for various classes of equines.

The requirements stated herein indicate the minimum amounts needed to sustain normal health, production, and performance of horses. Horses should be fed as individuals. In applying these recommendations, consideration should be given to the following factors: digestive and metabolic differences among horses that result in some horses being "hard keepers" (horses that need more feed per unit of body weight) and other "easy keepers" (horses that are easy to feed), and appropriate adjustments in feed intake to compensate for this variation; variation in production and performance capabilities of the animal and expectations of the owner; health status of the animal; variations in the nutrient availability in feed ingredients; interrelationships among nutrients; previous nutritional status of the horse; and climatic and environmental conditions.

Energy Requirements

The energy requirements are expressed as digestible energy (DE). Values for energy requirements are not based on metabolic body size, as there was no benefit from using metabolic body size ($kg^{0.75}$) over weight ($kg^{1.0}$) in determining the energy requirements of horses weighing 125 to 856 kg body weight. A deficiency of energy in the young horse results in a poor growth rate. In mature horses, it results in weight loss, poor condition, and performance. A lack of enough to eat is a common form of malnutrition with many horses.

Energy status can be determined by weighing animals regularly, and also by using subjective 'conditioning scoring' system to monitor the status of body condition. Based on body fitness with scores ranging from 1 (very thin) to 9 (very fat), most horses should be maintained at a score of at least 4 and not exceeding 7 (ICAR, 2013). Equine family consists of different types of domesticated animals having varied mature body weights, for example horses with 200kg, 400kg, 500kg, 600kg.

Environmental temperature has a large impact on the energy requirements for maintenance, especially if horses do not have a shelter.

Maintenance: Maintenance energy requirements of horses weighing 600 kg or less were estimated from the following equation (NRC, 1989).

DE, Mcal/day = 1.4 + 0.03 BW (BW = body weight)

The older horse can be treated as a maintenance animal. However, it needs to be monitored for weight gain because of decreased activity. Adjust the feeding accordingly.

A stalled horse has a lower requirement for energy. It is better fed with larger quantities of roughages to keep it occupied in eating or else stalled horse is likely to develop bad vices.

Gestation: The most important period during gestation is the last 90 days. The 1978 NRC report indicated that energy requirements during the last 90 days are 12% greater than for maintenance. The voluntary intake of hay will decrease as the foetus increases in size. Therefore, the energy density of the diet should be increased during the last 90 days of pregnancy. Estimates of DE requirements for the ninth, tenth and eleventh months of gestation were formulated by multiplying the maintenance requirements by 1.11, 1.13 and 1.20, respectively (NRC, 1989).

Lactation: The DE requirements of lactating mares depend upon the composition and amount of milk produced. Mares of light breeds may produce as much as 24 kg of milk per day at peak lactation, which occurs at about 8 weeks after parturition. But the average milk production is probably within the range of 12-18 kg daily. The mare converts the digestible energy in the feed into milk energy with about 60% efficiency. Horses are estimated to produce milk at 3 and 2% of their body weight during early lactation (1-12 weeks) and late lactation (13-24 weeks), respectively. Ponies have an average daily milk production of 4 and 3% body weight during early and late lactation, respectively.

The 1989 NRC report used the same assumption that it takes 792 Kcal of DE per kg of milk produced as used in the 1978 NRC report.

Growth: The DE requirements for growth of foals per kg gain are presented in Table 2. Energy requirements for maintenance and growth rate were calculated by using the following equation.

DE, Mcal/day = Maintenance DE + $(4.81 + 1.17 X - 0.023 X^2)$ (ADG)

ADG = average daily gain, kg; X is the age in months.

The DE requirement per kg of gain increases with the age of the foal. It is calculated as $4.81 + 1.17 X - 0.023 X^2$.

Nutrient Requirements for Different Physiological Functions

The nutrient requirements for maintenance (Table 3), of working horses (Table 4), of stallions (Table 6), of pregnant mares (Table7), of lactating mares (Table 8), for brood mares (Table 9) and for growth (Tables 10) are furnished as given by NRC (2007).

Work

Estimates of DE requirements for work are complicated because many factors that are difficult to quantitate can influence these requirements. These factors include condition and training of the animals, ability and weight of the rider, degree of fatigue, environmental temperature and diet composition. NRC (1989) furnished the energy requirements for light, medium and intense work, after reviewing the available research reports, as 25, 50 and 100% above maintenance, respectively, for ponies and light horses (200 – 600 kg).

Table 3 Nutrient requirements of horses for maintenance*

Category	DE (Meal)			CP(g)			Lys (g)			Ca	P
Maintenance (mature BW)	Min.[a]	Av[b]	Elev.[c]	Min.[a]	Av[b]	Elev.[c]	Min.[a]	Av[b]	Elev.[c]	(g)	(g)
200 kg	6.1	6.7	7.3	216	252	288	9.3	10.8	12.4	8.0	5.6
400 kg	12.1	13.3	14.5	432	504	576	18.60	21.70	24.80	16.0	11.2
500 kg	15.2	16.7	18.2	540	630	720	23.2	27.1	31.0	20.0	14.0

[a] Minimum maintenance applies to adult horses with a sedentary lifestyle, due either to confinement or to a docile temperament;

[b] Average maintenance applies to adult horses with alert temperament and moderate voluntary activity;

[c] Elevated maintenance applies to adult horses with nervous temperament or high levels of voluntary activity. * Source: NRC (2007)

For maintenance: DE (Mcal/day) = 1.4 + [0.03 × BW, kg]

For growth: DE (Mcal/kg BW/day = 56.5 X^{-0145}; (where, X = Age in months)

For desired ADG: DE (Mcal) for gain = (1.99 + 1.21 X - $0.021X^2$ × ADG; (where, X = Age in months)

The energy requirements for draft horses depend on many factors such as size of load and type of work. However, increasing maintenance requirements by 10% for each hour of field work should provide a reasonable guide. The energy required for work is presented in Table 4. There is a big difference in energy needs between various activities such as walking, slow trotting, fast trotting, cantering, galloping, jumping, racing at full speed, etc.

Protein Requirements

Horses require a regular intake of protein. They continually use protein either to build new tissues, as in growth and reproduction, or to repair worn out tissues. If adequate protein is lacking in a diet, the horse suffers a reduction in growth or loss of weight. Consequently, protein will be withdrawn from certain tissues to maintain the functions of the more vital tissues of the body as long as possible.

Protein is needed to form milk, muscle, hide, hoof, hair, hormones, enzymes, blood cells, and other constituents in the body.

It has been shown that animals are more resistant to infections if they are fed an adequate protein diet. This is because the compounds in the bloodstream that help resist disease are proteins. So, adequate protein in the diet is important to keep animals resistant to disease.

A protein deficiency results in a depressed appetite, which leads to inadequate consumption of total feed. In young horses, slow, inefficient growth and under-development occurs. Mature animals lose body weight. A

Table 4 Nutrient requirements of working horses

Work*														
Mature	DE (Meal)				CP (g)				Lys (g)				Ca (g)	P(g)
BW, kg	LT	MD	HV	VHV	LT	MD	HV	VHV	LT	MD	HV	VHV		
200	8.0	9.3	10.7	13.8	280.0	307.0	345.0	402.0	12.0	13.2	14.8	17.3	12.0–16.0	7.2–11.6
400	16.0	18.6	21.3	27.6	559.0	614.0	689.0	804.0	24.1	26.4	9.6	34.6	24.0–32.0	14.4–23.2
500	20.0	23.3	26.6	34.5	699.0	768.0	862.0	1004.0	30.1	33.0	37.1	43.2	30.0–40.0	18.0–29.0

*Type of work: LT-light, MD-medium, HV-heavy, VHV-very heavy; *Source:* NRC (2007)

The NRC (2007) suggested energy requirement for different works over and above the maintenance as below

Light work : DE (Mcal/d) = (0.0333 × BW) × 1.2

Moderate work : DE (Mcal/d) = (0.0333 × BW) × 1.4

Heavy work : DE (Mcal/d) = (0.0333 × BW) × 1.6

Very heavy work : DE (Mcal/d) = (0.0333 × BW) × 1.9

poor hair coat, reduced hoof growth, reduced conception rate, small and weak foals from pregnant mares and reduction in milk production in milch animals are some of the effects of protein deficiency. Protein deficiency and energy deficiency often occur together.

In terms of Crude Protein: Protein requirements are usually expressed as grams of CP required per day. Now more emphasis is placed on amino acid requirements rather than on protein needs since protein is not required *per se*. But, protein level is still used and is a good guide for meeting amino acid needs.

In horses, amino acids are absorbed predominantly from the small intestine while the predominant form of nitrogen absorbed from the hind gut is ammonia. The site of absorption also greatly influences the efficiency of protein utilization. Therefore, diet formulation for horses should be based on crude protein.

Protein Quality

Feeds that supply the proper proportion and amount of the various indispensable amino acids supply a "**good-quality**" protein whereas those feeds that furnish an inadequate amount of any of the indispensable amino acids are considered "**poor-quality**" protein sources. The diet that has the highest protein quality is the one that supplies all the indispensable amino acids needed in the proportions most nearly like those in which they exist in the body protein of the horse. Lysine is the first limiting amino acid in diets for growing horses, with threonine being the second limiting amino acid.

Protein is not stored for later use compared to other nutrients. Amino acids are not stored in the body as such. Body protein synthesis mechanism is governed by the completeness and balance of amino acids (simultaneous presence of all indispensable amino acids especially) supplied from the diet and those currently available in the body from amino acid synthesis. An incomplete mixture of amino acids is broken down and used as a source of energy, i.e., they are not held for any length of time in the tissues waiting for the arrival of the missing amino acid. This means that protein supplements should be mixed with the grain at the proper level so that the horse receives a well-balanced concentrate mixture each time it eats.

Dietary Protein Requirement

The dietary protein requirement of the horse is a function of the needs of the animal, the quality of protein available, and the digestibility of that protein.

Estimates of the **digestible protein (DP) requirements for**

maintenance of horses have ranged from 0.49 to 0.68 g of DP / kg BW/ day. A value of **0.60 g of DP / kg BW/ day** appears to be appropriate for most horses. If the horse consumes a forage diet with a digestibility of 46%, the CP requirement would be 1.3 g / kg BW/ day.

The 1989 NRC nutrient requirements for protein do not include a margin of safety. It is always better to feed a higher level of protein than required and is preferable to having a deficiency of protein. The protein needs of the horse decrease as it reaches mature size. Horses that are heavier at maturity usually have a higher protein requirement during early growth. When they reach maturity, however, all horses have about the same protein requirement. Protein requirements increase during the last one-third of pregnancy and during the lactation. CP requirements were calculated (see equations) assuming that (1) mares' milk contains 2.1 and 1.8% protein in early and late lactation, respectively; (2) digestible protein (DP) is used with an efficiency of 65% for milk production; (3) protein digestibility in typical lactation diets is 55%.

NRC (1989) recommendations are 5% above the 1978 recommendations for early lactation and 5% below the 1978 recommendations for late lactation.

It is reported that exercise has little or no effect on the protein requirement of the horse. The DP: DE ratio of working horses is same as that for maintenance. However, the increased DE intake needed for working horses provides adequate additional nitrogen to meet their requirements.

The protein levels recommended (Table 5) by Cunha (1991) are a little higher than those recommended in the 1989 NRC report. This provides a small safety factor to take care of many factors that may affect protein requirements. A number of studies have shown no harmful effects from feeding a reasonable amount of protein above the NRC requirement levels. Additional vitamins (A, D, E, thiamin, riboflavin, and B_{12}) and minerals (electrolytes) are needed for muscle metabolism and energy utilization.

Equations for calculating daily requirements (on DMB) as per NRC (1989)

I. Estimation of DE requirements, Mcal DE/day
A. Maintenance: 200-600 kg body weight DE = 1.4 + 0.03 W
  Greater than 600 kg of BW; DE = 1.82 + 0.0383 BW − 0.000015 BW^2

B. Stallions (breeding season):   DE = 1.25 (maintenance DE)
C. Pregnant mares: 9 months DE = 1.11 (maintenance DE)
    10 months DE = 1.13 (maintenance DE)
    11 months DE = 1.20 (maintenance DE)

Table 5   Recommended Protein Levels for Horses (Cunha, 1991).

S. No	Stage of life cycle	Percentage of protein in the total diet
1	Creep feed and feed for foals	16-18[a]
2	Weaned foals to 12 months	14-16[b]
3	Yearlings, long-yearlings, and two-year-olds	12-14[c]
4	Mares, (gestation and lactation) and breeding stallions	12-14[d]
5	Mature horses (idle and at work)	9-11[e]

[a] These feeds supplement the milk which the mare gives. The higher level protein would be used with poor milking mares.
[b] This is a critical time in getting a weaned foal started. A high-quality well-fortified diet with vitamins and minerals is needed.
[c] The faster growing and heavily trained animals would be given the higher level of protein and a higher level of vitamins and minerals.
[d] During early lactation, and with the heavy milking mares, the higher level of protein would be used.
[e] If the mature horses are idle, the lower level of protein is sufficient; with heavy work the higher level of protein would be used.

D. Lactating mares:
1. Foaling to 3 months: 1–12 weeks
200-299 kg of BW; DE = (maintenance DE) + (0.04 BW x 0.792)
300-900 kg of BW; DE = (maintenance DE) + (0.03 BW x 0.792)
2. 3 months to weaning: 13–24 weeks
200-299 kg of BW; DE = (maintenance DE) + (0.03 BW x 0.792)
300-900 kg of BW; DE = (maintenance DE) + (0.02 BW x 0.792)

E. Working horses: Light work DE = 1.25 (maintenance DE)
Medium/Moderate Work   DE = 1.50 (maintenance DE)
Intense Work   DE = 2.00 (maintenance DE)

F. Growing horses (4-24 months of age)
Not in training: DE = (Maintenance DE) + $(4.81 + 1.17 X - 0.023 X^2)$ (ADG)

In training: DE = 1.5 (Maintenance DE) + $(4.81 + 1.17 X - 0.023 X^2)$ (ADG)

ADG is average daily gain, kg day; X is the age in months.

II. Estimation of CP requirements, g/day
A. Maintenance: CP = (40) (Mcal of DE/day)
B. Stallion: CP = (40) (Mcal of DE/day)
C. Pregnant mares, 9 -11 months: CP = (44) (Mcal of DE/day)

D. Lactating mares

1. Foaling to 3 months:
200–299 kg of BW;

$$CP = \frac{(\text{maintenance DP}) + [(0.04 \text{ BW} \times 0.021 \times 1,000) / 0.65]}{0.55}$$

300–900 kg of BW;

$$CP = \frac{(\text{maintenance DP}) + [(0.03 \text{ BW} \times 0.021 \times 1,000) / 0.65]}{0.55}$$

2. 3 months to weaning:
200–299 kg of BW;

$$CP = \frac{(\text{maintenance DP}) + [(0.03 \text{ BW} \times 0.018 \times 1,000) / 0.65]}{0.55}$$

300-900 kg of BW;

$$CP = \frac{(\text{maintenance DP}) + [(0.02 \text{ BW} \times 0.018 \times 1,000) / 0.65]}{0.55}$$

E. **Working horses:** $\quad CP = (40)$ (Mcal of DE/day)
F. **Growing horses**
   Weanlings: $\quad CP = (50)$ (Mcal of DE/day)
   Yearlings and long yearlings: $\quad CP = (45)$ (Mcal of DE/day)
   2 year olds: $\quad CP = (42.5)$ (Mcal of DE/day)

Example for mare: The daily protein requirement of the 200-kg lactating mare during early lactation would be calculated as follows as per NRC (1989):

200 kg × 0.04 kg of milk produced × 2.1 % of protein in milk

= 0.168kg or 168 g of protein secretion

168 g ÷ efficiency of utilization coefficient (0.65)

= 258.46 g of protein for milk production

258.46 g + **maintenance DP** 200 kg x 0.6 g = 120 g

= 378.46 g of dietary digestible protein required

378.46 g ÷ apparent protein digestibility coefficient (0.55)

= 688.11g of dietary CP required

Dry Matter Intake

The upper limit to daily feed intake in adult mature horses is probably somewhere between 1.5 and 2.5% of body weight when expressed in terms of dry matter of feed. This is the reason why resting horses tend to put on weight. In growing horses, the upper limit in foals is approximately 4% of

Table 6 Nutrient requirements of Stallions*

Stallions	DE (Mcal)		CP (g)		Lys (g)		Ca (g)		P(g)	
Mature BW	NB	B	NB	B	NB	B	NB	B	NB	B
200 kg	7.3	8.7	288.0	316.0	12.4	13.6	8.0	12.0	5.6	7.2
400 kg	14.5	17.4	576.0	631.0	24.8	27.1	16.0	24.0	11.2	14.4
500 kg	18.2	21.8	720.0	789.0	31.0	33.9	20.0	30.0	14.0	18.0

* NB - Non-breeding, B – breeding; *Source*: NRC (2007)

Table 7 Daily nutrient requirements of pregnant mares (NRC, 2007)

Class of horses	BW (kg)	ADG (kg)	DE (Mcal)	CP (g)	Lys (g)	Ca (g)	P (g)
Pregnant mares (mature body wt. 200 kg)							
Early (< 5 months)	200	–	6.7	252	10.8	8.0	5.6
5 months	201	0.05	6.8	274	11.8	8.0	5.6
6 months	203	0.07	7.0	282	12.1	8.0	5.6
7 months	206	0.10	7.2	291	12.5	11.2	8.0
8 months	209	0.13	7.4	304	13.1	11.2	8.0
9 months	214	0.16	7.7	319	13.7	14.4	10.5
10 months	219	0.21	8.1	336	14.5	14.4	10.5
11 months	226	0.26	8.6	357	15.4	14.4	10.5
Pregnant mares (mature body wt. 400 kg)							
Early (< 5 months)	400	-	13.3	504	21.70	16.0	11.2
5 months	403	0.11	13.7	548	23.60	16.0	11.2
6 months	407	0.15	13.9	563	24.20	16.0	11.2
7 months	412	0.19	14.3	583	25.10	22.4	16.0
8 months	419	0.26	14.8	607	26.10	22.4	16.0
9 months	427	0.33	15.4	637	27.40	28.8	21.0
10 months	439	0.42	16.2	673	28.90	28.8	21.0
11 months	453	0.52	17.1	714	30.70	28.8	21.0
Pregnant mares (mature body wt. 500 kg)							
Early (< 5 months)	500	-	16.7	630	27.1	20	14
5 months	504	0.14	17.1	685	29.5	20	14
6 months	508	0.18	17.4	704	30.3	20	14
7 months	515	0.24	17.9	729	31.3	28	20
8 months	523	0.32	18.5	759	32.7	28	20
9 months	534	0.41	19.2	797	34.3	36	26.3
10 months	548	0.52	20.2	841	36.2	36	26.3
11 months	566	0.65	21.4	893	38.4	36	26.3

Table 8 Nutrient requirements of lactating mares (NRC, 2007)

Class of horses	BW (kg)	Milk (kg)/d	DE (Mcal)	CP (g)	Lys (g)	Ca (g)	P (g)
Lactating mares (mature body wt. 200 kg)							
1 month	200	6.52	12.7	614	33.9	23.6	15.3
2 months	200	6.48	12.7	612	33.8	23.6	15.2
3 months	200	5.98	12.2	587	32.1	22.4	14.4
4 months	200	5.42	11.8	559	30.3	16.7	10.5
5 months	200	4.88	11.3	532	28.5	15.8	9.4
6 months	200	4.36	10.9	506	26.8	15.0	9.3
Lactating mares (mature body wt. 400 kg)							
1 month	400	13.04	25.4	1228	67.80	47.3	30.6
2 months	400	12.96	25.3	1224	67.50	47.1	30.5
3 months	400	11.96	24.5	1174	64.20	44.7	28.8
4 months	400	10.84	23.6	1118	60.50	33.3	20.9
5 months	400	9.76	22.7	1064	57.00	31.6	19.7
6 months	400	8.72	21.8	1012	53.50	30.0	18.6
Lactating mares (mature body wt. 500 kg)							
1 month	500	16.30	31.7	1535	84.8	59.1	38.3
2 months	500	16.20	31.7	1530	84.4	58.9	38.1
3 months	500	14.95	30.6	1468	80.3	55.9	36.0
4 months	500	13.55	29.4	1398	75.7	41.7	26.2
5 months	500	12.20	28.3	1330	71.2	39.5	24.7
6 months	500	10.90	27.2	1265	66.9	37.4	23.2

Table 9 Nutrient requirement for Brood Mares (BM)*

Class of Mare	DE (Mcal)	TDN (kg)	DCP (kg)	Ca (g)	P (g)	Vit. A (1000 1U)
GSBM, DBM and Hafinger BM (mature BW 300-350 kg)						
Dry mares (maintenance)	12.9	2.9	0.22	16	10	9
Pregnant mares in last 90 d pregnancy	14.0	3.3	0.32	25	18	19
Mares in early lactation – 3 m to weaning. 6-8L/d	22.0	5.0	0.60	38	26	21
Mares in late lactation – 4 m to weaning, 3-4L/d	20.0	4.3	0.43	31	21	17

MABM, HBBM and TBE BM (mature BW 450 kg)

Dry mares (maintenance)	16.0	3.75	0.29	23	14	12.5
Pregnant mares in last 90 d pregnancy	18.4	4.17	0.39	34	23	25.0
Mares in early lactation- foaling to 3 months, 10-12 L/d)	28.3	6.43	0.84	50	34	27.0
Mares in late lactation – 4 months to weaning, 5-6 L/d	24.3	5.53	0.62	41	27	22.5

GSBM - General Service Brood Mare; MABM - Mountain Artillery Brood Mare; HBBM - Horse Breeding Brood Mare; DBM - Donkey Brood Mare; TBEBM - Thoroughbred English Brood Mare; Source: Raut(1998)

* Dry brood mares normally do no work. Hence their nutritive requirements are same as that for maintenance

Table 10   Daily Nutrient requirements for growth (NRC, 2007)

Class of horses	BW (kg)	ADG (kg)	DE (Mcal)	CP (g)	Lys (g)	Ca (g)	P (g)
Growing horses (mature body wt, 200 kg)							
4 months	67	0.34	5.3	268	11.5	15.6	8.7
6 months	86	0.29	6.2	270	11.6	15.5	8.6
12 months	128	0.18	7.5	338	14.5	15.1	8.4
18 months							
No exercise	155	0.11	7.7	320	13.7	14.8	8.2
Light exercise	155	0.11	8.8	341	14.7	14.8	8.2
Moderate exercise	155	0.11	10	362	15.6	14.8	8.2
24 months							
No exercise	172	0.07	7.5	308	13.2	14.7	8.1
Light exercise	172	0.07	8.7	332	14.3	14.7	8.1
Moderate exercise	172	0.07	9.9	355	15.3	14.7	8.1
Heavy exercise	172	0.07	11.2	387	16.7	14.7	8.1
Very heavy exercise	172	0.07	13	436	18.8	14.7	8.1
Growing horses (mature body wt, 400 kg)							
4 months	135	0.67	10.6	535	23.00	31.3	17.4
6 months	173	0.58	12.4	541	23.30	30.9	17.2
12 months	257	0.36	15.0	677	29.10	30.1	16.7
18 months							
No exercise	310	0.23	15.4	639	27.50	29.6	16.5
Light exercise	310	0.23	17.7	682	29.30	29.6	16.5
Moderate exercise	310	0.23	20.0	725	31.20	29.6	16.5

24 months							
No exercise	343	0.14	15.0	616	26.50	29.3	16.3
Light exercise	343	0.14	17.4	663	28.50	29.3	16.3
Moderate exercise	343	0.14	19.9	710	30.60	29.3	16.3
Heavy exercise	343	0.14	22.3	775	33.30	29.3	16.3
Very heavy exercise	343	0.14	26.0	873	37.50	29.3	16.3

Growing horses (mature body wt, 500 kg)

4 months	168	0.84	13.3	669	28.8	39.1	21.7
6 months	216	0.72	15.5	676	29.1	38.6	21.5
12 months	321	0.45	18.8	846	36.4	37.7	20.9
18 months							
No exercise	387	0.29	19.2	799	34.4	37	20.6
Light exercise	387	0.29	22.1	853	36.7	37	20.6
Moderate exercise	387	0.29	25	906	39	37	20.6
24 months							
No exercise	429	0.18	18.7	770	33.1	36.7	20.4
Light exercise	429	0.18	21.8	829	35.7	36.7	20.4
Moderate exercise	429	0.18	24.8	888	38.2	36.7	20.4
Heavy exercise	429	0.18	27.9	969	41.7	36.7	20.4
Very heavy exercise	429	0.18	32.5	1,091	46.9	36.7	20.4

Table 11 Nutrient requirements of Indian foals for growth (ICAR, 2013)

Age (months)	DE (Mcal)	TDN (kg)	DCP (kg)	Ca (g)	P (g)	Vit A 1000 IU	Total Feed Intake (kg)	Ratio Concentrate mixture	Hay	% DMI (kg)
Mature BW 300 kg										
6-12	10.90	2.50	0.37	23	17	5.6	3.24	65	35	2.3
12-24	11.00	2.55	0.25	18	13	7.7	4.00	50	50	1.8
24-48	11.10	2.52	0.21	15	10	8.0	4.25	40	60	1.6
Mature BW 400 kg										
6-12	13.00	2.96	0.43	27	20	7.4	4.20	65	35	2.2
12-24	14.10	3.20	0.33	23	16	10.5	5.25	50	50	1.7
24-48	13.90	3.16	0.27	20	13	11.0	5.35	40	60	1.5
Mature BW 500 kg										
6-12	15.60	3.55	0.52	34	25	9.2	5.00	65	35	2.1
12-24	16.90	3.85	0.42	29	20	13.0	6.25	50	50	1.6
24-48	16.45	3.75	0.33	25	17	13.0	6.60	40	60	1.5

BW, which falls as the horse ages. However, there is no reason why one should wish to satisfy the upper limits of appetite of equines if one can provide them with sufficient nutrients in a lesser bulk. This is particularly the case for high-performance horses. The weight of a horse's gut and content represents 10-20% of its body weight. This figure is subject to dietary manipulation and the lower it is the better would be anticipated athletic performance. Most of the weight is water. Horses with a high dry matter intake also have a high water intake.

The lower limit to daily feed intake is governed by two factors: nutrient, particularly energy requirement and minimum level of roughage consistent with proper digestive function. The minimum level depends upon the crude fibre level of the forage and the digestibility of the crude fibre. It is reported as 0.4 kg per 100 kg body weight when fed as hay. See Table 12 for a comprehensive guide on intake of concentrates, forages and total feed as % of body weight (NRC, 2007).

Table 12 Dry matter intake*

Category	DMI (% Body Wt)		
	Forage	**Concentrate**	**Total**
Growing horses			
Nursing foal (3 months)	0	1.0–2.0	1.0–2.0
Weaning foal (6 months)	0.5–1.0	1.5–3.0	2.0–4.0
Yearling foal (12 months)	1.0–1.5	1.0–2.0	2.0–3.5
Long yearling (18 months)	1.0–1.5	1.0–1.5	2.0–3.0
Two year old (24 months)	1.0–1.5	1.0–1.5	2.0–3.0
Mature horses			
Maintenance	1.5–2.0	0.0–0.5	1.5–2.5
Mares, late gestation	1.0–1.5	0.5–1.0	1.5–2.5
Mares, early lactation	1.0–2.0	1.0–2.0	2.0–4.0
Mares, late lactation	1.0–2.0	0.5–1.5	1.5–3.5
Working horses			
Light work	1.0–2.0	0.5–1.0	1.5–3.0
Moderate work	1.0–2.0	0.75–1.5	1.75–3.5
Intense work	0.75–1.5	1.0–2.0	1.75–3.5

* NRC (2007)

Relationship between Body Weight, Work Level and Appetite

The amounts of dry feed a horse needs to eat every day in order to maintain condition and body weight is given in Table 13. This will vary according to the horse's body weight and the amount of work it is doing.

Table 13 Relationship between Bodyweight, Work Level and Appetite*.

| Work level and Appetite | Body weight (BW), kg | | | | | |
	200	400	450	500	550	600
Resting, 1.5% BW	3 kg	6 kg	7 kg	7.5 kg	8 kg	9 kg
Light work, 2% BW	4 kg	8 kg	9 kg	10 kg	11 kg	12 kg
Moderate work, 2.5% BW	5 kg	10 kg	11.5 kg	12.5 kg	13.5 kg	14.5 kg
Intense work, 2.5-3% BW	6 kg	12 kg	13.5 kg	15 kg	16.5 kg	18 kg

* Source: Practical feeding of horses and ponies by Sarah Piliner (1998) pp. 60.

Once the dry matter to be fed is known, then the ratio between the roughage and concentrate in the dry matter is to be decided. A guide to the ratio of roughage to concentrates is presented in Table 14. The horse doing light work needs more hay and less energy feed, while the horse doing hard work needs less hay and a greater concentrate feed. Horses doing hard work may not be able to eat 3% of their BW, especially if they are fussy eaters, so their appetite should be calculated using 2.5% BW and energy-rich feeds used to provide the required energy levels.

Table 14 A Guide to the Ratio of Roughage to Concentrate*.

Work level	% Roughage	% Concentrate
Resting	90-100	0-10
Light (light competition)	75-80	20-25
Moderate (regular competition, e.g. one-day event horse)	65-70	30-35
Hard (hunting, advanced competition, e.g. three-day event horse)	55-65	35-45
Intense (racing)	40-50	50-60

* *Source*: Practical feeding of horses and ponies by Sarah Piliner (1998) pp. 60.

Formulation of Diets for Horses

The nutrient requirements of the horse in question are calculated firstly. Choose the feed ingredients depending on nutrient content, availability, price of feed ingredients, and preference of the horse owner. All diets for horses should contain adequate amounts of roughage. A good rule of thumb is that horses should be fed good quality roughage at least 1% of their body weight / day or be given access to a pasture for sufficient time to allow them to consume at least 1% of body weight of DM / day. The proportions of roughage and concentrate mixture are variable (see Tables 12 and 14) in feeding the horses to control energy intake, to maintain normal digestive tract fill, to minimize digestive dysfunction and to regulate consumption of feeds by horses that are fed in groups.

Feedstuffs

Concentrates

Bengal gram is the most popular feed of horses in the Indian subcontinent. It is usually fed as a single concentrate feed after soaking in water overnight.

Cereal Grains

Oats, barley and maize are the principal cereal grains for horses. Of the three, oats are preferred because they have the lowest energy and highest fibre levels. Oats require only simple, if any, mechanical processing. Oats can be fed whole, bruised or crushed because oat grains are quite soft and easily ruptured during mastication. Horses normally use their teeth to sufficient effect so that whole oats are nearly as well digested as those fed crushed or rolled. Oats contain approximately 5% oil (with high levels of unsaturated fatty acids), which is liable to rancidity once the grain is crushed. Crushed oats thus become progressively less palatable with storage and the rancidity is also associated with destruction of vitamin E. Naked oats are a competing alternative to hulled oats in equine nutrition. However, naked oat grain contains more ether extract, and crude protein compared to hulled oats. The crude protein, ether extract and crude fibre of oats, hulled oats and naked oats, respectively, are 12.4, 14.7 and 12 to 19%; 6.0, 7.2 and 8 to 11 and 8.9, 3.7 and 2.8 to 4.5%.

Barley and maize are hard grains and should not be fed whole. Barley may be rolled, flaked or boiled while maize is fed as flaked maize. The flaking process involves the use of heat and this gelatinises the starch, possibly rendering it slightly more digestible. Cooking increases the digestibility of the grain and makes it less 'heating' (see p. 307). However, this is not easy to explain since "heat" produced by digestion is greater for fibrous feeds. Wheat is the most likely cereal to cause colic because of its high gluten content since gluten leads to the formation of a doughy lump in the stomach. Hence, wheat should not be used except in very small quantities or in low levels in compound feeds.

Freshly harvested cereal grains may be associated with digestive disturbances and it is better to store them for a couple of months before use.

Maize Versus Oats

Horses performing high-intensity work (anaerobic) may need a higher level of grain such as maize to supply more starch and simpler sugars. However, caution is to be exercised regarding its level of incorporation because of digestive disturbances due to carbohydrate overloading. It was reported that substituting maize (higher in energy and lower in volume) for oats (lower in energy and higher in fibre and volume) decreased diet and intestinal tract volume and improved racing time.

Why are Oats Preferred over other Cereals?

Oats are considered to be a suitable feed for horses because of their good palatability, high fibre and oil content, and better protein quality (lysine content) compared with other cereals. However, the energy density of oats is rather low because of the high fibre content. Oat hulls contain fibre almost exclusively (84%) and the proportion of hulls in oats varies usually between 21% and 24%. In practice, various amounts of hull can be removed from conventional oats, which consequently influences the chemical composition and digestion of oat diets.

The horse's stomach is reasonably small and not an important site of bacterial digestion. But it still harbours a good population of lactobacilli, which produce lactic acid and gas by fermenting sugars and starch. A single meal of cereals may remain in the stomach for long periods awaiting the stimulus of further food being chewed in the mouth before being passed to the small intestine. The contents may ferment producing a lactacidosis and, in extreme cases, this can result in colic or even stomach rupture. Oats provide a more open textured material in the stomach due to their high fibre content and are thus the least likely to cause colic compared to other cereals.

The starch content in oats and hulled oats is 46-47% and 48-63%, respectively. Oat starch has been found more readily digestible in the small intestine compared to other cereals, for example, maize and barley. This is due to the different morphology of the starch granules of oats and higher amylase activity in the jejunum following the intake of oats.

Brans

Fibre in equine diets is important to maintain a stable hindgut environment that is less susceptible to acidosis. Wheat bran by tradition is a much favoured feed for horses. It has less energy and more fibre, protein and minerals than the wheat. But feeding high levels of wheat bran is associated with Big Head disease or Miller's disease or bran disease in mature horses due to its poor calcium to phosphorus ratio i.e. high in phosphorus and low in calcium. [Calcium deficiency results in the mobilization of calcium from the bone, which is replaced by a proliferation of fibrous connective tissue. This increases the size of the bone at that location (skull and jaw). Calcium deficiency in the growing horse most commonly causes leg problems such as enlarged joints, splints, and the epiphysitis syndrome]. Bran draws a lot of water into the gut (due to high fibre level) and thus has a laxative action.

Protein Supplements

Soybean meal is almost certainly the protein supplement of choice due to its high lysine content. Groundnut cake is the alternative. Linseed seeds are toxic and must be boiled in water before feeding. Linseed cake of expeller and *ghani* pressed type may be used instead. Feeding linseed produces a glossy coat (blooming hair coat) due to the relatively high level of unsaturated fat. The same effect can be achieved very much conveniently by incorporating any vegetable oil such as olive oil, maize oil, sunflower oil, etc. Solvent extracted linseed meal does not have any advantage over the other oilseed meals in giving the horse a glossier hair coat. In addition, linseed meal is low in lysine.

Other Feeds

Young grass is liked by the horses because the cell contents of young grass have high sugar content and most horses appear to have a sweet tooth. Molasses, molassed sugar beet pulp are used to reduce dust and to enhance the palatability of horse feeds. Beet pulp contains a high percentage of digestible fibre. Dried, molassed sugar beet pulp is the commonest alternative energy supplement to cereals. It is inferior to oats in protein but equivalent in energy. Addition of greater than 5-10% molasses will have too great a laxative effect.

Succulents such as carrots may be fed up to 2 kg per day. They are useful for adding variety to the diet and help to alleviate the boredom factor.

Roughages

A horse can eat fresh grass at 10% of its body weight every day. Requirements for maintenance as well as part of production can be supplied through *ad libitum* feeding of good quality fodders as a single feed or the mixture of fresh leguminous and cereal fodders in the ratio of 3:1. Lucerne leaf meal is a rich source of protein, calcium, phosphorus, carotenes and other micro nutrients. Lucerne, berseem, cowpea, oats and maize green fodders are excellent for horses. Their hays are also popular in feeding of horses. Green legumes may cause bloat in cattle, buffaloes or sheep, but not in horses. Pasture grasses such as *dub* (*Cynodon dactylon*), pongola, timothy and orchard grasses are popular. Straws and stovers are the poor quality fodders.

Soybean hulls or soyhulls are being used as a source of fibre in place of hay. Soyhulls are readily degraded in the equine digestive system by microorganisms in the caecum and large intestine. They contained 94.8% organic matter, 12.2-13.1% crude protein, 60.6-66.3% neutral detergent fibre, 43.7-49.0% acid detergent fibre, 2.25% lignin and 0.4% acid insoluble ash. Soyhulls are high in pectins and other soluble fibres but they contain relatively little starch. Therefore, soyhulls provide adequate energy without some of the common management problems associate with high-grain diets in both ruminants and horses. Soyhulls seem to be an acceptable replacement for up to 75% (as-fed basis) of the total forage in diets for horses (Coverdale *et al.*, 2004).

Hallway feeds, Kentucky (USA) are produced without steam flaking or micronising of ingredients. The pellets are of 2 mm (11/64 inch) and 13 mm (1/2 inch) size. The cube (13 mm pellet) is quite large and has additional advantages of better digestion because the horse has to chew the cubes. Hallway feeds are produced by using starch, fat and readily digestible fibre at varying level to meet the productive function of horses-from highspeed racing, eventing or endurance to pulling heavy loads.

Feeding the Foal

Feeding the foal (foal is young horse until it is weaned) starts *in utero* with feeding the pregnant mare a well-balanced diet to supply all the nutrients to the developing foal in the womb and to enable the mare to be a better milk producer after foaling. Mare's milk meets the foal's needs during the first 2 or 3 weeks of life.

Composition of mare's milk: Milk composition of mammalian species varies widely due to genetic, physiological and nutritional factors and environmental conditions. Gross composition of mare's milk in comparison to human and cow's milk (Malacarne *et al.*, 2002) is presented in Table 15. Milk represents the essential source of nourishment of mammals during the neonatal period. Hence it is physiologically and structurally correlated to the nutritional requirements of the newborns of each species. Mare's milk has noticeably less fat content compared to human and cow's milk, similar lactose content to that of human milk but higher than that of cow's milk and more protein and ash contents than those of human milk but less than those of cow milk. The energy supply of mare's milk is clearly lower than that of human milk and cow milk.

Table 15   Gross Composition of Mare's Milk in Comparison to Human and Cow's Milk*.

Constituent	Mare		Human		Cow	
	Mean	Range	Mean	Range	Mean	Range
Fat, %	1.21	0.5-2.0	3.64	3.5-4.0	3.61	3.5-3.9
Crude protein, %	2.14	1.5-2.8	1.42	0.9-1.7	3.25	3.1-3.8
Lactose, %	6.37	5.8-7.0	6.70	6.3-7.0	4.88	4.4-4.9
Ash, %	0.42	0.3-0.5	0.22	0.2-0.3	0.76	0.7-0.8
Gross energy, Kcal/kg	480	390-550	677	650-700	674	650-712

* Adapted from Malacarne *et al.*, (2002).

Antibodies are not provided to the foal by the mare during gestation because antibodies are too large to pass through the mare's thick placenta into the foal's bloodstream. Immunity for the foal is available only through the antibodies in the mare's first milk, the colostrum. One should help the foal suckle, if there is need to do so, as soon as possible after birth. A majority of normal foals will nurse within 1-2 h after foaling, while the most vigorous will nurse within 30-45 min. This is crucial because the intestinal tract is permeable to the colostral antibodies (through the special absorption cells in the duodenal lining) for about the first 24-36 h of foal's life. These special cells decrease rapidly over the first 24 hours of the foal's life. After 48 hours they are replaced with normal duodenal lining. This process of transfer of antibodies from the mare to the foal is called passive transfer.

Colostrum may be collected from the mares after their foals have suckled and it can be frozen for later use. During the needy times this colostrum should be slowly heated to body temperature and administer to the foal. This provides immune protection to the foal. Blood IgG levels below 400 mg/dl indicate a failure of passive transfer. Plasma transfusions can be used to raise the IgG levels in foals that are more than 24 hours old. Generally 1 litre of plasma is administered over a 30- to 60-minute period, depending upon the foal's vigour.

If the foal is restricted to milk alone, it soon becomes anaemic as milk is deficient in iron, copper, and possibly other nutrients. Total solids in milk decrease from 25.2 to 10% while lipids (0.7 to 1.3%) and lactose (4.6 to 6.5%) increase from the parturition to 4 months later. The crude protein in milk dropped from 19.1% shortly after birth to 3.8% 12h later and to 2.2%

2 months later. Other nutrients in milk such as gross energy (135 to 49 kcal/ 100 g), ash (0.72 to 0.27%), Ca (847 to 614 µg/g), P (389 to 216 µg/g), Mg (474 to 43 µg/g), Na (524 to 161 µg/g) and K (1143 to 370 µg/g) also follow the same trend. This is the reason why a good creep feeding programme is recommended at 3 weeks of age.

The creep feed is kept in creep, which is an enclosure with openings for the foals to get in but not the mares. Supplemental feed for suckling foals should be provided at least once daily, more often if warranted. The creep feed plus the milk the foal gets from its mother should be designed to provide a well-balanced diet. The creep feed given to the foal should be kept clean and fresh so that no mouldy or sour feed is consumed. The use of a creep feed helps to ensure that the inherited potential for growth and development is realized. At 5-6 weeks of age, a foal should be consuming creep feed at the rate of 0.5 % body weight. By weaning time, the foal should be consuming 2.27-3.64 kg of creep feed per day. Examples of creep feed are given in the Tables 16 and 16A. One of the most important advantages of creep feeding is to accustom foals to eating concentrates before they are weaned. Creep-fed foals are less susceptible to the stress of weaning.

Foals are weaned usually at 6 months of age. The nursing foal is assumed to be approximately 10% more efficient in utilization of DE than are mature horses.

Table 16 Creep Diet for Nursing Foal[a].

Feed	Percent in diet
Oats groats, rolled	15.00
Oats, rolled or flaked	20.00
Maize, barley, sorghum, rolled or a combination of them rolled or flaked	35.75
Soybean meal	15.00
Dried skim milk	05.00
Molasses	05.00
Dicalcium phosphate	02.00
Ground limestone	00.75
Trace mineralized salt[*]	01.00
Vitamin supplement	00.50

[a] Adapted from Cunha (1991); the ration should provide 18% CP, 0.9% Ca and 0.8% P.

[*] Trace minerals present are iodine 0.3 to 0.5, iron 40 to 80, copper 10 to 20, cobalt 0.2 to 0.3, manganese 30 to 40, zinc 40 to 80 and selenium 0.1 ppm; low levels are suggested for horses used for pleasure riding while high levels are meant for high-level performance horses that require a higher level of nutrition.

Table 16 A Composition of creep ration (ICAR, 2013)

Ingredients	Proportion (%)
Barley / oats / maize crushed	60.0
Wheat bran	5.0
Soybean / GN meal	30.0
Common salt	1.5
Dicalcium phosphate	1.0
Limestone	1.0
Brewer's yeast	0.5
Trace mineral mixture	1.0

Feeding schedule: It may be fed to foals only when 3 weeks old and on *ad lib* basis till the foal learns eating. Once it is habituated, feed can be provided 3 times a day. A good quality fodder (chopped oat hay) may be provided as mixed ration on 50:50 basis with concentrate to avoid overfeeding of concentrate that can cause epiphysitis and enterotoxaemia in some cases. **Scale of feeding/day**: 21 days to 2 months age – 0.8 kg; 2 to 4 months age – 1.3 kg; 4 to 6 months age –1.8 kg.

Feeding the Orphan Foal

An orphan foal may have to be hand-reared by using a nursing bottle, if a foster mother cannot be found. The foal should be taught to drink milk (mare's milk) from a bucket as soon as possible: first allow the foal to lick milk off the fingers and then immerse the fingers in the bucket; this will encourage the foal to follow the fingers and discover the milk.

A foal with proper care can be raised on cow's milk. In case the foal has not secured colostrum from its dam, hypodermic injection of horse serum is usually given. As mare's milk contains less fat and more sugar compared to cow's milk, the milk should be modified for a very young foal. Hence use the milk from cows in their first part of lactation and those giving milk with less fat content. It is suggested to add 150 ml lime water to 600 ml cow milk along with one teaspoonful of sugar. On the first day, the foal should be fed at hourly intervals with milk warmed to 100° F using nursing bottle. During the first two weeks, normal healthy foals should be fed every two hours and during the second two weeks they should be fed every four hours. They should then be fed four times a day until weaning. The amount and frequency of feeds needed will vary according to the size, age and health status of the individual foal, but initially foals should be fed about 150 ml. Each week the amount fed should be increased to the maximum that the foal will eat without scouring. Scouring without fever or any other signs of illness may indicate that the foal is being overfed and its diet should be adjusted accordingly.

The orphan foal should be introduced to solid feed as quickly as possible. This will encourage gut development in the foal, which facilitate early weaning from the bucket. Some solid feed need to be kept at the bottom of the pail to teach the foal to eat solid feed. Later balanced creep feed has to be introduced. The foal can be put on good pasture soon.

Feeding through Stomach Tube

If the foal is premature or lacks a normal suck reflex, it must be fed through a stomach tube until it has learned to suckle. A soft rubber tube is passed into the foal's nostril, down its throat and into its stomach. The foal's nostril should be greased and when the tube reaches the back of its throat the foal should swallow so that the tube passes down the gullet, not into the lungs. The person must listen to the end of the tube before putting any milk down the tube. If the tube is in the lungs a characteristic noise will be heard and the tube should be slowly withdrawn. Milk is then slowly poured into a funnel attached to the tube.

Feeding the Weanling (Horses that are 6 Months to 1 Year of Age)

One of the most critical times in the life of a growing horse occurs between weaning and about 1 year of age. Foals which have been given a creep feed and are already used to consuming concentrate mixture are better prepared for the shock of weaning. Studies indicated that light horses reached about 45, 66 and 88% of their mature weight at 6, 12 and 18 months of age. They also have about 83, 91 and 95% of their mature height at the withers at 6, 12 and 18 months of age. Therefore, during the first few months after birth the fastest growth and most elongation of bones occurs. After weaning the foal should be increased in concentrate mixture 1-1.5 kg and 1 kg forage per 100 kg body weight. The ration should provide 18% CP, 0.85% Ca and 0.75% P. The concentrate ration constitutes 65 to 70% of the total ration fed to the weanlings. The remainder of the ration would be a hay with at least 12% protein. It has been suggested that dietary imbalances may be the causative factors in a variety of developmental orthopedic diseases in young horses.

A very rapid rate of growth is associated with an increased incidence of bone and joint problems such as osteochondrosis, epiphysitis, cervical vertebra malformation and angular limb deformities.

Feeding the Yearling (Horses that are 1 to 2 Years Old)

If the horse reaches a year of age and is well grown, and has sound feet and legs, it has successfully passed a critical period in its life cycle. Weight gains will decrease during the second year of the foal's life. But the foal is still growing and should continue to be fed a high-quality ration. The horse should be placed on a feeding programme of 1 to 1.5 kg of forage and 1-1.5 kg of concentrate mixture per 100 kg of body weight. Concentrate mixture should contain 16% CP, 0.8% Ca and 0.65% P, while forage should have at least 10% CP. The level of feeding can vary considerably depending on how the horses are to be used, the kind and quality of ration, and the response of the horses to the feeding programme followed.

The long yearling (1.5 years to 2 year old) requires a little less protein, calcium, and phosphorus than the yearling. The roughage intake is about 60% of the total feed intake as compared to 40% concentrate. Long yearlings not required for racing or high-performance can be fed largely on roughage, but the roughage should contain at least 11% protein.

Composition of concentrate mixture for growing foals is presented in Table 17.

Table 17 Composition of concentrate mixture for growing foals (ICAR, 2013)

Ingredient	Proportion in young stock ration		
	6-12 months	**12-24 months**	**24-48 months**
Barley crushed	60	60	65
Toasted soybean / groundnut / cotton seed meal	25	20	12
Wheat bran	12	17	20
Common salt	1.0	1.5	1.5
Di calcium phosphate	1.5	1.0	1.0
Trace min mixture	0.5	0.5	0.5

Feeding for Performance

Feeding horses for racing, show, or performance is more complicated than feeding any other farm animal. These horses have widely differing feed requirements. Successful performance depends upon a combination of good stable management, feeding and exercise. While good feeding will not make a horse jump higher or run faster, poor feeding will undoubtedly damage a horse's ability to perform. Overfeeding or underfeeding will impair a horse's performance. A good feeding programme for the horse includes the actual feed and the feeder, who feeds the horse. The good feeder or more aptly the good trainer is one who can balance the horse's work and feed to produce an athlete ready to give its best.

A well-balanced feed is the first requirement and competent feeder is equally important. There is no substitute for dependability, regularity, alertness, hard work, and integrity of the person doing the feeding. There is a need for individual feeding and for a constant study of the peculiarities and needs of each individual horse. Some horses eat slowly, whereas others eat fast. Some will consume more feed than others. Some horses may like more concentrate or hay than others. Proper attention to these small details will mean the difference between developing a champion or just another horse.

Show horses and dressage horses are trained to have impeccable manners and to move freely and well. They need to be in very good condition with a gleaning coat, radiating good health. The show horse has to have enough stamina to remain at ease at the end of a long day while the dressage horse has to perform strictly controlled exercises. The work may be light work. The feeding regime must ensure that the horse is calm, well mannered and responsive in the ring.

The event horse has to be fit enough to gallop and jump at speed and yet disciplined enough to perform dressage and show jumping. The show jumper has to be well conditioned and responsive, without displaying excitable behaviour. Hence the event riders have to keep their horses happy mentally and physically by feeding as few concentrates as possible and leaving the horses out in the field every day. The hunter carries its rider for as long as 6 hours (40-48 km distance may be covered in a day), spending periods standing still interspersed with short periods of galloping and jumping over varied terrain. The animal may work like this twice a week. Obviously the hunter cannot eat enough on that day morning to supply the energy it will use up during the day. This means that it has to burn up body reserves which are then replaced over the next 2 or 3 days.

Feeding the High-level Performance Horse/ Race Horse

The high-level performance horse needs to be treated like an athlete and its likes and dislikes are to be taken care of while feeding, training, housing, and management. It is already stated that the energy needed for a strenuous effort, such as racing at full speed, is 70 times greater than that required for walking. This tremendous difference in energy requirement indicates the need for understanding how to provide energy for maximum racing speed and endurance.

The race horse is trained to compete at its maximum capacity during an approximate 1-3-minute racing period. This means that maximum availability and utilization of energy must occur during this short time. Diet must be manipulated to maximize the amount of energy available in the muscles during exercise or racing.

Feeding and training programmes are very important in maximizing energy storage and availability for optimum muscular activity and performance. H.M. Goodman and coworkers (1971 & 1973) showed that muscle glycogen and free fatty acids play a dominant role in supplying energy to the muscles for work in both unconditioned and conditioned horses. The conditioned horse adapts itself to utilize fat, in addition to glycogen, to meet the increased energy requirements of exercise and training. The unconditioned horse, however, is not able to oxidize or use fat as efficiently as the conditioned horse. The unconditioned one uses more muscle glycogen for exercise. Meyers *et al.* (1987) reported that adding 5 and 10% fat to the diet of the exercising horse had a sparing effect on muscle glycogen reserves. This glycogen reserve could later be mobilized to help defer fatigue in the exercising horse. The level of protein, vitamins and minerals used needs to be increased as the fat level in the diet is increased. Enhanced level of vitamin E appears to be beneficial with the unsaturated vegetable oil.

The use of 5-10% fat and a small increase in grain level in the diet may be beneficial for the high-level performance horse to increase energy density, reduce total feed intake, and decrease intestinal tract volume. It is reported that maximum bone strength does not occur in horses until they are 4-7 years old. But they are in training and performance much before this time. (See later for more information on the complexity of bone formation).

Sweating occurs as a horse runs or exercises. Any minerals that are lost in the sweat will increase their need in the diet. Sweat losses are influenced by temperature and humidity. The loss of sodium and chlorine appears to be of great concern since sweat contains 0.7% salt. Highly exercised horses in high temperatures and high humidity zones sweat considerably and become exhausted and fatigued. Similarly excess heat is generated during prolonged exercise. This heat must be dissipated by sweating. If the exercise or running is excessive and prolonged, there may be a significant electrolyte loss (salts dissolved in the body fluids). Hence there is a need so keep salt licks in horse stables though minerals are added to the diet. Electrolytes are to be given in water or feed during long distance endurance trails.

The need for magnesium, iron, selenium and iodine would be expected to increase with exercise. Magnesium is involved in energy release, iron is essential for the formation of haemoglobin in the red blood cells, selenium is important for muscle function, and iodine is necessary for general metabolism. Vitamin E is considered important for the exercising horse and stress increases the horse's need for B complex vitamins.

Horses being developed for racing must not be allowed to become fat. In developing a race horse, it is important that they receive the protein, energy, vitamins and other nutrients needed to develop the body of a well-trained athlete. They must also obtain adequate nutrition to perform to the maximum of their inherited potential. An example of ideal ration is furnished in Table 18. The ration should provide 18% CP, 0.95% Ca and 0.85% P. The concentrate mixture should be at a level of 40 to 50% of the total feed intake and this level can be increased during heavy training or racing. Roughage should be of high quality hay/ pasture. If the horse is standing in the stable without exercise, the concentrate part should be cut the night before the rest day to reduce the risk of 'tying-up' (azoturia) and then reintroduced over 2 days once work has resumed.

Table 18 Ration for Race Horses[*].

Feedstuffs	% in the ration
Oats, rolled	35.00
Maize, ground	10.75
Barley, rolled	12.50
Wheat bran	07.00
Alfalfa meal, 20% CP	08.00
Soybean meal, expeller 4-5% fat	15.00
Molasses	07.00
Dicalcium phosphate	02.00
Limestone	00.75
Trace mineralized salt	01.00
Vitamin supplement	01.00

[*] Adapted from Cunha (1991).

Slow release energy feeds that are broken down during exercise provide a continuous supply of energy to the working muscles. Hence high-digestible fibre sources such as sugar beet pulp, lucerne chaff and high fat diets are better than grain diets. Fibre in the diet traps water in the large intestine and acts as an essential reservoir of fluid which is used to replace sweat loss and to prevent dehydration during a ride. The provision of water to endurance horses is vitally important and they should be accustomed to drinking during the ride whenever possible. Electrolytes need to be given one or two days prior to ride in the feed and during the ride in water.

Feeding the Breeding Mare and Stallion

Filly is female horse until it is 3 years old and mare is female horse after 3 years age. Colt is male horse until it is 3 years old and stallion is male horse after 3 years age while gelding is castrated male horse. The breeding mare and stallion should be kept in a thrifty condition. Mares and stallions that become obese decrease in reproductive efficiency. Mares restricted in energy intake have impaired reproductive efficiency.

Feeding the Pregnant Mare

To have a foal every year most mares can be rebred within a few weeks of foaling and thus often gestation and lactation overlap. For breeding/gestation, the recommended maintenance needs for energy and protein should be sufficient during the breeding and early gestation periods. It is advised to increase the nutrient intake by 10 to 20% above the maintenance if mares loose the weight during lactation and enter the second trimester of gestation in sub-optimal body condition.

The most important period during gestation is the last 90 days. This is the period when growth rate of the embryo is the greatest. About 60-65% of the weight of the foetus is grown during this period. The products of conception accounts for 10-12% of the body weight of the mare. During the last 90 days of gestation, the mare will gain 50 kg weight at the rate of 0.55 kg per day. The gestation diet should have 11-12% protein. The foal weighs approximately 40-45 kg at birth. The concentrate mixture should supply 16% CP, 1.0% Ca and 0.9% P. The concentrate should form 35% of the total ration.

Feeding the Lactating Mare

A few days before the foaling mare should be provided a bulky diet to reduce potential constipation problems, and allowed 7 to 10 days after foaling to bring mares to full feed.

Proper nutrition is very critical since the mare needs to recover from parturition, produce enough milk, and rebreed successfully. The mare has to be fed enough balanced feed to produce milk as well as to maintain her body. An inadequate diet may account for much of the alternate year foaling that occurs because the mare fails to conceive while nursing the foal. Lactating mares should be fed 12-14% protein diet. Peak milk production usually occurs at 6-12 weeks after foaling. It then gradually declines until the foals are weaned at about 6 months of age.

Horses are estimated to daily produce milk equivalent to 3% and 2% of body weight during early lactation (foaling to 3 months) and late lactation (4 to 6 months of lactation), respectively (Cunha, 1980). A 500-kg mare may produce over 16 kg of milk /day.

During first 3 months of lactation feed intake increases and it is 37% over that of during the last 90 days of the gestation period. This is an increase from about 1.5 to 2.0% of body weight to 2.0 to 3.0% of body weight as DM intake. The concentrate part of the complete ration will be 45%. After 3 months, milk production decreases and accordingly the level of feed decreases. The dry matter intake is about 2.0 -2.5% of body weight and the concentrate mixture forms 40% of the total diet.

Feeding the Stallion

During the nonbreeding season, a high-quality pasture/forage will supply a large part of the feed for the stallion. Concentrate feeds should be fed in small amounts to supplement the forage and to keep the stallion in a trim, thrifty condition. A free choice mineral supply provides opportunity to obtain minerals not present in adequate amounts in the feed consumed.

Two or three weeks before the breeding season begins, the concentrate feed given to the stallion should be increased so that it will gain a little weight. This is similar to flushing practiced in ewes/sows and is important for the stallion to have good libido and fertile semen. During the breeding season the stallion should need more energy, protein, minerals, and vitamins. This is accomplished by feeding a higher level of concentrates in the diet. The concentrate mixture should be fed at the rate of about 1% DM of the body weight, the remaining being green and leafy forage or hay. The total diet should contain about 13% protein and the stallion should not be allowed to get too fat or too thin. The stallion should receive some exercise but excessive exertion may reduce libido.

Feeding Adult Horses

The energy requirements of mature horses at maintenance are low and can be met by feeding good quality roughages. However, salt and a balanced mineral supplement need to be provided free-choice. If good quality roughages are not available, some concentrates are fed to meet the nutritional requirements.

Horses have tremendous capacity for compensatory intake from the feeds of low energy content provided they are palatable. Mean voluntary intake of nonpregnant adult mares (about 530 kg BW) on a composite ration with about 2.27 and 2.06 Mcal ME per kg dry matter was, respectively, 2.07

and 2.46 DM per 100 kg BW (Raut *et al.*, 1982). However, this trend of feed intake was not seen in pregnant mares in their last quarter of gestation period and energy density of rations could not influence the feed intake significantly.

Systems of Feeding Horses

Stall feeding: The daily allowance of concentrate mixture is divided into 2 or 3 parts and fed to horses at 6-8 hours interval. Working horses are generally fed twice, while growing foals and lactating mares are fed three times in a day. Afterwards, mixture of cereal and leguminous fodders are offered.

Grazing: The animals are allowed grazing on pastures for 6-10 hours daily. Depending on the availability of herbage and the physiological stage of the animal, the supplements are offered.

Use of feeding bags: Working horses and ponies used for traction are required to be fed away from the home. The feeding bags are used to feed concentrate mixture. The concentrate is moistened and filled to half of the bag and tied behind the pole after putting the mouth of the horse to enable it eats comfortably. The bags are used for feeding the working and race horses in the intervals during the working hours. Buckets are also used for feeding the *tonga* ponies

Proper Bone Formation

It is estimated that only one in five Thoroughbred horses which start training get to the race track. Of those that get there, only one in five is still racing after one year. Feet and leg problems account for a large percentage of the horses that drop out along the way. Proper bone formation in horses is a very complex problem. It requires not only calcium and phosphorus, but other minerals, vitamins (A, D, and C), protein, hormones, and possibly other factors.

The ash in the bone contains about 36% calcium, 17% phosphorus, and 0.8% magnesium. In addition to Ca, P and Mg, copper, manganese, sodium, chloride, and possibly fluorine are concerned with proper bone formation. Proper protein nutrition is important in bone formation since bone contains about 20% protein. The weanling horse requires about 0.6-0.7% lysine. Bone is not static and is continually being re-formed throughout life in a continuous interchange of calcium and phosphorus between the bone, the blood supply, and other body systems. If more calcium and phosphorus leaves the bone than is being replaced, the bone will eventually become porous, weak, and may be pulled out of shape, deformed, or broken down by the weight of the horse and the pull of the body muscles.

A high-level performance horse is comparable to a human athlete but it has the disadvantage of training at a very young age compared to the human. If a human has a life span of approximately 77 years and horse a life span of 22 years, 2-year-old horse could be compared to a 7-year-old human. Most performance horses start training at about one year of age. This early age stress of training for high-level performance accounts for some of the breakdown which occurs in the feet and legs of horses. The pushing of young horses too early and too hard for high-level performance may result in damage to immature, partially ossified bones. When young horses are fed for rapid body and skeletal growth, they may develop bone abnormality and lameness problems. Further, proper attention has to be paid while selecting breeding stock, and avoid those with a tendency toward poor feet and legs.

Exercise Physiology

Energy is probably the most important nutrient needed by the high-level performance horse since the exercising muscle needs extra energy. Proper training for the specific task (racing, endurance riding, show jumping, polo activities, etc.) required enhances the capacity of the horse for energy utilization and performance. But storage and availability of the energy required for the different kinds of tasks the horse has to perform is also equally important. **Exercise, training and diet can influence energy storage**. The race horse may require as much as three times the maintenance DE requirement. The key to top performance is optimum conversion of the chemically bound energy (ATP) into the energy required for muscular contraction.

Energy Metabolism: The entire energy metabolic process is very complex and involves many complicated chemical reactions. Oxygen is needed to transform fat, cellulose, and VFA into ATP. Starch and other simpler sugars which are stored as glycogen can produce ATP in limited amounts without oxygen. ATP is the form of energy that is used for muscle contraction. Low-intensity work (aerobic) can utilize fats, VFA, and cellulose as energy sources. High-intensity work (anaerobic) can utilize starch and simpler sugars as energy sources. Most tasks the horse performs require a combination of aerobic and anaerobic work: low-intensity work involves the highest percentage of aerobic metabolism whereas maximum racing effort involves the highest level of anaerobic metabolism.

Muscle fibre types: The horse has three major muscle fibre types. They are slow-twitch, oxidative; fast-twitch, glycolytic and fast-twitch, oxidative-glycolytic fibres. The fast-twitch, glycolytic fibres are adapted for rapid contractions and can obtain energy efficiently by anaerobic metabolism. The slow-twitch fibres have slow contractions and obtain energy by aerobic metabolism. The fast-twitch, oxidative-glycolytic fibres have characteristics intermediate between slow and fast twitch and vary from primarily aerobic to primarily anaerobic.

The glycogen level and its decrease in horse muscle varies with the muscle fibre type and the kind of exercise. The slow-twitch and fast-twitch oxidative-glycolytic fibres are depleted after slow trotting exercise. The fastest rate of glycogen depletion occurs in the slow-twitch fibres. As glycogen is depleted, the capacity for exercise is decreased. The glycogen level of fast-twitch glycolytic fibres is not depleted at low-speed exercise until the other muscle fibres are depleted. The glycogen level of fast-twitch glycolytic fibres is depleted at maximum or submaximum high-intensity level of exercise after a period of time.

It is reported that there are significant variations in the distribution of muscle fibre types within individual muscles, between different muscles, and between the same muscle from adult and foetal origin in the pony. Further, it is found that different types or breeds of horses vary considerably in their musle fibre distribution. It is important that the muscle groups used for specific tasks be properly trained for the exercise they will perform.

Training and exercise are beneficial to proper bone development.

Adding Fat to the Diet of Exercising Horses

It would appear that horses developed for maximum racing performance might be benefited by the use of 5-10% fat in the diet. It is apparent that adding fat to the diet of exercising horses increases the caloric density and allows a reduction in total feed intake. A lowered feed intake minimizes the possible incidence of founder, colic, tying-up, and digestive disturbances which might otherwise occur with carbohydrate overloading.

The addition of fat to the exercising horse's diet has a sparing effect on muscle glycogen reserves. It may be due to a sparing effect on muscle glycogen or possibly to stimulation of muscle glycogen synthesis. Regardless of the exact mechanism of glycogen sparing effect, if a high-level performance horse can be conditioned to utilize fat as an energy source during aerobic work, the resulting increase in glycogen storage can add to the energy supply to the muscles of horses working in a state of oxygen debt. This could delay the onset of fatigue in the exercising horse.

Some Hints on Feeding Horses

- It is often quoted to feed the horse a little and often. The horse has to chew each mouthful of feed as it takes it. On fibrous feeds of low digestible energy, therefore, it has to spend a very substantial part of its day in eating enough to obtain sufficient nutrients. The physiological stimulus for gastric emptying would appear to be chewing of more food in the mouth. As the amount of roughages in the diet decreases, less time is spent for eating. Concentrate feeds increase leisure time and the stabled horse will spend its time displaying signs of boredom and inactivity, such as crib-biting, weaving, wind-sucking and other stable vices.

- It would seem prudent to limit meals of high dietary density (complete pelleted feed), those of concentrated carbohydrate sources, to no more than 0.5 kg DM per 100 kg body weight per meal and, if necessary for energy intake, to feed up to four meals per day.

- The timing of feeding in relation to work should be considered. Horses take approximately 40 min to eat 1 kg of hay and 10 min to eat 1 kg of cereals or concentrate pellets. It is unwise to work horses within 1.5 h of their completion of a concentrate feed. In the case of racehorses, no hay and only very small concentrate feeds should be offered on race days before the race. It may be necessary to muzzle some horses or to take other action to prevent them from eating their beds on such occasions. Hay deprivation on the day of a race means that hay will no longer be in the stomach and thus not impeding the diaphragm, it will be residing in the hind gut along with the large quantity of water required for its digestion; most of it will not have left the body until 36-48 h have elapsed.

- Feed the horse according to its condition. The rule of feeding according to condition is more easily said than practised and considerable experience is necessary. The horses are to be weighed periodically to know the effect of the feeding schedule followed. During times of less work, its intake of digestible energy should be reduced (see Table 9) by reducing the concentrate part of the total diet and increasing forage intake. By doing so the energy density of the total diet is reduced while leaving total dry matter intake constant. As workload increases, gradually increase the concentrate mixture at the rate of 0.25 kg/ day.

- Whenever the proportion of concentrates and roughage in the total diet are altered or changes in feed ingredients are effected to the reality of the animal's nutrient requirements, it is unwise to introduce new feedstuffs all of a sudden. Digestive enzymes can adapt to new feeds but only over period of days and not hours. Allow 7-10 days to change onto new feed.

- Some horses are greedy feeders and consume their concentrate feed without proper mastication. Such animals are subject to colic and digestive disturbances. Various strategies to slow down the eating need to be explored. These include diluting the energy of concentrate with bran, chopped hay, or placing large sized round stones in the feed box.
- Fats and oils are efficiently digested in the small intestine, so we can add extra 'non-heating' energy to the horse's ration by including oil. Substances such as potassium, magnesium, chromium, amino acids and B vitamins may be added to maintain calmness and reduce anxiety.

Characteristics of Horse's Droppings and Urine

Feed alone is not enough to keep a horse healthy; exercise, routine teeth care and deworming are also important. Horse's droppings and urine should be observed. Normal droppings contain 50-60% moisture; freely passed, without straining, as well-formed balls consisting of fine particles; colour varies from dark green to light green or yellow depending on the amount of green forage and concentrate feed without any offensive smell. Normal colour of urine is yellowish and cloudy; no excessive smell of ammonia; freely passed several times a day adopting the characteristic stance of staling. Dietary and other effects may reflect in the droppings and urine characteristics. Loose, cow-pat-like droppings may be due to inadequate roughage, green pasture; hard droppings may be due to dehydration; long pieces of hay or straw and whole grain in the droppings indicate that horse is greedy eater, bolting feed (swallowing feed quickly), sharp teeth. Strong ammonia smell in the urine indicate high protein in diet, dehydration; abnormal smell may be due to bladder infection or eating certain plants while grazing; reduced volume is due to dehydration; small and frequent urination may be due to urinary tract infection of mare in season.

Rules of Good Feeding

Sarah Pilliner (1998) listed these golden rules and these are as follows.

1. Feed according to work, condition and temperament
2. Feed only good quality feedstuffs
3. Feed plenty of roughage
4. Feed little and often
5. Make any changes gradually
6. Keep to the same feeding time every day

7. Feed something succulent every day
8. Leave 1 hour after feeding before work
9. Water before feeding
10. Keep utensils clean
11. Reduce the amount of feed on the horse's rest day

Gastrointestinal Related Disorders Associated with Microorganisms

A diet rich in starch increases the number of lactic acid bacteria, which produce high levels of lactic acid and VFA, specifically propionate.

Lactate is absorbed into the blood stream and causes lactic acidosis. It is also referred to as metabolic acidosis. *Streptococcus lutetiensis* was the most prevalent during the onset of laminitis. Laminitis may also be caused by excessive release of endotoxins as Enterobacteriaceae are lysed due to high lactic acid concentrations. Lactate-utilizing bacteria at this stage are overwhelmed by the influx in lactic acid production and those less tolerant to low pH will also die.

Lactic acidosis and endotoxaemia may lead to the onset of colic.

The amines produced within the digestive system may play a role in the onset of laminitis. Respiratory acidosis may also occur, i.e. when CO_2 is retained by the lungs and cardiac or peripheral circulation fails.

Excessive gas production is often caused by too much cereal in the diet. Symptoms are sweating and violent rolling. Concentrate feeds should be low in gluten (not too sticky). Hay and straw should not be cut too short, as all of these factors contribute towards the onset of colic.

Grazing in sandy soil areas may cause impaction and chronic inflammation of the intestine.

The build-up of gas in the intestine, usually caused by an impaction, restricts peristalsis that may lead to fermentation of feed within the stomach and small intestine and, in severe cases, twisting of the intestine and restriction of blood flow. In this case immediate surgery is required. The condition may be reversed by increasing the hay intake.

Feeding and Health-related Problems

Laminitis: Laminitis is defined as an inflammation of the lamina on the inner hoof wall. It affects the feet, causes extreme pain, a high fever, and the horse has a difficult time moving or walking. Founder is another name for laminitis. It may be due to many causes.

1. Avoid overfeeding or irregular feeding of concentrate grain mixture to horses. Whenever the quantity of concentrate is increased, it should be increased gradually.

2. Eating too much grain results in a high production of lactic acid in the horse's intestinal tract. The lactic acid damages the gut wall and allows bacteria to enter the blood. This results in endotoxemia (the presence of toxins in the blood), which affects the lamina by decreasing the blood flow to the lamina.

3. One of the reasons why laminitis is so complicated and enigmatic is its association with gastrointestinal disturbances, particularly a diet of lush grass at certain times of the year. Certain equine hindgut bacteria produce amino acid decarboxylase enzymes that convert free amino acids into monoamines. Therefore, amines formed and released from the gastrointestinal tract are hypothesized to act as the link between the ingestion of lush grass and the digital ischemia thought to precede laminitis. Equine caecal contents contain a range of amines (tryptamine is the most potent one) that are present in micromolar concentrations. Thus the monoamines could potentially induce laminar ischaemia and so trigger laminitis.

4. Colic can also cause laminitis by direct damage to the intestinal wall, such as with a torsion (twist of the intestine). The wall will die in that area and allow bacteria to get into the blood to cause laminitis.

5. After foaling see that mares completely expel their afterbirths. Retained afterbirths may cause uterine infection followed by laminitis.

6. Irregular feeding, quick changes in kinds of feed used, the use of mouldy, rancid, and wet feeds when the horse is used to dry feeds may result in indigestion. Indigestion may result in laminitis.

7. Avoid hard work and exercise on hard surfaces since this may bruise the laminae and cause laminitis.

8. In such cases, it is always safe to change the horse to a diet of good-quality hay.

A brittle, cracked hoof may result in case of deficiency of minerals and amino acids.

- Sulphur is a mineral involved in the chemical bonds that maintain the integrity of the internal hoof.
- Biotin improves the resilience of the hoof wall.
- Methionine and cysteine are the building blocks of keratin, the protein which makes up hoof and hair.
- Zinc is a mineral needed for hoof growth and skin condition.

- Calcium is needed for healthy bones and teeth and also has a role to play in hoof growth.

Colic

Colic refers to abdominal pain.

- The horse has a small stomach and if fed too much it cannot relieve the distended stomach by vomiting and thus colic may develop. If the distension is too great, the stomach may rupture and cause death.
- The small intestines are long and twisting and herniation through a body opening may occur and cause colic.
- The caecum and large and small colons are large in relation to the stomach. Impaction may occur in all the three and cause colic. Twisting may occur in the large and small colon, and some cases of colic may require surgery.
- Internal parasites play an important role in intestinal disturbances which may lead to colic.
- It appears that colic may be caused by obstruction in the digestive tract, digestive tract disturbance which usually produce gas, and parasite infestations which can be great enough to block the intestinal tract.
- Sand colic can result when horses ingest large amounts of sand while grazing impoverished pastures.

Thus colic can be complex and requires competent attention, prevention and treatment.

Feeding and Management Suggestions which may Minimize Colic

- Feed at regular times daily and avoid sudden diet changes. A necessary diet change should always be done gradually.
- Horses that are greedy or fast eaters are to be slowed down. This can be achieved by keeping mineral blocks or smooth rocks. Improper chewing of feed may cause colic. Hence check the teeth of the horse.
- Feed should have optimum level of fibre to avoid impaction of feed in the stomach or other digestive disturbances. Do not feed horse 2 hours before and one hour after hard work.
- Water should always be made available since inadequate water intake causes colic. The hot, tired horse should be cooled out slowly and allowed only small quantities of water until its thirst is satisfied.

- The droppings of the horse should be observed frequently and watched for consistency and unusual odour.
- Feed mangers should be kept clean. Mouldy or rancid feed may cause digestive disturbances or colic.
- Horses need adequate exercise. Colic problems are much less in such horses.
- Horses sweat greatly and it contains 0.7% salt as well as other minerals. Hence salt and minerals should be available in the stalls for free choice consumption.

Lactation Tetany

Tetany is a condition in which there are localized, spasmodic contractions, twitching, or cramps. It is due to a fall in the plasma calcium concentration that may occur in the lactating mare as a result of the loss of calcium into the milk. Lactation tetany in a mare is prevented in subsequent lactations by feeding a low-calcium ration during the last 2 to 5 weeks before foaling; switch to high calcium ration, immediately following foaling.

A low-calcium ration stimulates the parathyroid gland, so that it is able to respond more rapidly and effectively to a fall in the plasma calcium concentration and mobilize more calcium more rapidly from the bone to prevent tetany. The low-calcium ration also increases the efficiency of intestinal calcium absorption, which is very important to meet the extra calcium needs of lactation. (Tetanus or lockjaw is a disease caused by the bacterium *Clostridium tetani*).

Tying-up or Exercise-related Muscle Problems or Azoturia

Azoturia is also known as 'Monday morning' disease or exertional rhabdomyolysis. It is normally observed in horses that are fed on a ration with good amount of concentrates even on rest days. The day after a rest day such horses exhibit this condition where the muscles of the loins and hindquarters seize up leading to stiffness and pain. The signs vary from slight hind leg stiffness to severe pain and total reluctance to move. Treatment involves reduction of pain and inflammation. Vitamin E and selenium supplements may aid muscle strength and reduce the incidence of azoturia. Prevention is better by following these tips: reduce the concentrates if the horse has no work; warm up and cool the horse properly; leave the horse out in the field for grazing as much as possible; make any changes in the diet gradually, etc.

Hypomagnesaemic Tetany

Feeding fertilized spring grass may cause hypomagnesaemic tetany (grass staggers) in animals due the very poor availability of magnesium.

Quidding or Dropping Half-chewed Feed

Quidding or dropping half-chewed feed out of the mouth may be observed in some horses. This may be due to sharp edges of molar teeth. The sharp edges on outside of upper molar and inside of lower molar can lacerate the tongue and cheeks and make eating painful. The signs of sharp edges include very slow eating, bolting the feed i.e.; swallowing feed quickly, loss of condition of the animal.

Osteochondrosis

It is reported that osteochondrosis (cartilaginous hypertrophy) in foals is clinically similar to lameness that has been associated with a simple copper deficiency. Horses with the genetic predisposition for fast growth and those that are fed heavily for faster growth are frequently prone to develop osteochondrosis. A high incidence of osteochondrosis, epiphysitis, and other skeletal disorders are found in grazing horses, where forages and feeds are deficient in copper and zinc. But all such cases are not attributed due to deficiencies of copper and zinc. (The place where bone growth occurs is **epiphysis**. Inflammation of the epiphysis is called **epiphysitis**. The mineral imbalance in the milk may result in epiphysitis, causing enlarged joints and crooked legs, or in a decreased growth rate).

Osteochondrosis (OC) is a disorder frequently diagnosed in horses. OC prevalence is very high: a prevalence of 25 to 40% is no exception in warm-blood breeds, although cold blood horses also suffer from this disorder. OC is a disturbance in the process of ossification that occurs in young animals. It is a dynamic disorder and lesions may repair or get worse during the first months until 12 months of age. It starts at birth or possibly even before. At an age of five months, prevalence is at its highest. Regression of lesions is joint dependent, but no further substantial reduction in osteochondrosis is observed after an age of 12 months.

Several factors do influence bone formation, and irregular ossification leads to the formation of loose fragments. Irrespective of a good genetic background, bone development depends on minerals such as calcium, phosphorus and magnesium, trace elements such as copper, zinc, and manganese, and vitamins such as vitamin D and K. Studies conducted by Counotte et al. (2014) revealed that magnesium-supplementation and more exercise of the foal could lower the osteochondrosis prevalence significantly; mainly the osteochondrosis prevalence of the knee joint was very low after supplementation of magnesium.

Heaves

Heaves or pulmonary emphysema results in a loss of elasticity in the lungs, and an accumulation of air in the lung tissue since it cannot be expired properly. The horse coughs, has difficulty breathing, and may show a nasal discharge. Heaves may occur when horses consume dusty, musty, mouldy feeds or when they are exposed to dusty bedding; some horses may be allergic to the hay or some horses are more susceptible than others.

Enteroliths

Enteroliths are also known as calculi or stones. The presence of nidus (nails, pins, needles, pebbles, etc) and adequate concentrations of ammonia, magnesium and phosphorus are needed for calculi formation. Calculi found in the intestines of horses are primarily composed of magnesium, ammonium and phosphate. The elimination of a nidus from the feed by making sure clean feeds are used is a very important way of preventing calculi formation. Some horses pass small calculi in the faeces and never develop any problems. In some cases, enteroliths can grow large enough to block the intestines and cause serious damage.

Wood Chewing

It is known that animals, which are short of minerals will eat dirt and chew wood and other objects. Therefore, the first step is to prevent this from occurring and to make sure the diet is adequate in minerals. Mineral requirements are a complex matter and much remains to be learned. As soils decline in fertility, new minerals may need to be added to horse diets. Further, plants do not need selenium, iodine, and cobalt, while sodium is essential only for certain plants. Declining soil fertility, increased horse productivity, and intensified and confined conditions increase the need to supply adequate minerals in the diet. Mineral interrelationships, availability, chemical and physical form of minerals, mineral processing methods, acid-base balance affect the mineral needs of the horse.

Some horses chew each other's tails when they are fed only a completely pelleted diet. This may be due to a lack of enough roughage. It could be due to a lack of some minerals, or it could be due to some other deficiencies.

Boredom may also cause wood chewing. Keeping horses in a small stall or area could cause wood chewing. The wood chewing may be a manifestation of dissatisfaction with the close surroundings and the lack of a paddock for exercise, running, and something to do, see, and explore. Simply, wood chewing may be a bad habit similar to nail biting in humans.

Thumps or Synchronous Diaphragmatic Flutter (SDF)

Synchronous diaphragmatic flutter, that is contraction of the diaphragm in synchrony with the heart, may occur owing to electrolyte losses as a result of physical exertion. Here a decrease in the plasma concentration of calcium, chloride and/or potassium is observed.

Prussic Acid Poisoning and Cystitis

Immature sorghum, sudangrass and sudan-sorghum hybrids contain a glycoside which may breakdown to prussic acid or hydrocyanic acid in the digestive tract. This cyanogenetic glycoside is also present in the second growth following periods of drought, frost, or heavy trampling. Prussic acid poisoning is very rapid. Sometimes the first sign of trouble is finding horses dead or dying. Prussic acid poisoning results in abnormal breathing, trembling muscles, spasms or convulsions, nervousness, respiratory failure, and death.

The sorghum-sudan hybrids and sudangrass hybrids may also cause a disorder known as cystitis (urinary tract inflammation). This disease causes continuous urination and incoordination in gait, and the mares appear to be constantly in heat. Animals seldom recover after the incoordination or dribbling of urine occurs. Hay made from such grasses will not produce the disease. Hence, one needs to exercise caution if sudan or sorghum-sudan hybrid pastures are used for horses.

Nitrate Toxicity

Horses are less susceptible to nitrate toxicity than are ruminants. Intakes of excessive amounts of nitrates may result in acute toxicity. Ingested nitrates are converted to nitrites. Nitrites are absorbed and convert blood haemoglobin to methaemoglobin. This compound prevents the blood from picking up oxygen from the lungs. This compound gives the blood a chocolate-brown colour. Clinical signs of acute nitrate toxicity are usually observed within one-half to four hours after excessive nitrate ingestion. These signs include colic, diarrhoea, frequent urination and signs of hypoxia (inadequate oxygen). Hypoxia causes a rapid, weak pulse, increased depth and rate of respiration, laboured breathing, incoordination, muscle tremors, weakness and a dark bluish tinge to body tissues (cyanosis), noted particularly on the mucous membranes of the mouth. Acute nitrate toxicity is treated by methylene blue given intravenously (10 mg/kg BW) at several-hour intervals. Methylene blue assists in converting methaemo-globin to haemoglobin.

Purified Diets for Horses

The term purified or synthetic diet is used interchangeably. They both refer to a diet that consists of purified ingredients instead of grain, protein supplements, and other feeds (see the table 19).

Table 19   Example of a Purified Diet.

S. No.	Ingredients	Supplies
1	Casein (vitamin free)	Protein
2	Glucose	Carbohydrates
3	Cornstarch	Carbohydrates
4	α-cellulose	Fibre or roughage
5	Corn oil	Fat
6	Dicalcium phosphate	Calcium and phosphorus
7	Salt	Sodium and chlorine
8	Individual minerals as mineral salts	Magnesium, iron, copper, cobalt, manganese, zinc, potassium, sulphur, iodine, and selenium
9	Individual vitamins as synthetic vitamins	A, D, E, K, C, B_1, B_6, B_{12}, pantothenic acid, niacin, riboflavin, choline, inositol, p-aminobenzoic acid, biotin.

Purified diet ingredients are used to know exactly what the diet contains. Purified diet method makes it possible to subtract a vitamin, mineral, fat, carbohydrate, protein, or amino acid (if synthetic amino acids are used instead of casein in the diet) or to vary the level of protein, energy, minerals, and vitamins and to determine their effect on the test animal. This cannot be done with a natural or practical diet consisting of maize, barley, oats, soybean meal, linseed meal, lucerne meal, bone meal, and salt.

However, one needs to be careful in applying nutrient requirement data obtained with purified diets directly to practical diets. This is because the feeds in the purified diets are much more digestible than those in the practical diet. The nutrients in practical diets are in their natural state and they are in different forms from those fed in purified diets. These result in a difference in availability and in requirements between purified and practical diets. Further, the two types of diets may have different effect on the synthesis and requirements of certain nutrients by the intestinal tract microorganisms present in the horse. Hence, there is a need to conduct experiments with practical diets as well. In case of pigs, it was revealed that a big difference can occur in the nutrient requirements obtained with a purified diet (Zinc, 18 ppm; Vitamin D, 45 IU/lb feed) as compared to a practical diet (Zinc, 50; Vitamin D, 227).

Purified Diet Composition

The composition of purified equine diet is presented in Table 20. It does not contain selenium and it should be added. This diet was readily pelleted. It was also consumed by suckling and weanling foals at a level in excess of 2.5% of body weight and resulted in 1 kg gain per day. The blood values were within normal ranges and resulted in the passage of formed stools.

Nutrition of Donkeys

Population wise Pakistan, Ethiopia, China and Mexico had donkeys in descending order with Mexico hosting 3.3 million donkeys as per the census of 2004. Studies conducted by R.A. Pearson and colleagues (2001) and D.G. Smith and colleagues showed superior ability of donkeys to retain food particles for longer time in the digestive tract compared with other equines; digestive efficiency of donkeys is superior to ponies and horses. Comparative studies of the intake and digestion of forage feeds by donkeys and horses have shown that, while differences between the two species are small on good quality and highly-digestible forages (such as lucerne), on low-quality forages (such as barley and oat straws) donkeys are better able than horses to digest the high-fibre, low-protein materials. This may account for their ability to maintain weight in the dry season compared to the horse.

Aganga and Tsopito (1998) reported that donkeys are grazers as well as browsers; the teeth and lips of donkeys permit them to graze close to the ground and thus they can graze short vegetation efficiently. This could explain why during the dry season donkeys are able to maintain live weight even when the amount of vegetation available for grazing is sparse. Moreover, the donkey differs from the horse because its narrow muzzle and mobile lips promote greater selectivity in feeding, which allow them to maximize feed quality rather than quantity. The donkey may use a selective feeding strategy, searching for high-quality bites when foraging over a

Table 20 Composition (%) of Purified Equine Diet (Stowe, 1969).

Component	
Casein, vitamin free, kg	16.00
Glucose, kg	40.00
Cornstarch, kg	25.00
Cellulose, kg	13.00
Cottonseed oil, kg	1.00
Dicalcium phosphate, kg	2.40
Sodium chloride, kg	1.00
Potassium carbonate, kg	1.415
MgO, g	65.0
Zn SO_4. $7H_2O$, g	8.8
Mn SO_4. H_2O, g	8.0
Fe SO_4.$7H_2O$, g	4.5
Cu SO_4. $5H_2O$, g	2.00
Co Cl_4. $6H_2O$, g	0.6
KI,	0.5
Inositol, g	40.0
Choline chloride, g	24.0
Niacin, g	4.476
p-aminobenzoic acid, g	2.200
Thiamin HCl, g	1.544
Riboflavin HCl, g	0.455
Calcium pantothenate, g	0.455
Pyridoxine, g	0.356
Folic acid, g	0.207
Menadione, g	0.037
Vitamin A, g (250 IU/mg)	1.760
Vitamin D_2, g (500 IU/mg)	0.110
Vitamin E, g (222 IU/g)	20.000
Total ration	100 kg

Stowe, H.D., 1969. J. Nutrition 98: 330.

heterogenous pasture or rangeland, but when provided with homogenous hay employing an alternative strategy of maximizing intake (Aganga *et al.*, 2000).

Survival Advantage of Donkeys over Cattle

Maintenance costs: D.G. Smith and R.A. Pearson reviewed the factors that affect the survival of donkeys in semi-arid regions of sub-Saharan Africa.

Donkeys appear to have a survival advantage over cattle. Results of several studies showed that donkeys have two energetic advantages over cattle that may affect their ability to survive drought conditions (Smith and Pearson, 2005). 1. Although the energy cost of standing per kg of live weight is higher in donkeys than in cattle, the live weight of adult donkeys (150-200 kg) is much lower than that of adult cattle (250-500 kg) kept by small-holders in sub-Saharan Africa. The daily maintenance requirements for energy of donkeys (18-24 MJ/day) are therefore much less than those of cattle (24-48 MJ/day); donkeys only need to consume around half the daily amount of net energy compared to cattle in order to survive. 2. The energy cost of walking in donkeys is about half that of cattle and donkeys expend much less energy in foraging than do cattle. A donkey that typically forages for 16 h per day will expend approximately 26% less energy per kg of live weight than a cow that spends typically 10 h per day foraging.

Water requirements: Experimental studies conducted to compare the ability of donkeys and Zebu cattle to tolerate dehydration revealed that donkeys were only slightly more able to tolerate long-term water deprivation than zebu cattle. Donkeys appear more able to tolerate thirst than are ponies. A greater ability to tolerate thirst, to re-hydrate rapidly and to maintain appetite may give donkeys a survival advantage during times of drought over less thirst-tolerant animals. The ability to withstand dehydration and tolerate thirst should not be equated with an overall lower water requirement. Donkeys require as frequent access to water as any other type of livestock; donkeys that had free access to water drank more than those that had access only every 48 or 72 h.

Nutritional factors: Standard texts on donkey nutrition give conflicting estimates of the voluntary dry matter intake (DMI) of donkeys. McCarthy (1989) estimated daily DMI of between 1.75% and 2.25% of body weight, while Fielding and Krause (1998) estimated daily DMI of between 2.5% and 3% of body weight. A summary of published studies showed that it ranges between 0.9% and 2.5% of live weight (Smith and Pearson, 2005). The analysis of published results also revealed that donkeys and, to a lesser extent, ponies are able to maintain intakes of poor-quality forages that would cause a depression of feed intake in cattle. In terms of drought survival, donkeys have an advantage over cattle in that they have a low DMI requirement, which they can maintain when feed quality is low, but are as efficient at extracting nutrients as cattle.

Foraging behaviour: The foraging behaviour of donkeys may give them three advantages over cattle in drought survival (Smith and Pearson,

2005): 1. Donkeys are able to select a diet that is of better quality than that of cattle from the same area of rangeland. 2. Donkeys spend longer foraging during the day, which gives them more time to find feed of better quality. 3. Donkeys have a lower DMI requirement and therefore can more easily satisfy this requirement with feed of better quality.

References

Aganga, A.A. and Tsopito, C.M., 1998. A note on the feeding behaviour of domestic donkeys: a Botswana case study. Applied Animal Behaviour Science, 60, 235-239.

Aganga, A.A., Letso, M. and Aganga, A.O., 2000. Feeding donkeys. Livestock Research for Rural Development, 12, 1-7.

Coverdale, J.A., Moore, J.A., Tayler, H.D. and Miller-Auwerda, P.A., 2004. Soybean hulls as an alternative feed for horses. Journal of Animal Science, 82, 1663-1668.

Cunha, T.J., 1991. Horse feeding and nutrition. 2nd ed., Academic Press.

Fielding, D. and Krause, P., 1998. Physiology, nutrition and feeding. In D. Fielding and P. Krause (eds.), Donkeys, MacMillan Education, London, 14-31.

Lewis, L.D., 1982. Feeding and care of the horse. 1st ed., Media, P.A: Williams & Wilkins.

Malacarne, M., Martuzzi, F., Summer, A. and Mariani, P., 2002. Protein and fat composition of mare's milk: some nutritional remarks with reference to human and cow's milk. International Dairy Journal, 12, 869-877.

McCarthy, G., 1989. The principles and practice of feed rationing for donkeys. In E.D. Svendsen (ed.), The Professional Handbook of the Donkey, 2nd edn., Donkey Sanctuary, Sidmouth, 54-63.

Parker, R., 2003. Equine Science. 2nd edition, Thomson and Delmar Learning.

Pathak, N.N., 1987. Feeding of equines. In: Advanced Animal Nutrition for Developing Countries (ed) U.B. Singh, Published by Indo-Vision Private Ltd., Ghaziabad, pp. 450-459.

Pearson, R.A., Archibald, R.F. and Muirhead, R.H., 2001. The effect of forage quality and level of feeding on digestibility and gastrointestinal transit time of oat straw and alfalfa given to ponies and donkeys. British Journal of Nutrition, 85, 599-606.

Pilliner, S., 1998. Practical feeding of horses and ponies, Blackwell Science Ltd, United Kingdom.

Raut, B., Ranjhan, S.K. and Pathak, N.N., 1982. Indian Journal of Animal Science, 39, 1045.

Smith, D.G. and Pearson, R.A., 2005. A review of the factors affecting the survival of donkeys in semi-arid regions of sub-Saharan Africa. Tropical Animal Health and Production, 37 (Suppl. 1), 1-19.

Subcommittee on Horse Nutrition, National Research Council. 1989. Nutrient Requirements of Horses, 5th Revised Edition, Washington, D.C., National Academy Press.

11

Efficiency of Feed Conversion to Animal Products in Farm Animals and Poultry

Milk, meat and eggs are foods of superior nutritive value. The most successful human diet in terms of the optimum nutrition of people is one that contains animal products. Wittwer (1975) reviewed the potentials for increasing food production and pointed out that animals can either add to the total supply or be directly competitive. For example, poultry, swine, dogs, cats and other pets compete for human food supply. In contrast, most of the milk and meat produced in the world by cattle, buffaloes, sheep and goats result from grazing nonarable land and from the use of waste byproducts and crop residues. Thus ruminants add to human food supply. Of course, poultry provide eggs and swine provide ham and bacon. Out of the world's land area of about 13.4 billion hectares is only 10% arable, 22% permanent pastures and meadows, 30% forests and the remainder 38% nonproductive.

Domestic ruminants utilize much of the pastures and meadows and some of the forests to produce meat and milk. In many countries animals provide traction power to produce and transport crops.

Two centuries ago, English clergyman and pioneer economist Thomas Malthus argued that population growth inevitably outpaces food output unless checked by moral restraint, disease or famine. Efficiency and productivity are key to feeding our growing population while minimizing agricultural use of land, water, energy and other resources. Animal nutrition plays a critical role in this effort. Properly nourished animals are healthier, grow faster, use feed more efficiently and produce meat, milk and eggs that are more nutritious.

Efficiency of Production

	Efficiency of Production/ha/year	
	Energy (MJ)	Protein (kg)
Dairy cow (milk)	12,000	150
Potato	1,80,000	220
Sugarcane (the most efficient crop in terms of energy production, yield 18 tonnes/ha)	3,00,000	–
Pea	15,000	325

Plant Production Versus Animal Production

Observe the data presented in respect of dairy cow and potato, sugarcane and pea crops.

Plant production is far more efficient in terms of edible energy and protein per acre of land than animal production.

This shows that a typical high protein, low energy crop like peas produce 25% more energy and more than twice as much protein than obtained by the production of milk. This example depicts that production of food from animal source is inefficient.

Why is Production of Food from Animals Inefficient?

Plant production is inherently more efficient than animal production because it is carried out mainly by green plants which capture solar energy to synthesize carbohydrates, fats and protein from CO_2, H_2O and inorganic nitrogen. Farm animals, on the other hand, depend on the consumption of the very same carbohydrates, fats and proteins produced by green plants and convert them into edible tissue, milk and eggs with an efficiency that does not exceed about 26% for protein and 18% for energy but may be very low for both.

Animals convert only a portion of the feed nutrients they consume to human food. For this reason protagonists of vegetarianism say a much larger population could be fed if humans ate plant products directly rather than feeding the plant products to animals and using their (animal) products for food. But animal products (milk, meat and eggs) supply good quality proteins and other important nutrients vital to the health and well-being of humans.

In addition, man has had an appetite for meat and animal products through the years. Hence it is essential to use certain animals as 'mediators' for food production from the plant products. Because of the low efficiency of animal production and the fact that it requires added investment and operating expenses, food from animal sources is considerably more expensive than food from plants.

Precision animal nutrition is considered as one of the biggest contributors to animal welfare. Enhancing animal welfare through precision animal nutrition (see page No. 366) and livestock and sustainability of global food system are briefed in this chapter.

Biological Factors that Affect the Overall Efficiency of Animal Production

1. *Efficiency of production of animals as producers of human food:* Estimated percentage overall efficiency of converting fodder into edible animal products (Wedin *et al.* (1975) J. Anim. Sci., 41: 667-686)

Animal Species	Crude Protein	Energy
	%	
Non-ruminants		
Broilers	23	11
Turkeys	22	9
Layers	26	18
Swine	14	14
Ruminants		
Dairy cattle	25	17
Beef cattle	4	3
Mutton (Sheep one lamb/year)	4	2.4
twins		3.4
triplets		4.2

These values indicate that the efficiency of conversion of plant products to edible animal products varies from about 2 to 18% for energy and from 4 to 26% for protein.

2. *Rate of production:* Within each animal species and product, the efficiency of feed conversion depends primarily on the rate of production and the level of feeding, which are closely related (Table 1). At an increased rate of production the feed intake of the animal increases and the proportion of feed expended on maintenance decreases. This is beneficial since feed consumed for maintenance produces no product.

Obviously, as the level of feed intake increases, in terms of multiples of the maintenance requirement, from one to two, three, four and so on, the proportion of the ration expended on maintenance and wasted decreases from one to 1/2, 1/3, 1/4, and so on. At the same time, the proportion of the ration which supports production increases in a curvilinear fashion from zero to 1/2, 2/3, 3/4 and so on. The gross efficiency of production increases proportionately as the rate of production increases.

Table 1   Feed Intake of Producing Animals in Terms of Multiples of the Maintenance Requirement.

Class of stock and level of production	Feed intake in multiples maintenance
Dairy cow (550 kg wt)	
Producing 13 kg milk/day	2.0
Producing 30 kg milk/day	4.0
Steer (300 kg)	
Daily gain 400 g/day	1.4
Daily gain 700 g/day	1.7
Daily gain 1000 g/day	2.0
Pig (50 kg)	
Daily gain 750 g/day	2.3
Poultry (1.0 kg)	
Daily gain 27 g/day	1.5
Poultry (1.4 kg)	
Laying 40%	1.33
Laying 80%	1.67

3. *Gastrointestinal physiology: ruminants versus monogastrics:* The efficiency of all animal production is limited by the incomplete digestion and transformation of feed into tissue, milk and eggs. In ruminants, microbial fermentation further limits the efficiency of conversion of the combustible energy of feed. A great proportion of the diet undergoes an added transformation into microbial matters and into volatile fatty acids (VFA). Although the VFA are efficiently absorbed, the heat increment in ruminants is relatively high. As a result, the ME or NE content of most of the diets is lower in ruminants than in monogastric species. Science behind the methane formation and the methane mitigation practices are detailed later (page No. 367).

On high-protein diets ruminal digestion may well reduce the quantity and quality of protein in the digesta. Rumen microflora converts poor quality protein and even nonprotein nitrogen into high quality protein.

4. *Type of animal product: Meat versus milk and egg production:* Meat production is considerably less efficient than milk and egg production. The reasons are :

   (a) Only part of the carcass of animals is edible. A variable but large proportion of offal (skin, hair, bone, feathers, blood, intestine, body fat, etc.) reduces the amount of edible meat, although all the offal may be converted into useful byproducts. On the otherhand, milk and eggs (except the shell) are edible products.

   (b) The other reason for the low efficiency of meat production is related to the rate of production. Animals raised exclusively for meat consume a lower multiple of their maintenance requirement than lactating ruminants or egg-laying hens.

5. *Sex of the animal:* The males of all the farm species are more efficient meat producers than the females. Males grow faster than females. Males are also leaner than females and produce less offal fat.

6. *Fertility:* Regular conception and normal pregnancy in animals minimize the periods of low production, especially the duration of the dry period.

   Prolificacy (high fecundity) in pigs greatly increases their overall efficiency. Sheep and goats are intermediate in prolificacy among farm mammals. Twins and triplets are common in goats and in some breeds of sheep. Beef cow at best produces one offspring a year and this considerably reduces the relative overall efficiency of beef cattle husbandry.

   In the domestic fowl, prolificacy surpasses the level required for maximizing the efficiency of meat production and is the condition which permits egg production to be a highly efficient system of animal production.

7. *Age and weight:* Young animals have more lean mass and less body fat. The amount of fat increases with age. The overall efficiency of meat production decreases when meat animals are raised longer beyond a specific age. Optimal slaughter time varies with the genetics

of breed and with the environment, including diet, climate and husbandry.

As the protein and fat laid down in the body varies with the age of the animal the feed efficiency also varies. For example, feed efficiency for growing (20-35) Large White Yorkshrie (LWY) pigs is 3.13 to 3.35 while for finishing (35-65 kg) LWY pigs it is 3.82 to 4.13 for feeds with varying energy and protein ratios.

Feed Efficiency for Milk Production

Efficient dairy production is characterized by high milk production per animal and aims at efficient conversion of feed energy and nutrients to human-edible food, such as milk and meat. Dairy efficiency is defined as yield of milk per unit of dietary dry matter (DM) consumed. It is not commonly measured in dairy herds as is feed conversion to weight gain in swine, beef, and poultry. Variation between animals in feed conversion efficiency (FCE) may have genetic components, allowing selection for animals with greater efficiency and reduced environmental impact. Feed efficiency for milk production depends on diet and other environmental factors and on the genetic ability of the cow to utilize these inputs to produce milk. Greater daily milk yield, high quality forages and improved feed digestibility increases dairy efficiency. Animals in early lactation have higher dairy efficiency. Inclement environmental / weather conditions, animals in late lactation, animals of first lactation have low dairy efficiency.

The most promising approach is by improving productivity and efficiency through better nutritional management (Gerber et al., 2013). High concentrate and lipid supplementation is considered the most effective in lowering methane production per unit of energy intake. A myriad of other supplements and additives are currently being investigated to mitigate the methane emission. The biological mechanism is to shift rumen fermentation towards propionogenesis, whereas fibrous diets result in a preferential production of acetate, butyrate and methane.

The data on the effect of breed (purebreds, crossbreds, buffaloes, graded buffaloes and nondescript animals, tables 2, 3 and 4), feed processing, total mixed ration versus conventional ration and precision feeding on feed conversion ratio has been furnished in the following for clarity.

Efficiency of Feed Conversion in Indian Dairy Animals

V.D. Mudgal *et. al.* (2003) presented data on efficiency of feed conversion in Indian Dairy animals based on research work conducted at NDRI, Karnal for full lactation milk output. Feed intakes were high quality forages 80% and

Table 2 Purebred Holstein cows, USA, UK

S.No	Feed dry matter per kg milk yield	Source
1	0.54 to 0.87	T R Dhiman et al., 1993, J Dairy Sci, 76, 1945
2	0.55 to 0.91	T R Dhiman and L D Salter 1993, J Dairy Sci. 76, 1960
3	0.65 to 0.73	T R Dhiman et al., 2001, Anim Feed Sci Technol, 90, 169
4	Early lactation = 0.53 to 0.56; Mid lactation = 0.71 to 0.75; Late lactation = 0.94 to 1.09	R M Kirkland and F J Gordon, 2001,Livest Prod Sci 72,213.

Table 3 Crossbred cows, India

S.No	Feed dry matter per kg milk yield	Source
1	0.95 to 1.04	S K Chouraba et al., 2003, Indian J Anim Sci73, 1353.
2	0.85 to 0.87	Puranik et al., 1997, Indian J Anim Sci 67, 146.
	2.03 to 2.07	S Radotra and V S Upadhay, 2002, Indian J Anim Sci72, 815.
4.	1.94 to 2.15	R C Saha et al., 2002, Anim Nutr Feed Tech., 2, 83.
5	2.42 to 2.84	K S Rao et al., 1999, Indian J Anim Nutr., 16, 155.

Table 4 Buffaloes, India

S.No	Feed dry matter per kg milk yield	Source
1	3.44 to 3.85	D P Tiwari and B R Patle, 1997, Indian J Anim Nutr., 14, 98.
2	2.80 to 3.22	D Nagalakshmi et al., 2004, Anim Nutr Feed Tech., 4, 23.
3.	1.60 to 1.82	A K Mishra et al., 2007, Indian J Anim Sci 77, 405.

concentrate mixture 20%. The percent TDN output/input for crossbred cows (Karan Swiss), Sahiwal cows, Murrah buffaloes and well-fed desi cow, respectively, were 25, 28, 19 and 6; the data for percent protein output/input were 24, 24, 15 and 4.5. It is evident that high yielding animals were most efficient in converting feed nutrients to milk nutrients.

The quantity of dry mater intake consumed per litre milk yield was also calculated and the values were 1.09, 1.10, 2.09 and 5.98 for Karan Swiss cows, Sahiwal cows, Murrah buffaloes and non-descript cows, respectively.

Effect of Feed Processing on Feed Efficiency

B.V.S. Reddy and coworkers from ICRISAT, Patancheru, India identified Sweet sorghum [*Sorghum bicolour* (L.) moench] as a potential alternative raw material for bioethanol and bioenergy. It can produce stalk to a tune of 54-69 t/ha. The bagasse produced after juice extraction from stalks can be used as animal feed. The feed value of the sweet sorghum bagasse is not less than that of non-sweet stem, which is the mainstay of the feed market in and around Hyderabad, India (Blummel et al., 2009).

Venkata Seshaiah et al. (2013) studied the effect of differently processed sweet sorghum bagasse based complete rations on cost economics in graded Murrah buffaloes (450 kg; average 3 lactations) [Buffalo Bulletin, 32 (3) 231-238]. The results revealed that sweet sorghum bagasse can be used as an alternative roughage source to sorghum straw and the expander-extruder pellet bagasse based complete ration found to be efficient and gave higher profits (Table 5).

Table 5 Effect of feeding differently processed sweet sorghum bagasse based complete rations on feed conversion ratio and cost of milk production in lactating graded Murrah buffaloes

Parameter	Straw SSM	Chopped SSBC	Mash SSBM	Pellet SSBP	SEM
Feed intake, kg	12.04[a]	11.76[b]	12.13[a]	12.16[a]	0.10
Feed conversion ratio, kg /kg milk yield	2.28[b]	2.27[b]	2.19[b]	1.76[a]	0.01
Cost of feed, Rs/d	96.62[a]	75.56[c]	79.15[b]	81.78[b]	0.22
Cost of feed/kg milk, Rs	18.26[a]	14.61[b]	14.29[b]	11.83[c]	0.07

Each value is the average of six observations; [a,b] Values bearing the different superscripts in a row differ significantly (P<0.05); SEM: Standard error of means; SSM: Sorghum straw and concentrate mixture in 50:50 ratio processed into mash form; SSBC: Chopped sweet sorghum bagasse and concentrate mixture in 50:50 ratio in complete ration; SSBM: Sweet sorghum bagasse and concentrate mixture in 50:50 ratio complete ration in mash form; SSBP: Sweet sorghum bagasse and concentrate mixture in 50:50 ratio complete ration in 16 mm expander-extruder pellet form.

Effect of total mixed ration vis-à-vis conventional ration on feed efficiency: From the data presented in the Table, it can be concluded that feeding of maize stover based TMR supplied adequate nutrients and showed a positive tendency in improving milk yield thus reducing the cost of milk production (Table 6).

Table 6   Effect of feeding conventional and total mixed ration (TMR) on feed efficiency and cost economics in graded Murrah buffaloes in a 120-day on-farm lactation trial*

Parameter	Conventional ration (20kg green fodder, 4kg paddy straw & 3kg Concentrate Mixture)	TMR (Maize stover & Concentrate Mixture 60:40)
Total dry matter intake (kg/d)	11.00 ±0.14	11.19 ±0.10
Milk Yield (Kg)**	6.02 ±0.13	6.73 ±0.10
6%FCM (%)**	5.53 ±0.10	6.51 ±0.12
Feed efficiency (kg DMl/kg 6% FCM)**	1.99 ±0.07	1.70 ±0.10
Total cost of feed (₹ Id)	61.40 ±0.21	62.30 ±0.19
Cost of feed /kg 6% FCM (₹)**	11.10 ±0.39	9.57 ±0.58

* K Raja Kishore, D Srinivas Kumar, J.V. Ramana and E Raghava Rao (2013) Animal Science Reporter; TMR had 12.8% CP, 42.5% CF, 58.9% NDF & 33.7% ADF; " Values in the rows differ significantly (P<0.01)

Precision Animal Nutrition and Feed Efficiency

The primary objective of raising livestock and poultry is to produce good quality animal products in the form of milk, meat and eggs to the consumers as a profitable enterprise with least contribution to climate change in a precision animal nutrition mode (Reddy and Krishna, 2009). It is well documented worldwide that imbalanced nutrition is a major factor, in addition to shortage of feed, responsible for low livestock productivity. Balanced nutrition contributes to improving animal output as well as to reducing both the cost of production and the emission of greenhouse gases per unit of animal product.

Feeding a balanced ration can increase net daily income by 10-15 percent for those having one-two cows and/or buffaloes and can reduce enteric methane emissions by 15-20 percent per kg of milk produced (FAO, 2012).

Enhancing Animal Welfare Through Precision Nutrition

Maintaining healthy animals is a key component of animal welfare. Feed has a fundamental influence on productivity, health and welfare of the animal. Feed quality influences animal product quality and safety, and the environment. To achieve balance among these parameters, the animal's nutritional requirements must be properly met. That is where precision animal nutrition matters.

Production systems and animal welfare: In intensive production systems, animals are being pushed towards maximizing productivity. Here animals receive inappropriate or excessive diets which might compromise their health and welfare (for example occurrence of metabolic diseases, increased excretion of N, P, ammonia, etc into the environment). In extensive and smallholder systems in developing countries, animal productivity and animal welfare are compromised by inadequate nutrition. An array of management-related factors such as housing and bedding, restraining systems, space and crowding, transport conditions, stunning and slaughter methods, castration of males and tail docking affect welfare (FAO, 2013). That means on-farm animal husbandry practices are intrinsically linked with animal welfare.

Precision animal nutrition is considered as one of the biggest contributors to animal welfare. Sufficient dietary fibre is important to prevent feather pecking in birds. Ensuring good rumen health in ruminant animals is key for the maintenance of efficiency and productivity, and thus herd profitability.

Livestock and sustainability of global food system

Livestock is the largest land use sector on Earth. The livestock sector occupies 30% of the world's ice-free surface and contributes 40% of global agricultural gross domestic product. It uses the vast areas of rangelands, one-third of the fresh water and one-third of global cropland as feed (Herrero et al., 2013b). The ever-increasing human population (more than 9 billion by 2050), together with increasing demand for livestock products (caused by urbanization, increasing incomes and nutritional and environmental concerns) is exerting a great pressure on the global food system.

The livestock sector contributes significantly to global warming through GHG emissions (see page no. 369). Livestock sector is also responsible for environmental (nutrient) pollution and land degradation. At the same time, livestock is an invaluable source of nutrition (critically important proteins and micronutrients) and livelihood for millions of poor people. Livestock also provide nutrients for crops. There is growing recognition that the following are essential for the sustainability of the global food system (Herrero et al., 2013a; Herrero et al., 2013b).

- Improvement in resource use efficiency
- Improvement in environmental performance of livestock systems
- Establishment of sustainable levels of consumption of animal-sourced foods

Global Livestock Systems

Livestock production systems (LPS) vary substantially and this heterogeneity of livestock production systems offer great opportunity to exploit the large mitigation potential inherent in the diverse production systems. Herrero et al. (2013b) provided the first systematic quantification of global livestock systems in terms of feed use, feed conversion efficiency, land productivity, and non-CO_2 emission intensity. They distinguished eight production systems for ruminants and two production systems for monogastrics. In simple terms, they vary from extensive rangeland systems to mixed crop-livestock to industrial livestock systems. In terms of livestock productivity, these may qualify as low-input low-output systems (extensive rangeland systems) to more efficient and productive livestock systems (industrial livestock systems).

Havlik et al. (2014) investigated the role of livestock production system transitions (LPSTs) in achieving climate policy targets (i.e. decreasing emission of GHGs). Transitions to more efficient livestock production systems present an attractive mitigation opportunity for reducing CH_4 and N_2O emissions per unit of livestock product while simultaneously increasing productivity. Hence sustainable intensification of livestock production systems might become a key climate mitigation technology (Havlik et al., 2014).

Science behind Methane emissions and its mitigation measures

Methane emissions by the ruminant animals are not only an environmental hazard but represent also a loss of energy from the animal. In dairy cows, the CH_4 energy loss (% of gross energy intake) is about 5.3 to 6.1% (Benchaar et al., 2013; Hassanat et al., 2013). Methane emission from ruminant depends on the diet composition and quantity of feed consumed. The methane production (Haque et al., 2014) ranges from 13.9 to 14.2 g/kg energy-corrected milk, 18.7 to 19.6 g/kg dry matter intake and 438 to 447 g/day.

Methane and carbon dioxide are natural byproducts of fermentation of carbohydrates (Figure 1) and, to a lesser extent, amino acids in the rumen and the hindgut of farm animals. Methane is produced by highly-specialised methanogenic prokaryotes, all of which are archaea (Methanogenic archae). The vast majority of methane production occurs in the reticulorumen and exhaled from the nose and mouth. Only 13% of total enteric methane is produced in the hindgut of sheep and only about 11% is excreted through the anus (Murry et al., 1976). If hydrogen is allowed to accumulate in the rumen, it depresses digestion, so the archae remove it as methane.

Methods to estimate methane production: (1). Traditional respiration chamber method (Blaxter and Clappert, 1965): Open circuit respiration chamber can measure with high accuracy but only on few animals and not in their natural environment. (2). Sulfur hexafluoride (SF_6) tracer technique (Johnson et al., 1994): This method has been standardized and used by NDDB workers to measure methane in dairy animals in different parts of India at field level. (3). The newly developed CO_2-method (Madsen et al., 2010): It is a pertinent technique to get measurements on many animals within a short time and evaluating differences between feeds with a reasonable precision.

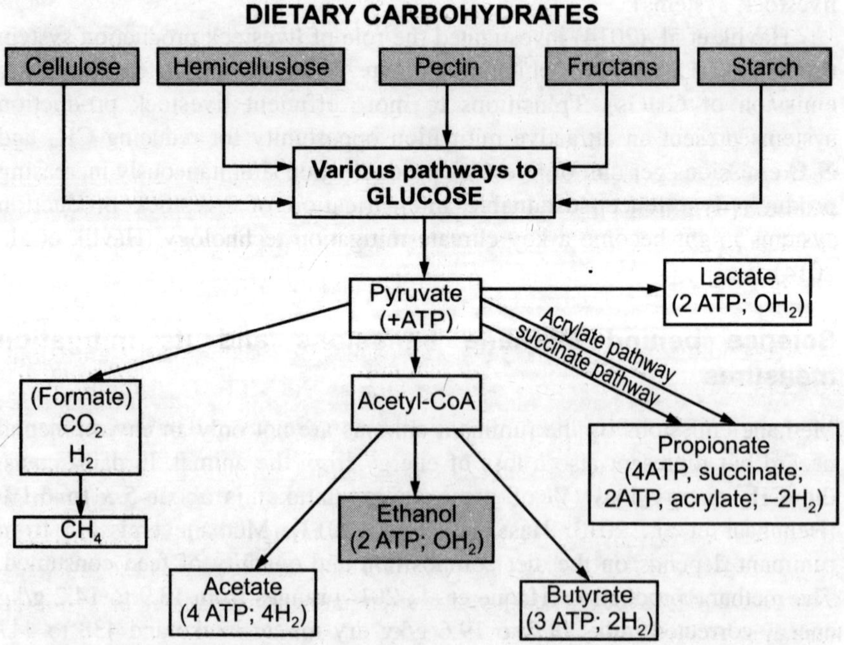

Figure 1 Simplified from Van Soest, 1994 and Russell and Wallace, 1997

Figure represents a simplified fermentation pathways and end-product formation from carbohydrates in the rumen environment. The general stoichiometry of the reactions (Van Soest, 1994) is as follows.

Glucose + ammonia = Microbes + Methane + Carbon dioxide + VFA

The basic problem in anaerobic metabolism is the storage of oxygen (i.e. as CO_2) and disposal of hydrogen (H_2) equivalents (i.e. as CH_4). Methane is the most important "2H" sink, the next being the VFA, propionate. Considering that acetate, propionate, butyrate, CO_2 and CH_4 are the only fermentation products and that all fermentation products are formed from plant carbohydrates with the monomer formula $C_6H_{12}O_6$ (glucose), the amount of glucose moles fermented may be described (Wolin, 1960) as

Glucose = 0.5 acetate + 0.5 propionate + butyrate; one mole of glucose yields 0.61 moles of methane (Hristov et al., 2013).

Mitigation of Greenhouse Gas Emissions in Livestock Production

Animal production is a significant source of greenhouse gas (GHGs: methane, CO_2 & N_2O) emissions worldwide. Livestock sector emits about 18% of total global anthropogenic GHG emissions (Steinfeld et al., 2006). In a recent report entitled 'Tackling climate change through livestock: A global assessment of emissions, and mitigations opportunities' (FAO, 2013), it is stated that GHG emissions associated with livestock supply chains add up to 14.5% of all human caused GHG releases. The main sources of emissions are: feed production and processing (45% of the total), outputs of GHG during digestion by cows (39%), and manure decomposition (10%). The remainder is attributable to the processing and transportation of animal products.

Depending on the accounting approaches and scope of the emissions covered, estimates by various sources such as TPCC, FAO, EPA or others' place livestock contribution to global anthropogenic GHG emissions at between 7 and 18 % (Hristov et al., 2013). The current analysis was conducted to evaluate the potential of nutritional, manure and animal husbandry practices for mitigating methane (CH_4) and nitrous oxide (N_2O) – i.e. non-CO_2 – GHG emissions from livestock production. These practices were categorized into enteric methane, manure management and animal husbandry mitigation practices.

Enteric Methane Mitigation Practices

- Increasing forage digestibility and digestible forage intake (chemical treatments of low-quality feeds, strategic supplementation of the diet, ration balancing and crop selection for straw quality are effective mitigation strategies)
- Inclusion of dietary lipid/concentrate feed or strategic supplementation of concentrate to all-forage diets; processing of grain to increase its digestibility: These should not compromise digestibility of fibre.
- Several feed supplements have a potential to reduce methane emission from ruminants. These include nitrates, ionophors, dietary (condensed) tannins, some direct-fed microbials such as yeast-based products.

Overall, improving feed quality and the overall efficiency of dietary nutrient use is an effective way of decreasing GHG emissions per unit of animal product.

Manure Management Mitigation Practices

- Manure storage is a source of methane emission and a source of nitrous oxide.
- Decreased digestibility of dietary nutrients is expected to increase fermentable organic matter concentration in manure, which may increase manure methane emissions.
- Feeding protein close to animal requirements following the phase feeding of protein as per the life stage is an effective manure ammonia and nitrous oxide mitigation practice. Rumen degradable protein and bypass protein need to be fed in a balanced way to avoid ammonia losses and optimize animal productivity in ruminants. Decreasing total dietary protein and supplementing the diet with synthetic amino acids is an effective ammonia and nitrous oxide mitigation strategy for non-ruminants.
- Diets for all species should be balanced for amino acids to avoid feed intake depression and decreased animal productivity.

Animal husbandry mitigation practices: Increasing animal productivity can be a very effective strategy for reducing GHG emissions per unit of livestock product. For example, improving the genetic potential of animals and achieving that potential through proper nutrition and improvements in reproductive efficiency, animal health and reproductive lifespan are effective and recommended approaches for improving animal productivity and reducing GHG emission intensity.

12

Body Composition of Animals

Significance of Body Composition of Live Animals

Knowledge of body composition is necessary in nutritional and clinical studies.

1. *Nutritional evaluation:* In many nutritional studies on the effect of diet on the performance, growth rate and feed efficiency are the criteria used. But changes in the body composition are of importance, since it has been shown that changes can occur while growth remains unaltered. The measurement of weight and size of body in nutritional studies do not reflect the true picture of body composition. e.g. infantile growth consists of more water, protein and bone minerals and less fat. Weight gains do not provide a good basis for evaluating nutritional adequacy whereas body composition would yield information on the nature of such gains, muscle, bone or fat.

2. *Evaluating leanness in farm animals:* Body composition is also important in evaluation programme of animals of superior muscle development for breeding purposes and in evaluating changes in the body while on special hormonal or other physiological treatments.

3. *Clinical implications:* Information on the effect of undernutrition or injury on body composition (electrolyte balance and body water) is useful as a tool for diagnosing and following treatment effects in a number of pathological conditions.

4. *Exercise and physical training:* Body composition changes during physical training provide useful data of information for evaluating the effectiveness of the dietary regimen.

Determination of whole body composition: Measuring body composition by direct method i.e. slaughter method is laborious and the data (of body composition) on a given animal can be obtained only once, although what is desired is information on its changing body composition due to the ration fed or treatment. Hence body composition estimation by indirect methods is quite popular since it facilitate to know the body composition of the living animal.

Determination of the whole body composition using chemical analyses or comparison at slaughter cannot be used on valuable animals or when sequential studies of the same subject are required. Therefore, during the period 1980-2000 many efforts have been made to find non-destructive methods to predict in *vivo* body compostion in different species.

Let us study various indirect methods available.

Indirect Methods for Estimating Body Composition

1. *Chemical methods:* The principle employed is that lean body mass of animal (i.e. empty body weight less weight of fat) is reasonably constant in composition. This means that if the weight of water in the living animal can be measured, the weight of protein, fat and ash can then be calculated by using the multiple regression equations.

   Body water can be determined by 'dilution' techniques. These involve the injection of compounds known to go into solution in body water and the quantitative determination of dilution of a marker used, after equilibrium has been reached. The marker substances most commonly employed are antipyrene and its analogs (N-acetyl-4-aminoantipyrene, 4-aminoantipyrene) and water containing radioactive isotopes of hydrogen, tritium, or its heavy isotope, deuterium. One difficulty with these techniques is that the markers mix not only with actual body water, but also with the water present in the gut (in ruminants as much as 30% of total body water may be in the gut contents).

   A second chemical method for estimating body composition *in vivo* is based on the concentration of potassium in the lean body mass. Lean muscle mass can be estimated from whole body counting of ^{40}K to calculate protein.

2. *Densitometric methods:* The composition of the carcass is often estimated without dissection or chemical analysis from its density or specific gravity. Fat has an appreciably lower specific gravity than bone and muscle, and the fatter the carcass the lower will be its specific gravity. The specific gravity of carcass is determined by

weighing it in air and in water, but this method has technical difficulties which make it imprecise.

Hydrodensitometry is a commonly used reference method in humans for measuring body fat mass or fat - free mass. This method assumes a constant density of the fat - free mass as 1.1 kg/L and that of the fat mass as 0.9 kg/L. Body density is calculated from weight in air and from underwater weight (submerged to neck in a sitting position) with simultaneous determination of the residual lung volume by the dilution. Body fat is calculated from body density.

3. *Dual-energy X-ray absorptiometry (DEXA):* This is a novel, noninva-sive technique available for the *in vivo* measurement of body composition. This method is widely used for the measurement of bone mineral and soft tissue composition in small animals. Body composition of humans is determined by the Lunar DPX whole body X-ray densitometer at medium scan mode.

4. More advanced *in vivo* techniques such as ultrasonic scanning for fat measurements (Scanogram), computerised tomography (CT) scanning, nuclear magnetic resonance spectroscopy (NMRS) can be used in breeding studies selection for dressing percentage and carcass quality among young bulls. It seems such high investment in equipment appears to be justified in view of favourable cost/benefit ratios.

5. Another non-invasive technique, total body electrical conductivity (TOBEC), has been shown to accurately predict lean body mass or weight of total body water in mammals such as swine, rat, humans, rabbits, etc. This technique is cheaper and easier to use than X-ray computerized tomography or nuclear magnetic resonance. Moreover, it needs less preparation than ultrasound, which required the shaving of the animal. However, it showed only medium accuracy in predicting body fat in birds and in anaesthetized rabbits.

The studies conducted on female rabbits (steady state awake animals) revealed that TOBEC is a non-invasive, safe and quick procedure and appears to be accurate in predicting body water and body energy in reproducing rabbits at different physiological states (Fortun-Lamothe et al., 2002). However, this method is not accurate in predicting the body proteins and ash content of rabbit does.

13

Foodstuffs, Nutrients and their Functions

Proteins

The term protein is a collective one which embraces an enormous group of closely related but physiologically distinct members.

Elementary composition of proteins: In common with the fats and carbohydrates, the proteins contain carbon, hydrogen, oxygen and a large but fairly constant percentage of nitrogen. Most proteins also contain sulfur and a few contain phosphorus and iron. A typical protein has carbon 51-55, hydrogen 6.5-7.3, nitrogen 15.5-18.0, oxygen 21.5-23.5, sulfur 0.5-2.0, phosphorus 0.0-01.5% and iron.

Proteins are polymers of amino acids which vary in relative amount and kind from protein to protein. There are some 20 to 22 different amino acids present in proteins. The classification of amino acids is described in Chapter 4 of *Principles of Animal Nutrition and Feed Technology*. In 1955 the work of Sanger and associates culminated in the determination of the complete primary structure of the hormone polypeptide insulin (Molecular wt. 6000), a brilliant achievement for which Sanger received the Nobel prize.

Amino Acids and Protein Quality

The recognition that the nitrogen present in the body had its origin in nitrogen compounds present in the food dates primarily from the work of Francois Magendie published in 1816. After it became established that proteins were the nitrogen compounds essentially concerned, Magendie produced the first evidence that all proteins were not of equal value through his famous "gelatin report" published in 1841. This finding stimulated growth and nitrogen balance studies by German, Swiss and Danish scientists as to why gelatin was inferior.

The first satisfactory explanation as to why proteins differ in nutritional quality was proposed around 1870 by L. Hermann, a German Physiologist who stated that digestion produce units (amino acids now) and all these units were needed in the food. In 1876 Escher (a Swiss physiologist), fed dogs a purified diet containing gelatin, which caused them to lose weight. Weight was maintained when tyrosine was added. Amino acid analysis of proteins by Abderhalden in Germany provided the basis for more meaningful studies by Kauffmann who showed that gelatin was deficient in cystine besides tyrosine. Willcock and Hopkins in England, using purified diets, showed that mice receiving zein (maize protein) as the sole protein ingredient died, while those receiving casein (milk protein) lived.

In 1909 Osborne and Mendel in USA began their classic purified diet studies with rats using pure proteins. They found that certain proteins which caused nutritive failure could be rendered satisfactory by the addition of missing amino acids. Young rats lost weight on zein as the sole protein, but grew when lysine and tryptophan were added and maintained body weight on tryptophan supplementation.

Later Rose and Harper detailed the essential-nonessential or dispensable-indispensable amino acids.

Classification of Proteins

I According to Solubility and Structural Conformation

1. Fibrous Proteins (insoluble in water) e.g. collagen, elastin and keratin
2. Globular proteins (soluble in water or water containing certain salts) e.g. albumins and globulins (immunoglobulins, haemoglobin, lactoglobulins, myoglobins)
3. Intermediary (have fibrous structure but a solubility of the globular form) e.g. myosin of muscle and fibrinogen of blood.

II According to Composition

1. Simple proteins
2. Conjugated proteins

   (a) nucleoproteins (ribosomes; RNA)

   (b) lipoproteins (VLDL; phospholipid, cholesterol, neutral lipid)

   (c) glycoproteins (g globulin; galactose, mannose, hexosamine)

   (d) phosphoproteins (casein of milk, phosphate)

   (e) haemoproteins (haemoglobin, cytochrome c, catalase; iron protoporphyrin)

(f) flavoproteins (succinic dehydrogenase, D-amino acid oxidase; FAD)

(g) metalloprotein [(ferritin; Fe(OH₃), cytochrome oxidase; Fe and Cu, alcohol dehydrogenase; Zn, xanthine oxidase; Mo and Fe]

III According to Biological Function

1. Enzymes e.g. hexokinase, lactate dehydrogenase
2. Storage proteins e.g. ovalbumin, casein, ferritin, gliadin, zein
3. Transport proteins e.g. haemoglobin, haemocyanin, myoglobin, β_1-lipoprotein, ceruloplasmin
4. Contractile proteins e.g. myosin, actin
5. Protective proteins e.g. antibodies, fibrinogen, thrombin
6. Toxins e.g. ricin, gossypin
7. Hormones e.g. insulin, growth hormone
8. Structural proteins e.g. glycoproteins, α-keratin, collagen, elastin, mucoproteins

Nutritional Classification of Proteins

	Group	Limiting essential amino acids
I	Complete proteins e.g. Egg protein Promote good growth	Nil
II	Partially complete proteins e.g. Wheat proteins Promote moderate growth	Partially lacking in one or more EAAs
III	Incomplete proteins e.g. Gelatin, zein Do not promote growth	Completely lacking in one or more EAAs

Functions of proteins: Proteins are vital to any living organism. They are the important constituent of tissues and cells of the body. They form the important component of muscle and other tissues and vital body fluids like blood. The proteins in the form of enzymes and hormones are concerned with a wide range of vital metabolic processes in the body.

Proteins supply the body building material and make good the loss that occur due to wear and tear. Proteins as antibodies help the body to defend against infections. Thus proteins are vital to the living process and carry out a wide range of functions essential for the sustenance of life.

If the diet does not contain adequate carbohydrate and fat to provide energy, dietary protein may be broken down to provide energy which is a wasteful way of using proteins.

Foods or feeds with the same protein content have different values in nutrition, i.e. they differ in protein quality. Those proteins whose assortment of amino acids more nearly approximates the needs of the animal are of high quality and those who do not are of low quality. In a facetious vein, pig protein would be the best protein to feed pigs; nutritionally sound but economically disastrous.

Maize protein (zein) is very low in lysine and rich in leucine. Proteins of soybean meal, milk solids, whey or fish meal are much higher in lysine (Table 1). Relatively little difference exists with respect to valine. Evaluation of feeds for protein quality is dealt elsewhere (Refer Chapter 15 of *Principles of Animal Nutrition and Feed Technology*).

Table 1 Essential Amino Acid Content of the Proteins of Certain Feeds (as a % of total Protein).

Amino acid	Tankage	Meat meal	Blood meal	Fish meal	Milk	Egg	Cereal[a]	Animal[b]
Arginine	5.9	7.0	3.7	7.4	4.3	6.4	4.8	5.7
Histidine	2.7	2.0	4.9	2.4	2.6	2.1	2.1	3.3
Lysine	7.2	7.0	8.8	7.8	7.5	7.2	3.1	7.7
Tyrosine	2.9	3.2	3.7	4.4	5.3	4.5	4.8	3.9
Tryptophan	0.7	0.7	1.3	1.3	1.6	1.5	1.2	1.1
Phenylalanine	5.1	4.5	7.3	4.5	5.7	6.3	5.7	5.4
Cystine	-	1.0	1.8	1.2	1.0	2.4	1.7	1.2
Methionine	-	2.0	1.5	3.5	3.4	4.1	2.3	2.6
Threonine	3.0	4.0	6.5	4.5	4.5	4.0	3.4	4.5
Leucine	7.7	8.0	12.2	7.1	11.3	9.2	7.1[c]	9.2
Isoleucine	2.7	6.3	1.1	6.0	8.5	8.0	4.3	4.9
Valine	5.4	5.8	7.7	5.8	8.4	7.3	5.2	6.6

[a]Average based on wheat, corn, rye and oats.
[b]Average based on tankage, meat meal, blood meal, fish meal and milk.
[c]Corn is not included in this average. Of its protein 22% is leucine.
Source: Applied Animal Nutrition by Crampton and Harris.

Animal proteins are the mainstay of protein quality in rations for non-herbivorous animals. SBM, because of its higher BV, has replaced much of animal proteins.

Meat, milk and fish proteins are relatively rich in lysine, though they are likely to be short of methionine and cystine compared to egg protein. This can be overcome by fortification of the diet with pure methionine or vitamin B_{12} or both. Isoleucine level of meat meal, fish meal and milk is at least 50% higher than that of cereal protein. But blood meal (and consequently tankage, which contains blood) is low in isoleucine. Blood meal (and tankage) are valuable supplements to the plant proteins.

Proteins of cereals and pulses have a mutually supplementary effect in human nutrition. A combination of cereal and pulse in the ratio of 5:1 has been found to give an optimum combination. Cooking/heat treatment improves the digestibility of proteins of vegetable foods (particularly pulses). Low digestibility of plant proteins is due to the presence of trypsin inhibitors which are destroyed on cooking. On excessive heating, the lysine in proteins reacts with reducing sugars in foods and renders part of the lysine unavailable due to the 'maillard reaction'. (Refer textbook 'Principles of Animal Nutrition and Feed Technology' page No. 298)

Dietary fibre or Nonstarch polysaccharides (NSP): Cellulose, hemicellulose, gums, pectins and lignins comprise non-digestible carbohydrates in humans. It is already explained that these structural carbohydrates are not digested by the mammalian enzymes but by microbial enzymes. These are designated as dietary fibre or unavailable carbohydrates and most of them are voided as such and thus contribute to the bulk of stools. These are necessary for mechanism of digestion and elimination of waste. The fibre (insoluble fibre e.g., cellulose) stimulates the contraction of the muscular walls of the digestive tract and thus prevents constipation.

Lack of adequate dietary fibre (e.g. refined foods) leads to constipation and colon cancer in humans. Dietary fibre is of two types: soluble and insoluble. Gums, mucilages, etc. (soluble fibre) in the diets have been shown to lower blood cholesterol in hypercholesterolemic subjects and blood glucose in diabetics (delays absorption of glucose). e.g. oat bran (soluble fibre) intake at 3 g a day has been reported to reduce cholesterol by 5 to 6 mg per 100 ml blood. Vegetables (leafy vegetables), fruits, condiments, spices and unrefined cereals are comparatively rich in fibre. The daily diet of an adult person should contain at least 40 g of dietary fibre.

Addition of fibre to low fibre diets decreases the incidence of diverticulitis and constipation. High fibre diets also appear to reduce the incidence of appendicitis, cancer of colon and heart disease. There is only one downside to this story, and that is flatus, better known as "wind". A bit of wind is a small price to pay for a happy gut.

Cereal-legume based Indian diets provide around 55-85 g fibre per day, But caution is on the absorption of minerals since fibre and phytates form insoluble complexes with calcium, iron and zinc. Also refer 'chapter on Poultry Nutrition' in this textbook for more details on NSP. Refer textbook Principles of Animal Nutrition and Feed Technology page No. 23 to 31.

Classification of Lipids

I Saponifiable (yield soaps, salts of fatty acids, on alkaline hydrolysis)
1. Acylglycerols (Backbone : glycerol)
2. Waxes (nonpolar alcohols of high molecular weight)
3. Phosphoglycerides (glycerol 3-phosphate)
4. Sphingolipids (sphingosine)

II Nonsaponifiable (these do not contain fatty acids)
1. Terpenes
2. Steroids
3. Prostaglandins

Phospholipids: Phosphoglycerides and sphingolipids are phospholipids. Phosphatidic acid (glycerol, two fatty acids and a phosphate group) is parent compound of phosphoglycerides. Phosphatidyl choline (lecithin), phosphatidyl ethanolamine (cephalin), phosphatidyl serine are examples of phosphoglycerides. Sphingolipids or sphingomyelins are derivatives of the basic compound sphingosine. Sphingosine with a long saturated or monounsaturated fatty acid (18 to 26 carbon atoms) is called a ceramide.

Glycosphingolipids: These are neutral and acidic. Neutral glycosphingolipids are sphingolipids with one or more neutral sugar residues as their polar head groups. The simplest one is cerebroside. e.g. galactocerebrosides (cerebroside of brain); sulfatides are sulfate esters of galactocerebrosides. Acidic glycosphingolipids (gangliosides) have sialic acid.

Fats in the Diet

Fats in the diet can be of two kinds: The visible fat and invisible fat.

Visible Fat

1. Solid fats e.g. animal fats like butter and ghee. These contain vitamins A and D.

2. Liquid fats e.g. vegetable fats like groundnut oil, mustard oil, coconut oil, safflower oil, and til oil. Vitamins A and D are not present in these oils. Vegetable oils contain vitamin E, which protects the oil from oxidation.

3. Hydrogenated vegetable oil known as "Vanaspathi". Vitamins A and D can be added at a level of 700 IU and 50 IU, respectively.

These fats are triglycerides of fatty acids, both saturated and unsaturated. Saturated fatty acids predominate in animal fats while unsaturated ones dominate in vegetable oils.

Invisible Fat

Some amount of the fat is present in other food items like cereals, pulses, oilseeds, milk, egg, meat, etc. This invisible fat is believed to contribute significantly to the total fat and EFA content of the diet depending upon the foodstuffs present in the diet (Table 2). Diets containing nuts, oilseeds, soybean and avocado pear and animal foods have a higher amount of invisible fat.

Table 2 Some Data on Average Fat Content (g/100 g Edible Portion).

Foodstuff	Content (g /100 g)
Rice, Wheat, Ragi, Jowar	2-3
Maize	5
Bajra	6
Blackgram, Rajmah, Greengram, Lentil, Redgram	2
Cowpea	3
Bengalgram	7
Soyabean	20
Fenugreek seeds	10
Green leafy vegetables	0.4
Groundnuts, Seame, Mustard	40

Cholesterol

Cholesterol is a constituent of animal foods (Table 3). It is absent in plants. It is synthesized in the body. Hence it is not a dietary essential. Average cholesterol should be around 180 mg per 100 ml blood plasma for healthy Indians. Excess cholesterol in blood gradually deposit under the lining of blood vessels, resulting in a condition known as "atherosclerosis" in which the blood vessels are narrowed and hardened. The coronary arteries supplying blood to the heart are affected and coronary heart disease results.

Table 3 Fatty Acid Composition and Cholesterol Content of Animal Foods[*].

Item	Fat g/100 g	Saturated fatty acid g/100 g	Cholesterol mg/100 g
Cow milk	4	2	14
Buffalo milk	8	4	16
Butter	80	50	250
Ghee	100	65	300
Cheese	25	15	100
Whole egg	11	4	400
Egg yolk	30	9	1120
Chicken without skin	4	1	60
Chicken with skin	18	6	100
Mutton	13	7	65
Pork	35	13	90
Beef	16	8	70
Prawns/Shrimps	2	0.3	150
Lean fish	1.5	0.4	45
Fatty fish	6	2.5	45

[*] Values vary depending on the dietary regimen of the animal.

Factors that Influence Elevation of Blood Cholesterol

These are related to human beings specifically, but may be applicable to animal feeding as well.

1. *Quantity of fat:* The quantity of fat that should be included in a well balanced diet is not known with certainty. The following points must be kept in view in deciding the desirable level of fat in the diet:

   (a) The minimum amount of fat to meet the EFA requirement.

   (b) The amount needed to promote absorption of fat soluble vitamins.

   (c) To provide palatability to food.

   (d) The undesirable effect of excessive intake of fat.

2. *Quality of fat:* Animal fats have high proportion of saturated fats (Table 3). Butter, ghee, coconut oil and hydrogenated vegetable oils have been shown to cause considerable elevation of blood cholesterol when consumed in large amounts. The PUFA present in oils like groundnut oil, safflower or sunflower oil (refer Table 4 and 5) have been shown to prevent an increase in serum cholesterol on a high fat diet and are thus considered antiatherogenic. These suppress formation of clot in the blood. However, high levels of PUFA have

Table 4 Major Fatty Acid Composition of Vegetable Oils and Milk Fat.

OILS	Major fatty acid (%)							
	C 12:0	C 14:0	C 16:0	C18+ C18:1	C 18:2	C 18:3	C 20:1	C 22:1
1. Coconut	42.7	26.1	8.5	5.9	1.2	0.17	-	-
2. Mustard	-	-	2.5	9.9	13.9	12.1	6.7	55.0
3. Dalda (hydrogenated)	-	-	16.1	81.9	2.0	-	-	-
4. Cottonseed	-	0.8	18.1	23.4	57.7	-	-	-
5. Soybean	-	-	12.0	42.3	45.7	-	-	-
6. Sunflower	-	-	6.8	34.3	59.0	-	-	-
7. Safflower	-	-	7.7	12.4	80.0	-	-	-
8. Groundnut	-	-	10.5	47.1	40.3	0.4	1.8	-
9. Milk fat*	2.6	10.8	36.8	34.3	1.3	0.8	-	-

* Milk fat also contains C4, C6, C8, and C10 fatty acids (total 12-15%).

Table 5 Fatty Acid Composition of Common Fats and Oils (g/100 g).

Source of fat/oil	Saturated	Monoun-saturated	Linoleic	Alpha linolenic
Coconut, Palmkernel, Red palm oil, Palm oil, Ghee	45-90	7-44	2-10	< 0.5
Groundnut, Sesame, Rice bran oil	15-22	40-50	25-40	< 0.5 -1.5
Safflower, Sunflower, Cottonseed, Corn oil	12-22	17-25	50-70	< 0.5-1.0
Mustard oil	8	70	12	10
Soybean oil	15	27	53	5.0
Vanaspathi/dalda	24	19	3	< 0.5

undesirable effects due to formation of excess free radicals and consequent tissue damage. The content of healthful fatty acids, linoleic and linolenic are given in Table 6 and 7. Alpha linolenic (n-3) and other n-3 PUFA are useful for maintaining a healthy heart (Refer Chapter 4 of *Principles of Animal Nutrition and Feed Technology* for more details).

LDL (low density lipoprotein) cholesterol is a strong atherogen. HDL (high density lipoprotein) cholesterol scavenge cholesterol from blood and tissues and deliver to the liver where it is processed for excretion. It is good cholesterol. Aerobic exercise increases HDL cholesterol while weight lifting and other exercises reduce LDL cholesterol.

TABLE 6. Linoleic Acid (n-6) Content of Common Foodstuffs.

Name of the foodstuff	Linoleic acid (g/100 g edible portion)
1. Green leafy vegetables	0.04
and other vegetables	0.06
2. Blackgram, Rajmah, Ragi, Rice	0.1-0.5
3. Coconut (fresh), Cowpea, Greengram, Redgram, Lentil, Wheat	0.6-1.0
4. Jowar (milo), Maize (corn),	1.5-2.0
5. Bengalgram, Fenugreek seeds	3.5
6. Dry chillies, Cumin seeds, Coriander seeds, Mustard	5.0
7. Soybeans, Cashewnuts, Groundnuts	8-10
8. Almonds, Sesame	14-16

TABLE 7. Alpha-linolenic Acid (n-3) Content of Common Foodstuffs.

Name of the foodstuff	Alpha linolenic acid (g/100 g edible portion)
1. Rice, other vegetables, Ragi, Jowar, Maize	0.01 to 0.05
2. Bajra; Greengram, Lentil and Redgram; Green Leafy Vegetables (GLV); Wheat, Bengalgram, Dry Chillies, Cumin seeds, and Coriander seeds; Groundnuts	0.1 to 0.2
3. Almonds, Cashewnuts, Sesame	0.3 to 0.4
4. Cowpea; Blackgram and Rajmah	0.5 to 0.7
5. Soya	1.0
6. Fenugreek seeds	2.0
7. Mustard seeds	3.5

3. *Mode of consumption of fat:* At the same level of total daily intake, consumption of smaller amounts of fat a number of times (frequently) during a day has been shown to cause less elevation of blood cholesterol content as compared to consumption of the same at one time of the day.

Egg and Cholesterol

Today's egg has more protein and less fat. Most of these changes have likely resulted through genetic selection. Cholesterol values for today's egg (213 mg) are also reported to be substantially lower than those observed in 1976 (USDA, 1989). The differences in cholesterol are postulated to be largely due to improved analytical methods. The NRC's Food and Nutrition Board's committee on Diet and Health (1989) has recommended that dietary cholesterol should be less than 300 mg per day. Although the egg has been targeted as a rich source of cholesterol, the egg provides an essential source of linoleic acid and the proportions of saturated: monounsaturated: polyunsaturated are balanced relative to the ratios suggested by the American Heart Association. The average composition of hen's egg is presented in Table 8.

TABLE 8. Average Composition of the Hen's Egg.

	Per kg Whole egg	Per egg of 57 g	Proportion of nutrient in edible part of egg
Gross constituents (g)			
Water	668	38.1	1.00
Protein	118	6.7	0.97
Lipid	100	5.7	0.99
Carbohydrate	8	0.5	1.00
Ash	107	6.1	0.04
Amino acids (g)			
Arginine	7.2	0.41	0.97
Histidine	2.6	0.15	(assumed for all
Isoleucine	6.4	0.36	amino acids)
Leucine	10.1	0.57	
Lysine	7.9	0.45	
Methionine	4.0	0.23	
Phenylalanine	6.0	0.34	
Threonine	5.5	0.31	
Tryptophan	2.2	0.13	
Valine	7.6	0.44	
Major minerals (g)			
Calcium	37.3	2.13	0.01
Phosphorus	2.3	0.13	0.85
Sodium	1.2	0.066	1.00
Potassium	1.3	0.075	1.00
Magnesium	0.8	0.046	0.58
Trace elements (mg)			
Copper	5.0	0.3	1.00
Iodine	0.3	0.02	
Iron	33	1.9	traces of minor
Manganese	0.3	0.02	elements in shell
Zinc	16	1.0	
Selenium	5.0	0.3	

Source: Animal Nutrition by McDonald *et al.* 1995.

Mineral content of hen egg (58 g): calcium, 1.98 g; phosphorus, 0.115 g; sulphur, 0.114 g; chlorine, 0.088 g; sodium, 0.073 g; potassium, 0.067 g; magnesium, 0.027 g; iron, 1.1 mg; copper, 0.067 mg; manganese, 1 to 4 ppm; selenium, 25 to 914 µg/100 g.

Egg (contents) has no carbohydrate, calcium and vitamin C. Egg is a store of balanced protein, easily digestible lipids, low-energy source, important source of sulphur, phosphorus, iron and vitamins-biotin (B_8) and folic acid (B_9).

Fertile Egg Versus Nonfertile Egg: No scientific proof exists that fertile eggs are more nutritious than nonfertile eggs except that possibly the developing embryo might provide more nutrients. Fertile eggs are more expensive to produce and deteriorate more rapidly than do nonfertile eggs.

Organic/Green eggs: Eggs produced by hens raised traditionally in their natural environment are referred as organic/green eggs. Such eggs may be promoted as much safer (since no residues of antibiotics, hormones, etc. are possible to present) and more nutritious than those produced by hens on the usual commercial rations. Of course, there is no reason for concern about eating eggs produced by hens on commercial rations. Organic eggs are no higher in nutritive value than regular eggs. If the ration for hens on an organic diet is not so well balanced, the nutritive value of organic eggs tends to be lower. Egg production from organic diets is lower and such eggs are much more expensive.

NUTRITIONAL POTENTIALITY OF IMPORTANT FOODSTUFFS

Foodstuffs may be grouped or classified in different ways: Three food group system, five food group system and eleven food group system.

Nutritional classification of foods: They have been broadly grouped under three heads from the nutritional point of view:
1. Energy yielding foods, 2. Body building foods, and 3. Protective foods.

1. *Energy yielding foods:* Foods rich is carbohydrates and fat are called energy yielding foods. Cereals, roots and tubers, dried fruits, sugar and fats are included in this group.

2. *Body building foods:* Food rich in proteins are called body building foods. Milk, meat, fish, eggs, pulses, oilseeds and nuts and low-fat oilseed flours are included in this group.

3. *Protective foods:* Foods rich in proteins, vitamins and minerals are termed protective foods. Milk, eggs, liver, green leafy vegetables (GLV) and fruits are included in this group.

   (a) Foods rich in vitamins, minerals and proteins of high B.V. e.g. milk, eggs and liver

   (b) Foods rich in certain vitamins and minerals only e.g. GLV and fruits.

Dietary factors that modify nutrient requirements

- Absorption of nutrients from diets predominantly based on plant foods is often inferior to that from diets based largely on foods of animal origin.
- Many inhibitory factors present in plant foods like tannins, phytates and antitryptic factors interfere with the intestinal absorption of nutrients such as proteins, phosphorus, iron, zinc, beta-carotene and vitamin B_{12}.
- There are close interrelationships between metabolism of nutrients. Some well-known interrelationships are energy-protein, energy-B vitamins (B_1, B_2 and niacin), protein-B_6 vitamin, tryptophan-niacin, ascorbic acid-iron, beta-carotene-retinol, etc.

There are inter-individual differences in nutrient requirements even between individuals of the same age, sex and body weight. The coefficient of variation in nutrient requirements between individuals is currently assumed to be around 12.5%.

Specific Foods that are Particularly Helpful for Immunity

Immunity Nutrients: Immune system (neutrophiles, etc.) is a voracious user of vitamins and minerals. So feed your immune system with the vitamins and minerals it needs to protect you from bacterial and viral invasion. While every vitamin and mineral plays a part in this fight, there are five critical immunity nutrients that help you to strengthen your defences. They are copper, zinc, vitamin C, folate and vitamin B_{12}.

Foods rich in certain minerals and vitamins support immune function. Factors that cause stress in modern life such as environmental pollution, radiation, pesticides and insecticides and even some medications create an overabundance of oxygen free radicals in the body. These are highly destructive molecules that have had one of their paired electrons ripped off, and are in search of grabbing an electron from a healthy molecule, leaving it damaged. When this happens, a chain reaction occurs.

Free radical damage spreads in tissues, resulting in heart disease, cancer (due to damage to DNA), senility, arthritis, cataract, and emphysema. Researchers now believe that most of the aspects of degenerative ageing are due to free radical destruction.

To help combat this inner oxidation from free radicals an increased intake of foods rich in antioxidants is recommended. Antioxidant nutrients supply that renegade free radical molecule with the electron it is desperately seeking, and stop the chain reaction of damage.

Antioxidant nutrients: Vitamins C and E and β-carotene, minerals such as zinc, copper, manganese and selenium. Vitamins C and E inhibit the LDL-cholesterol from oxidizing and damaging the lining of the coronary vessels where platelets clump together, causing clots that lead to heart attacks. Several new studies show how angina and myocardial infarction (heart attack) are reduced with increased beta-carotene and Vitamin E intake.

Garlic has healing effect. A natural antibiotic, garlic is also proven to have immune enhancing benefits, and improves high blood pressure, helps fight tumour formation. Garlic is a decongestant, antiprotozoal and insecticidal. Eating raw, garlic kills bacteria and prevents heart disease.

Antioxidant nutrient	Rich sources
β-carotene (vitamin A precursor)	Leafy dark green vegetables, yellow and orange vegetables, carrot, sweet potato, broccoli, spinach, turnip, beet, papaya, apricot.
Vitamin C	Citrus fruits, most fruits and vegetables, kiwi, broccoli, greens, tomato, pomegranate.
Vitamin E	Whole grains, vegetable oils, leafy dark greens, sweet potatoes and organ meats.
Vitamin B$_6$	Leafy dark greens, potatoes, nuts and whole grains.
Vitamin B$_{12}$	Fish, dairy products, eggs, organ meats, chicken and pork.
Folic acid	Leafy dark greens, legumes, fish.
Calcium	Dairy products, leafy dark greens, salmon.
Copper	Organ meats, seafood, legumes, nuts, fruits.
Iron	Poultry, fish, meat, liver, leafy dark greens (spinach), dried fruit, molasses.
Magnesium	Dark green vegetables, dairy products, whole grains, seafood.
Manganese	Whole grains, nuts, leafy dark greens, shell fish and milk.

Selenium	Broccoli, mushrooms, cabbage, celery, cucumber, onion, garlic, brewer's yeast, grains, fish, brazil nuts are a good source.
Zinc	Whole grains, yeast, wheat bran and germ, sunflower seed, seafood, meat. Oysters are rich sources.

"Let your Food be your Medicine"

Sprouts are basically young, new plants, alive, green and growing. Almost any edible seed can be sprouted. It is best to choose legumes. Any whole grain available can be used to sprout. Soak the seeds for overnight. Pour off the water into another container and use it. This water is rich in minerals, vitamins, etc. Tie it in a muslin cloth and hang. The seeds should be wet. Hence it is regularly rinsed. Sprouting takes 36 to 48 hours. But to get complete benefit, sprouts should be allowed to 'grow' to a sufficient length. It should be kept for four to five days, after being regularly rinsed. On the fifth day, the sprouts should be placed in the sun. This turns them green.

Nutritive value of a seed is increased. Nutrients are in a more digestible form. Protein content is increased.

Vitamin B content jumps from three-fold to ten-fold over the dry seed. Vitamins A, E and K are increased. Vitamin C is actually created while the seed is sprouting. Minerals like Ca, Zn, Fe can be obtained very well. Sprouts are also high in fibre.

Sprouts help in curing ulcers, blood clots and other degenerative diseases. They retard the mutation process (i.e. the process that leads to undesirable hereditary changes). They help in anaemia, infertility, and breast milk flow.

Sprouts make a vitamin rich substitute for fruits and vegetables. They also provide a complete food in a predigested form from which nutrients are easily and efficiently assimilated by the body.

Nutrients for Blood Production and Cell Growth: Folate, vitamin B_{12}, iron and zinc are especially required because of their key role in the synthesis of cells, including red blood cells. Folate deficiency is the most common cause of megaloblastic anaemia (Anaemia in which red blood cells are immature and therefore large) in infants and children.

Folic acid plays a key role in preventing birth defects in newborns. In adults, folic acid also helps reduce levels of homocysteine, and so may play a role in preventing heart disease.

Information on Foodstuffs that are used in Animal Feeding

Tomatoes are a rich source of lycopene, beta-carotene, folate, potassium, vitamin C, flavonoids and vitamin E. Many of these nutrients may function individually, or in concert, to protect lipoproteins and vascular cells from oxidation, the most widely accepted theory for the genesis of atherosclerosis. This hypothesis has been supported by *in vitro*, limited in vivo, and many epidemiological studies that associate reduced cardiovascular risk with consumption of antioxidant-rich foods. Other cardioprotective functions provided by the nutrients in tomatoes may include the reduction by LDL cholesterol, homocysteine, platelet aggregation and blood pressure. Because tomatoes include several nutrients associated with theoretical or proven effects and are widely consumed year round, they may be considered a valuable component of a cardioprotective diet.

Soya has been found to have a therapeutic role in menopausal woman: The phytoestrogens, isoflavones especially help regulate the hormonal balance. Soya helps to reduce cholesterol. It is an excellent source of high quality protein and bone building calcium. It has plenty of fibre.

Banana is a good source of carbohydrate. Banana and papaya contain pectin, which helps in bowel movements. Dried fruits like raisins and dates are rich in iron.

Green Leafy Vegetables (GLV) are rich in several antioxidants that protect the cells from free radical damage. GLV may help keep the brain younger and more active. Fenugreek and amaranth have 3 to 4 times more vitamins C and E than even spinach. Coriander and green chillies are sources of vitamin C and β-carotene.

Low-oxalate containing GLV as calcium sources: Coriander leaves, 184 mg; fenugreek leaves, 395 mg; mint, 200 mg; ponnaganti, 510 mg; drumstick leaves, 440 mg; curry leaves, 830 mg; gogu leaves, 172 mg; betal leaves 340 mg (120 mg P) per 100 g. Ragi grain has no oxalate while horsegram has oxalate 417 mg/ 100 g.

Examples of fatty fish include mackerel, rohu, catla, rawas, sardines, hilsa. Salmon, herring, whitefish, tuna, sardines, mackerel contain omega 3 fatty acids in descending order.

Refining of vegetable oils (removal of small amounts of free fatty acids, colouring matters and odorous compounds) has no much nutritional consequences; deodourisation step also removes part of the sterols, and a small portion of the tocopherols.

Ginger eases digestive complaints. It has ability to increase blood circulation and that includes circulation below the belt. It has cardiovascular stimulating effects. It may play a role in lowering blood pressure and improve blood flow.

Asafetida and garlic are known to have antibacterial property. Turmeric and cloves contain powerful antioxidants. Turmeric has anticancer properties.

Soluble fibre reduces triglyceride absorption, increase bile acid output and decrease LDL and total cholesterol.

Low-calorie, nutrient-dense diets make lean muscles.

Calcium rich foodstuffs include gingilly seeds, ragi grain, rajmah, soybean, *agathi* leaves, amaranth and fenugreek leaves and milk. The oxalic acid present in certain foodstuffs (Table 9) form insoluble calcium salt making it unavailable for absorption.

Table 9   Some Foodstuffs Oxalic Acid Content Wise in Descending Order.

Foodstuff	Content, mg/100 g
Gingilly seeds	1700
Amaranth (tender) GLV	772
Plantain green vegetable	480
Horsegram grain	417
Almond, cashewnut	300-400
Amla fruit	296
Tamarind leaves, tender	196
Gogu, curry leaves	
Drumstick leaves,	
Drumstick vegetable	101
Beet root	40
Seethaphal, mango fruits	30
Bajra grain	21
Potato	20
Tomato ripe	4
Tomato green	2
Cow milk	2

Cereals and millets have phytates (Table 10), which interfere with iron absorption.

Table 10   Some Foodstuffs Phytin Phosphorus Wise in Descending Order.

Maize grain	85% of P as Phytin P
Wheat grain,	80% of P as Phytin P
Wheat flour	
Coriander seed	81% of P as Phytin P
Jowar grain	77% of P as Phytin P
Ragi grain	74% of P as Phytin P
Curry leaves,	
Drumstick leaves	60% of P as Phytin P
Rice, bajra,	
All pulses and	
legumes, Guava fruit	40-50% of P as Phytin P
Fenugreek seeds,	
Pepper,	
Drumstick vegetable,	
Plantain green,	30-40% of P as Phytin P
Potato, Papaya ripe,	
Pomegranate	
Banana ripe,	10% of P as Phytin P
Chillies dry, Rohu fish	

The presence of calcium carbonate in the drinks damaged the teeth. Continuous intake of milk adulterated with caustic soda, urea, etc lead to slow poisoning and nervous disorders, nausea and other gastrointestinal problems.

β-Carotene

Some Vegetables and Fruits (β-carotene content wise in a descending order).

Drumstick leaves	(20000 μg/100 g)
Agathi leaves	
Fenugreek leaves	
Curry and gogu leaves	
Carrot, mint leaves	
Ponnaganti, coriander leaves	
Mango fruit	
Pumpkin, green chilies	
Papaya, tomato	
Orange, Cherries red	(140 μg/100 g)

Absorption of β-carotene

For practical purpose only about 50% of β-carotene in foods is considered to be absorbed. The availability of β-carotene from the GLV and vegetables vary from 25-50% depending on the fat content of the diet. Taking both absorption and availability into consideration, one unit of β-carotene in foods is assumed to yield only 0.25 units of retinol in the gut mucosa. The requirement of β-carotene is therefore 4 times the requirement of retinol.

Nutritional Manipulation for Quality Animal Products

Designer products are being developed by feeding nutraceuticals to animals and birds. In case of ruminant animals certain protection measures are to be undertaken to keep the nutraceutical out of bounds of rumen fermentation while in monogastrics and birds the nutraceutical can be added straight to the diet. Nutraceuticals refer to products designed for specific health benefits that fit into a category between nutritional products and pharmaceuticals. A nutraceutical is any substance that is a food or a part of a food that provides medical or health benefits, including prevention and treatment of disease. Dietary flax, oats, pearl millet, marine microalgae supplementation in poultry and swine feeding enhances the healthful properties of eggs and meat. Many more are being added to the list.

Nutraceuticals include omega 3 fatty acids (ALA, EPA, DHA), antioxidants (lutein, vitamin E, tocopherol), CLA, selenium. Docosahexaenoic acid (DHA) boosts the immune system and helps brain development. Antioxidant lutein protects against cancer. Conjugated linoleic acid (CLA) has anticarcinogenic, hypocholestorolemic and antiatherogenic effects. Ruminant animals naturally produce this fatty acid (CLA) during fermentative digestion. Humans and other monogastrics do not have the ability to synthesize CLA and must obtain from the diet.

Diet Manipulation to Produce Designer Eggs and Designer Meat

- Feeding of fish oil (menhaden oil) up to 3% in chicken layer diets increased total n-3/omega-3 fatty acids (alpha linolenic acid, EPA, DHA) in eggs.
- Hens fed 3% oat bran or 3% cottonseed hulls had decreased egg cholesterol.
- As rapeseed increased in the diet, the percentage of saturated fatty acids in the eggs decreased, and polyenoic n-3 fatty acids increased (including long-chained polyenoic fatty acids not present in the

rapeseed oil) [Treated rapeseed was fed to laying hens at 7.5, 15 or 22.5% of the diet. Rapeseed decreased egg production and feed efficiency in hens fed at 22.5% of the diet].

- Chicken hens receiving flax seed in the diet produced eggs with 415 mg (normal egg has 125 mg) omega-3 acids (Dr. Sheila Scheideler at Nebraska, USA). Consumption of such eggs improved the ratio of omega-3 acids to omega-6 acids (linoleic, archidonic, etc) [Alpha-linolenic acid is a plant version of omega-3 acid and a concentrated source is flax seed (linseed)].

- Feeding of copper supplements to swine diets alter the amounts of saturated and unsaturated fatty acids in the muscle.

- Feeding of copper sulphate (250 mg/kg diet) to broiler chickens improved growth rates and feed utilisation. Reduced plasma cholesterol levels and decreased breast muscle cholesterol were observed in copper-supplemented birds at 42 days of age.

- Feeding 3% garlic powder resulted in lower levels of plasma cholesterol, liver cholesterol, blood reduced glutathione and breast and thigh muscle cholesterol as noticed when growth promoting levels of copper was fed. Both garlic and copper alter lipid and cholesterol metabolism though the mechanism is different.

Fatty Acid Profiles: Omega-6 and Omega-3 Fats in eggs

The fatty acid content of eggs can be modified by changes in the hen's diet. The ratio of polyunsaturated to saturated fats in egg lipid is 0.59. It is much better than that recommended by most health associations. It has been emphasised the importance of correct ratio of two families of polyunsaturated fatty acids (PUFA) in the diet i.e., omega-6 and omega - 3. There is gross dietary imbalance in omega-6 and omega-3 fats. Desirable ratio between n-6/omega-6 and n-3/omega-3 fatty acids is 6:1. The reader may refer Appendix II for the examples and data. Hence 'omega-3 fat' enriched foods are needed.

High levels of omega (n)-6 PUFA are found in evening primrose oil, corn oil, soybean oil, sunflower oil while fatty fish, linseed or flax seed, rapeseed are rich sources of omega (n)-3 fats. By modifying the diet of hen towards higher n-3 fatty acid content, the n-3 fatty acid content of eggs can be increased. Chicken has somewhat unique ability to divert increased quantities of alpha linolenic acid (18:3 n-3) into the egg when its diet has high levels of this nutrient.

Enriched Eggs or Designer Eggs

Epidemiological studies have related the high habitual intakes of fatty fish with a low incidence of ischaemic heart disease in the Eskimo population of Greenland and the Japanese population. The 25% population of vegetarians and some proportion of nonvegetarians do not consume fish (consumption of fatty fish is still less), while majority consume eggs. So efforts have been made to enrich eggs with n-3 fatty acids so that the enriched egg would be an alternative source for those who do not eat fish or who cannot regularly eat fish. Designer eggs are available since 1995 in Brazil, Germany, Australia, New Zealand, etc. The new egg is said to have 40% less cholesterol, 29% less saturated fat, higher vitamin E and omega-3 fatty acid content. Omega-3 fatty acid enriched eggs are creating interest among health-conscious consumers.

In view of the current interest in having higher levels of selenium in our diets as a means of combating old age, cancer and infertility, it has been suggested that one way to do this would be to increase the selenium content of eggs. It has been reported that by feeding natural selenium (selenium yeast) to layers, the selenium content of the egg can be increased significantly. Similarly organic selenium may be included in layer diets.

Designer egg containing enhanced levels of omega-3 free fatty acids, folic acid, vitamin E and tocopherol has much to offer in terms of dietary supplementation of omega-3 fatty acids and biological antioxidants for the well being of mankind. Such enriched eggs with tocopherols as well as with essential free fatty acids are stable from autoxidation and maintain their quality during storage or processing.

Food Additive Sweeteners

In the US Sucralose is available under the brand name 'Splenda'. Sucralose is made from sucrose by swapping three of its hydrogen - oxygen groups with chlorine atoms. The molecule's geometry is retained while the sweetening power is enhanced by 600 times. Refer Chapter 12 of *Principles of Animal Nutrition and Feed Technology* for more details. Although its molecules snap into those sweetness taste receptors, they differ enough in structure from sugar to go unnoticed by the digestive enzymes, which need a specific fit to break down food. That's why Sucralose - sweetened products are safe for diabetics.

Aspartame, acesulfame potassium, saccharine, cyclamate, alitame, etc. high intensity synthetic sweeteners are available to meet the demand for alternative food choices comprising low calorie, low sugar and low fat food products. These artificial sweeteners are nontoxic. These are granted GRAS status in many countries abroad. These gained the approval of FAO/WHO Codex Alimentarius.

Natural Sweeteners

Demand for non-saccharide sweeteners is increasing due to rise in the number of diabetic patients. The plants found mostly in the Himalayas can provide a new source of non-saccharide sweeteners. The plant derived sweeteners do not have any adverse impact on health which is a common problem of synthetic sweeteners. Herbal non-saccharide sweeteners-terpenoids, steroidal saponins, dihydrochalcone, dihydroiso-coumarin are 100 to 10,000 times sweeter than sucrose and are good for health.

Sweeteners in Soft Drinks

In June 1999 Government of India issued a notification permitting the use of the two artificial sweeteners aspartame and acesulfame - K (Potassium) (ASK) in combination [The PFA Rules, (1954) already permit the use of each of these individually] in sweetened carbonated water and soft drinks subject to a minimum level of 5 percent sucrose, or sugar content, to allow the benefit of the synergistic sweetener enhancement.

Low-calorie "Diet" Soft Drinks"

Low-calorie "Diet" soft drinks (e.g. Diet Pepsi, Diet Coke) are available in India since June 1999 with the necessary amendment was made to the PFA Act. Coca-Cola and Pepsi-Cola provide around 230 calories of energy packed in a 330 ml can and can make people grow belly. Health conscious people prefer "Diet" drinks. Diabetics may prefer a Diet drink to the original cola. Government wanted the companies to add on the packages of 'Diet' a tag line: "Not recommended for children" since they had no nutritional value. Similarly diet drinks are not to be taken by phenylketoneurics (product contains phenylalanine, which in large amounts can lead to mental retardation). Diet drinks are claimed to have 1 calorie energy.

Lathyrism

Lathyrism is a crippling disease characterised by paralysis of the leg muscles occurring mostly in adults consuming large quantities of seeds of *Lathyrus sativus* or other lathyrus species over long periods. In India, the disease occurs in Madhya Pradesh, Bihar and Uttar Pradesh.

Types of lathyrism: Two types of lathyrism have been reported to occur in animals and human beings, *viz.*, Osteolathyrism and neurolathyrism. Accordingly skeletal deformities, paralysis of muscles of the legs are observed sometimes resulting in convulsions and death in severe cases. *Lathyrus sativus* seeds have been implicated for a long time as responsible for lathyrism. This disease is mainly of the neurological type. The main neurotoxic substance was recently obtained in crystalline form and its structure was established as beta oxalylamino alanine (BOAA).

Prevention: There are three possible approaches for the eradication of the disease.

1. Treatment of the seed by leaching out the toxic factors in hot water.
2. Education of the public on the dangers of consuming untreated *L. sativus*.
3. Cultivation of other pulses in place of *L. sativus*.

14

Rabbit Nutrition

Rabbits have traditionally been raised for fur, wool, meat, as laboratory animals in biomedical research or as pets. Europe tops the world in rabbit production while Korea and China are principal players in Asia. The popularity of rabbitry (Rabbitry is rearing of rabbits) started picking up since the 1960s. The French are the heaviest consumers of rabbit meat in the world (about 6 kg a year). France produces at least 2.5 times more than the second producer, Italy.

As an industry, rabbit farming is gaining popularity in cooler and temperate parts of India such as Jammu and Kashmir, Himachal Pradesh (Garsa (Killu), parts of Uttarakhand (Gharwal CSWRI, and Kumaon regions) and Nilgiri hills of Tamil Nadu. The average wool production per animal per year has gone up to 700-800 g (German Angora Breed), whereas broiler production has touched 3-4 weeks age under Indian conditions (Archana Phull and Phull, 2003).

Attributes of Rabbits for Efficient Food Production

Rabbits have a number of attributes that suggest that they could become increasingly important as sources of animal protein for human nutrition. Meat rabbits have a rapid growth rate, and can be raised on low concentrate diets consisting largely of forages and agricultural byproducts. They have a high reproductive potential; females are biologically capable of producing a litter every 32 days, giving a potential yield of 11 litters per year (gestation period is 31 days).

1. Rapid growth rate: Growth of fryer rabbits is 40 to 45 g/ day.
2. High reproductive potential: Rabbits have the highest reproductive capacity of any livestock species. Does will rebreed within 24 hours

of parturition (Kindling). This is known as postpartum breeding. However, such intensive production is not currently recommended. Does should be rebred 7 to 35 days after kindling in commercial system.

3. High proliferation: Average litter size is 7. A doe can produce 30 to 50 offsprings (kits) in a year. Birth weight is 60 g.

4. Rabbits have a high feed conversion ratio and their meat is low in fat and cholesterol. They eat forages and fibrous agricultural byproducts that are not normally consumed by monogastrics and man.

5. Rabbits can be adapted to any set of circumstances, backyard rearing or commercial farming. They are suitable to urban agriculture as they can be raised on small tracts of land.

The rabbit should be lifted by the skin behind the ears, the scruff. The rabbit is then held and supported by placing the other hand under the hindquarters. Young rabbits are usually transferred quickly from hutch to basket by its pelvis or the skin on their back. Rabbits are susceptible to heat stress as they do not have sweat glands. They can be raised at 30° to 32° C.

Rabbits and Hares

Hares are different from rabbits. Hares are born fully haired with eyes open and can run within a few minutes of birth.

The important breeds of rabbits are German Angora, White Angora, Newzealand White, White giant and Soviet chinchilla. Flemish Giant is a popular broiler rabbit. Angora rabbit is for fur. The new born kits/ bunnies are hairless with closed eyes. They start developing hair 4 days after birth and open their eyes after the 10th day.

Some Characteristics of the Digestive Physiology of the Rabbit Digestion and Metabolism - Peculiarities

Rabbit is a nonruminant herbivore. It is a hindgut fermenter. Digestive system is well adapted for the digestion of the large quantity of forage typical of herbivorous diet. Caecum, a blind pouch branching off from the small intestine, is the major site of microbial fermentation. It is followed by colon, rectum and anus. Caecum is characterized by its enormous size. Its length, including the appendix, is as great as or in excess of the length of the body. The caecal mucosa forms a spiral fold along the length of the caecum and this increases its internal surface. The volume of the caecum and of the colon increases linearly to become the largest digestive compartment from 5 to 6 weeks of age (40% of the total digestive volume). The motility of the caecum consists of extremely vigorous peristaltic and antiperistaltic contractions. The highest bacterial counts (10^9-10^{10}/g) are found in the caecum. Protozoa, which are present in the caecum of some herbivores such as the horse and the guinea pig, have not been found in the rabbit caecum (Hernicke, H., 1977). Microorganisms ferment the nutrients reaching the caecum. Most of the digesta (80% or more) is contained in the stomach and caecum.

The bacterial flora of the caecal contents synthesise all B-vitamins. Bacteria utilize the urea available in caecal contents as nitrogen source and multiply. Fermentation of the diet releases volatile fatty acids and can provide up to 40% of the animal's energy needs. It has been shown that the caecal mucosa can also absorb water, electrolytes and amino acids.

Ingestive Behaviour

During the first 3 weeks of life the young are fed only once in every 24 hours by their mother. Five to 15 ml of milk are sucked by the newborn within 2 to 3 min. Rabbit milk contains 20-24% fat. Adult domestic rabbits, on the contrary, are more continuous eaters and they take one or two meals every hour throughout the 24-hour period.

From 16 to 18 days, young rabbits begin to eat small quantities of solid feed in addition to their mother's milk. Before 25 days of age, a rabbit eats around 25 to 30 g solid feed. The water intake of the young rabbit is closely related to intake of solid feed. The feeding behaviour thus changes quickly as the young rabbit moves from a single meal of milk per day (from birth to 15 days old) to a large number of solid and liquid meals more or less alternating and taking place irregularly throughout the day: from 25 to 30 solid or liquid meals in 24 h (Gidenne and Fortun-Lamothe, 2001). Caecotrophy (see p. 403) begins in the young rabbit at about 3 weeks of age, i.e. when the animals begin to eat solid food in addition to their mother's milk. Thus at 25 days of age it is possible to collect caecotrophes in sufficient quantity for an analysis of microbial activity 'in situ'. In view of this feeding pattern less variation in digestive function and intermediary metabolism is expected; nevertheless, caecotrophy strongly influences the digestive and metabolic systems.

Gastric Functions

(a) **Functions of the stomach itself:** The gastric lipase secreted by a small area of the stomach wall around the cardia reaches its maximum production in the 30-day-old rabbit. It then decreases rapidly between

30 and 60 days and this continues until 180 days. It is not measurable in the adult. In the suckling rabbit specific lipases degrade the milk fat to medium chain fatty acids.

In the very young rabbit (1st week of life) the stomach wall secretes a pepsin the optimum pH of which is around 1·8 to 2·4 and another peptidase, rennin or chymosin, with an optimum pH of 3·4 to 3·8. From 21 days, the optimum pH of the pepsin falls to about 1·2 to 1·8, and rennin is no longer detectable in the 45- to 60-day-old rabbit. This endopeptidase is responsible for the coagulation of milk in the stomach by breaking the kappa-casein chain. The secretion of pepsin only becomes quantitatively important from the age of about 30 days.

The gastric pH is thus a useful criterion, because it influences the activity of enzymes such as salivary amylase and the proteolytic enzymes of the gastric juice. It also plays a role in solubilization and digestion of minerals. It is reported that secretion of hydrochloric acid begins at 16 days of age and is completely established by 30 days, after which the gastric pH does not change.

The gastric pH falls sharply during the period around weaning (from 4·6 at weaning age of 29 days to 1·8 at 36 days and to 1·6 at 42 days). However, there are variable reports. Apart from the possible effect of weaning age or feeding, these variations might be due to the location of measurement: when the rabbit practices caecotrophy, the pH of the fundus is almost neutral while the caecotrophes are being stored, whereas the pH of the antrum always remains very acid (< 3 after weaning).

After weaning, the rabbit stomach is always full as a result of the animal's continuous food intake and it cannot be emptied by fasting alone. It is also necessary to prevent reingestion of faeces. The stomach contents are tightly packed and much more solid than in other mammals.

(b) **Functions of caecotrophes within the stomach:** Soft faecal pellets are stored in the fundic region of the stomach where they remain intact for several hours. The soft faecal pellets consist of a bacterial concentrate within a mucus envelope. Within the stomach, they act as small incubators. The bacteria can thrive and produce amylase since they are protected by the mucus coat. This amylase diffuses into the stomach contents and may have a role in starch degradation because of its lower sensitivity to stomach acidity.

Establishment of Intestinal Flora

T. Gidenne and L. Fortun-Lamothe from France reviewed in 2002 the digestive capacity and nutritional needs of young rabbits. Until the end of the 1st week of life, the anterior part of the digestive tract of the young rabbit is virtually sterile (unlike that of the pig or the rat). During the first 2 weeks the stomach flora is absent in 75% of rabbits and very sparse in the small intestine. This situation is due to the bacteriostatic role of the C_8 and C_{10} fatty acids, which are prevalent in rabbit's milk (0.45 to 0.55 of the fatty acids) and are liberated by the young rabbit's gastric lipase. Feeding the rabbits with artificial milk based on cows' milk, without C_8 or C_{10} fatty acids, leads to the development of an abnormal intestinal flora. Thereafter the stomach flora increases slightly, and contains about 10^4 to 10^6 bacteria per g from the 30th day; a low level (100 to 1000 times less than in the rat), when one considers that the rabbit eats its own caecotrophes containing 10^7 to 10^9 bacteria per g. In the small intestine, the establishment of bacteria is faster and more abundant (10 to 100 times) than in the stomach.

The facultative anaerobic bacteria present before weaning are absent thereafter. Individual variation declines after weaning (28 to 30 days) and the flora stabilizes at 10^6 to 10^8 bacteria per g of contents. The caecum and the colon harbour an abundant flora (10^7 to 10^9 bacteria per g) from the 1st week, and thereafter the total number of bacteria remains permanently high (10^9 to 10^{10} per g). The facultative anaerobic flora is simple in the rabbit, dominated by *streptococci* until 14 days of age. Enterobacteria appear when solid feeding begins. The absence of the genus *Lactobacillus* in the rabbit flora is noteworthy and original.

The strictly anaerobic, non-sporulating bacteria, especially gram-negative bacteria (*Bacteroides*) dominate the digestive flora in every segment of the intestine. Sporulating bacteria are 100 to 1000 times less numerous than the *Bacteroides* and belong to the genera *Clostridium*, *Endosporus* and *Acuformis*.

The *Streptococci: S. faecium, S. faecalis* are nearly always absent from the stomach. In the small intestine, caecum and colon, their number reaches a maximum in rabbits aged 7 to 14 days and then declines with age.

Escherichia coli is generally absent in 2- to 3-day-old rabbits. This type of bacteria appears in specific pathogen free rabbits at 7 days reaches a maximum at the end of the 3rd week (up to 10^7 per g) and then falls sharply. This trend is practically independent of the feeding regimen of the young: milk followed by solid food, or given exclusively milk until 42 days. However, ten to 20% of 15- to 22-day-old rabbits have no detectable *E. coli* and this proportion reaches 30% in older rabbits (studied up to 49 days).

The bacteria involved in fibrolysis (hydrolysis of cellulose, xylans, pectins, etc.) only become established after 15 days of age, when solid feeding begins and a fibrous substrate enters the caecum. Then the fibrolytic flora increases slowly. Some of the strains involved in fibrolysis have been identified in the caecum: *Eubacterium cellulosolvens, Bacteroides sp.* (cellulose), *Bacteroides ruminicola, Butyrivibrio fibrisolvens* (pectins and xylans). However from 42 days of age xylanolytic and pectinolytic bacteria become established at a higher density than the cellulolytic bacteria.

So long as the rabbits are given only milk, the cellulolytic flora does not appear, even in rabbits of 35 to 42 days old. Hence, an exclusively milk diet until 42 days results in the absence of cellulolytic flora. It also produces a fermentative profile specific to a proteolytic metabolic activity, associated with a very low VFA concentration and a high pH. On the other hand, the removal of milk from 18 days of age by early weaning is followed 4 days later by a high concentration of VFA and a lower caecal pH compared with animals of the same age that are receiving only milk. For this reason, it seems necessary to offer young rabbits (from 18 to 20 days of age) a diet suited to their digestive capabilities, which will favour the establishment of a balanced caecal ecosystem.

Digestion of Food and Development of the Digestive Capacity

The development of the enzymatic system needed for the digestion of foods depends mainly on two kinds of factor: **ontogenetic factors** related to the age and the growth of the individual, and **nutritional factors** (Gidenne and Fortun-Lamothe, 2002). The development of the ability to digest starch depends primarily on ontogenetic factors. Several authors have suggested that the digestive tract of the young rabbits is not mature enough to digest starch until 35 days of age. The enzymatic system needed for the digestion of proteins (at least those of milk) is already effective at the time of birth in the stomach (pepsin) and pancreas (trypsin, chymotrypsin). The development of the trypsic and chymotrypsic activity of the pancreas is linear between 25 and 52 days of age, and seems to depend mainly on ontogenetic factors. The capacity of rabbits to digest fats is well developed from birth, as the lipids in the milk (10 to 25% on fresh basis) are their main source of energy.

The flora of the caecum and colon possesses numerous enzymic activities, which enable it to degrade the digesta that has escaped intestinal absorption: proteolysis, ureolysis, amylolysis, fibrolysis (pectins, cellulose, etc.). The degradation products are mainly ammonia and short-chain fatty acids (volatile fatty acids; VFA). The caecal concentration of these end products controls the acidity (pH) of the caecal medium, thus reflecting the fermentative activity of the flora. The fermentative activity, characterized mainly by the VFA concentration, is almost nil at 2 weeks of age and then increases rapidly with the start of ingestion of solid food, hence the fall in pH. The latter is also reinforced by the slight fall in ammonia concentration with age. A qualitative change in the fermentation is also observed: an increase in the proportion of butyrate with age (at the expense of acetate), whilst propionate remains stable. The whole tract (or faecal) digestibility is high at 25 days of age whichever nutrient is considered.

Although the development of the digestive capacity of the young rabbit is essentially under the control of ontogenetic factors, several research workers stated that the nutritional composition of the diet consumed around weaning could affect the development of intestinal digestive capacities and more particularly microbial activity in the caecum. The caecal fermentative parameters are also indicators of the health of the animals and their susceptibility to infection. It appears that a good supply of fibre before and after weaning has a favourable effect on health status. The ingestion of solid food before weaning seems to depend on numerous factors: the amount of milk available with the doe and the total quantity of food consumed before weaning, which is influenced by the factors such as palatability (aromatic compounds) perhaps, nutritional composition (such as simple sugar content) or the physical quality of the pellets (size, diameter and hardness).

Soft Faeces and Hard Faeces

The rabbit produces two types of faecal pellet, one soft type and the other hard type. Separation of digesta on the basis of particle size occurs in the hindgut. Peristaltic action rapidly moves large particles, primarily lignocellulose, through the colon to excrete them as hard faecal pellets. Antiperistaltic action moves small particles and solubles into the caecum, where they undergo fermentation. At intervals, the caecal contents are expelled as "soft faeces" and consumed by the rabbit directly from the anus without mastication. They are stored in the fundic region of the stomach where they remain intact for several hours. This reingested material provides microbial protein, vitamins and small quantities of volatile fatty acids (VFA are absorbed in the caecum and large intestine). The amino acids provided by microbial protein make only a minor contribution and diet must supply the additional amino acids.

Caecotrophy

Caecotrophy is the eating of faecal like pellets produced in the caecum. This is also called as coprophagy, sometimes called refection. Coprophagy is usually practised by the domestic rabbits as young as 3 weeks of age at night and wild rabbits during the day time while they are in burrows. Rabbits have a very strong physiological urge to carry out caecotrophy. This practice is sometimes called pseudo-rumination. Caecotrophy is a very important part of the rabbit's digestive processes. It recycles some unabsorbed nutrients as well as returning protein and vitamin B rich bacteria for enzymatic digestion in the small intestine. **Rabbits are caecotrophes rather than coprophags.**

A dietary supply of vitamins A, D and E is necessary. Bacteria in the gut synthesize vitamin K and vitamin B group in adequate quantities. Disease and stress may increase the daily vitamin requirements. Oxidation destroys vitamins A and E more readily than the other vitamins.

Level of Fibre

Better-feed efficiency for growth is possible by lowering the level of fibre/ lignocellulose (ADF) and increasing that of starch. However, a low supply of lignocellulose increases the frequency of digestive problems and thus reduces the digestive safety of the diets. In rabbit breeding, specific or non-specific enteropathy is always a major problem, leading to large losses of animals: about 30% from birth to slaughter in France, based on the production records of around 850 rabbit farms. Further, rabbits have a short reproductive life (< 10 months) for the doe.

Rabbits digest fibre poorly because of the selective separation and rapid excretion of large particles in the hindgut. Of forage eaters such as guinea pigs, horses, sheep, goats and cattle, the rabbit has the poorest ability to digest fibre the reason being that rabbits take about 30 hours only for the majority of food to pass through the digestive system [The average crude fibre digestibility in the rabbit is 0.14 compared with 0.22 for pigs, 0.33 for the guinea pigs and 0.41 for the horse (Maynard and Loosli, 1968)]. They need a generous amount of fibre (about 15%) in the diet to promote intestinal motility and minimize intestinal disease. Fibre may also absorb toxins of pathogenic bacteria and eliminate them via the "hard faeces". Diets low in fibre promote an increased incidence of intestinal problems. e.g. enterotoxaemia. High fibre diets (> 20% CF) may result in an increased incidence of caecal impaction and mucoid enteritis.

Proportions of VFAs in the caecal contents are of the order 60 to 70% acetic, 15 to 20% butyric and 10 to 15% propionic acid. The ratios are influenced by the level of fibre in the diet, a high (14.7%) fibre level tending to increase acetate and reduce propionate and butyrate when compared with a low (6.1%) dietary crude fibre. The production and absorption of VFAs appears to take place in the caecum and proximal colon only.

Role of Dietary Fibre in Rabbit Feeding

The rabbit is a monogastric herbivorous animal and its digestive physiology is well adapted to high intake of plant cell walls. Therefore, dietary fibres (Current levels of fibre in a complete feed used for the growing rabbit: CF 14-18%; ADF 16-21%; NDF 27-42%) are the main constituent of a rabbit feed even in intensive production. In general, cellulose is slowly hydrolysed by the enzymes of the host digestive tract (mainly composed of bacteria and protozoa according to animal species), while hemicellulosic and pectic fractions are generally more rapidly hydrolysed and fermented and the lignins remain largely undigested. These general facts are also proved in rabbit, since whole tract digestion of cellulose remain inferior to that of hemicelluloses (see Table 1).

Table 1 Whole Tract Digestibility Coefficient of Fibre Fractions (%) in the Growing Rabbit (Gidenne, 2003)

Class of dietary fibre	Mean	Range
Lignin (ADL)	10-15	−13 – + 50
Cellulose (ADF – ADL)	15-18	4–37
Hemicellulose (NDF – ADF)	25-35	11–60
Uronic acids (water soluble and insoluble)	70-76	30–85

T. Gidenne reviewed the role of fibres in rabbit feeding for their digestive health (Gidenne, 2003). Because the retention time in the caeco-colic segment is relatively short (8–12 h), the rapidly fermentable cell-wall oligosaccharides should play a key nutritional role for the rabbit digestive processes than for digestive health and sanitary status. Therefore, ingredients rich in pectins and hemicelluloses (e.g., brans and pulp) are particularly well digested by the rabbit.

Supplying dietary fibre to the growing rabbit is essential to avoid digestive disturbances. Its digestive 'security', however, is reached if attention is paid to respect a balanced fibre supply for low and highly digested fibre classes (Gidenne, 2003). Cellulose and lignins that are poorly digested play a key role in reducing the incidence of diarrhoea in the growing rabbit. Incorporating fibre sources rich in digestible fibre (brans and pulp) in the rabbit feeds covers a double interest. When it replaced sources of starch or protein, digestible fibre is highly utilised for growth, and it improves the digestive health of the animal, if a correct supply in lignocellulose is respected. Because of their high digestibility, digestible fibre may also have another nutritional role in stimulating the activity of the caecal flora in the young.

Gidenne *et al* (2001) evaluated the performance and digestive response of the growing rabbits (New Zealand white X Californian hybrid) fed diets containing same amount of ADF but change in the nature of the ADF (this reflected in diets with reduction of ADL and increase of cellulose). Total tract apparent digestive coefficients were determined at 42 to 48 days of age using 6-day collection period. Retention time in the whole tract was measured over a 4-day period following oral administration of ([141]cerium-labelled cell wall particles) the marker. The nature of the lignocellulose affected the performance and health of the rabbits. Foods containing lignocellulose with low lignin proportions caused higher mortality and morbidity rates and slower rate of passage in the gastrointestinal tract. In contrast, a high intake of lignins (over 5 g/day) reduced the health risk due to digestive troubles and stimulated the transit of digesta through the digestive system. An intake of lignin (ADL) of about 6 g/day appeared to ensure a good growth performance and health status.

Enterotoxaemia

Rabbits are very susceptible to the development of digestive disturbances. Enterotoxaemia is caused by proliferation in the caecum of bacteria that elaborate very potent toxins. *Clostridium spiroforme* is the causative microbe. Diets high in fermentable starch and low in fibre provoked increased enteritis incidence in fryers, while diets low in starch and high in fibre had protective effects. It was proposed that enterotoxaemia was caused by carbohydrate overload of the hindgut, providing a substrate allowing the proliferation of pathogens. A critical factor leading to enterotoxaemia is a drop in the caecal pH. The upset in normal gut flora is referred as dysbiosis. This indicates that the VFA produced in the caecum are important metabolites since they aid in the control of pathogenic organisms by helping to maintain an optimum pH in the caecum.

Copper sulfate has been shown to prevent enterotoxaemia. It was reported that copper sulfate at 250 ppm concentration in the medium inhibits growth of and toxin production by *C. spiroforme*.

Ascorbic acid inhibits toxin production. Commercial feed additives such as Lacto - Sacc (microencapsulated lactic acid bacteria and yeast culture) and Acid - Pak 4 – Way (Buffer pack containing microencapsulated bacteria, organic acids, and enzymes) are helpful in preventing enterotoxaemia.

Intestinal Microbiota - Role of Probiotics, Prebiotics and Postbiotics

Bacteria that colonize the gastrointestinal (GI) tract are collectively termed the intestinal microbiota. This bacterial community is important for extracting energy by fermenting the indigestible carbohydrates to short-chain fatty acids (SCFAs). Recent studies showed a wide range of functions in the GI tract including development of the immune system, defence against pathogens and inflammation. Identification of links: gut-brain, gut-lung and gut-liver highlighted the importance of the microbiota. Microbiota-derived metabolites have been detected in circulation. Thus, the intestinal microbiota playS an important role in a wide range of functions and whole body homeostasis (Klemashevich et al., 2014).

Alterations in the intestinal microbiota composition and function (i.e.dysbiosis) have been correlated to several diseases including obesity, diabetes, cancer and asthma. Therefore, an emerging approach for combating the onset or progression of these diseases is the restoration or 'strengthening' of the intestinal microbiota.

Introducing probiotics or adding prebiotics are the diet-based approaches employed for manipulating the intestinal microbial community. Advances in high-throughput sequencing and metabolomics have led to the emergence of postbiotics that can be used directly and specifically to manipulate microbiota function.

Diet-derived Postbiotics

An emerging approach to strengthening the microbiota is to first identify the molecules that are depleted in a particular disease, and then supplement the diet with either the depleted molecule or a precursor molecule that can be converted to the bioactive molecule by the microbial community. This approach is especially attractive as these postbiotics are an important class of functional molecules used by the microbiota to modulate human health.

Amino acid derivatives transformed by the gut microbiota make up one class of compounds that are potential postbiotics; example, indole that can be derived from tryptophan. SCFAs are another class of bioactive and beneficial molecules produced by the microbiota.

Conclusions: Manipulation of the microbiota through probiotics and prebiotics has shown great potential for treating a broad range of human diseases. Potentially more effective approaches, such as mixtures of prebiotics and probiotics or 'synbiotics', are emerging as our understanding of the role the microbiota plays in health and disease increases. Recent advances in metagenomics have begun to establish the phylogenies of microbes in human intestines. It is expected that the growing volume of genomic information will further accelerate the discovery of new probiotic strains as well as the development of food-derived prebiotcs and postbiotics for treating human disease.

Dietary Antioxidants in Rabbit Nutrition

Dietary antioxidants protect tissues against oxidative damage. There are a variety of stress factors that can disturb normal cell functions, initiating chain reactions that can compromise cell integrity and induce excessive production of reactive oxygen species. This could result in damage to the cell structures, including proteins, lipids and DNA, and induce physiological and pathological changes in the animal resulting in poor performance. Alpha-tocopheryl acetate and vitamin C are the most widely used dietary antioxidants in practical rabbit nutrition. The effect of selenium as antioxidant in most rabbit studies is doubtful (Abdel-Khalek. 2013). Alpha-tocopheryl acetate supplementation at the rate of 200 mg/kg diet could increase α-tocopherol content of muscles and could minimize their oxidative rancidity. Thus the supplemental antioxidants improve the functionality and protection against oxidative rancidity of the meat.

Acidification of Drinking Water in Rabbits

A commercial mixture of organic acid was added to ground water (control) in groups: pH 5.0, pH 4.3 and pH 3.6 by 0.55 g/kg, 0.85 g/kg and 3.3 g/kg, respectively (Zhu et al., 2014). The effect of drinking water acidification on the performance of weaned rabbits (5-week old) was studied for an experimental period of 35 days. The most appropriate pH of acidified drinking water was found to be 4.3 based on maximal positive effect on ADG, final weight and FCR.

Dietary Fructooligosaccharides (FOS)

Urinary N excretion was lowered by FOS feeding in rabbits (Min et al., 2013). Studies with ^{15}N-urea venous administration revealed that FOS in the diet increased the transfer of blood urea N to the caecum for bacterial synthesis, thereby increasing nitrogen utilization compared to glucose-fed rabbits.

NUTRIENT REQUIREMENTS AND FEEDING OF RABBITS

Nutrient requirements of rabbits during different lifestages are presented in Table 2. Tobin (1996) reported energy requirements in terms of ME per kg metabolic body weight. They are as follows: maintenance 418.4 KJ, growth 798-882 KJ, early and late gestation 567 and 840 KJ and lactation 1260 KJ. Rabbits require essential amino acids in the diet, as the bacterial protein obtained via coprophagy is inadequate. NRC (1977) recommended arginine 0.6%, lysine 0.65% and methionine plus cysteine 0.6% as a percentage of the diet to support growth and provide a safety margin for those at maintenance.

Table 2 Nutrient Requirements of Rabbits fed ad *libitum** (Percentage or amount per kg of diet).

Nutrient	Maintenance	Growth	Gestation	Lactation
Digestible Energy, kcal	2100	2500	2500	2500
CP %	12	16	15	17
DCP %	9	12	11	13
TDN %	55	65	58	70
Crude fibre % **	14	10-12	10-12	10-12
Fat % **	2	2	2	2

* Nutrient Requirements of Rabbits, NRC 1977.
** May not be minimum but known to be adequate.

Nutrient requirements as provided by ICAR (2013) are furnished in Table 2 A.

Table 2A Nutrient Requirements of Rabbits*

Nutrient	Growth	Maintenance	Gestation	Lactation
Digestible energy (kcal)	2700	2200-2300	2700	2700
Crude Protein (%)	18	14	18	19
Arginine (%)	0.6	0.6	0.6	0.6
Lysine (%)	0.7	0.5	0.7	0.7
Meth. & Cyst (%)	0.6	0.4	0.7	0.7
Digestible CP (%)	12-14	10-11	12-14	12-14
Crude Fibre (%)	12	12-14	12	10-12
ADF (%)	16-18	16-18	16-18	16-18
Fat / lipids (%)	2-4	2	2	2

* Source: ICAR(2013)

Feeds for Rabbits

Green roughages such as lucerne, berseem, cowpea, Stylo, siratro (legumes) and tender green grasses are relished by rabbits. Root crops such as carrots and turnips are favourites.

Digestibility of roughages in rabbits is lower than that in the ruminants. Consequently the TDN values in the feeds for rabbits are lower. For concentrate feeds there is no difference in the nutritive value for rabbits and ruminants. Normally 50 to 70% of DM requirements are supplied through roughages and the remaining with the concentrate mixture depending upon the physiological stage of rabbits. Complete pellet feed is popular.

Feeding large amount of cabbage or rapeseed produces goitre in rabbits as well as in other species. Cottonseed meal should be limited to no more than 5-7% of the diet since rabbits are sensitive to gossypol. Subabul has a toxic amino acid, mimosine. In rabbit feeding subabul leaves should not be fed more than 10% of the total DM intake (while in ruminants subabul can be incorporated up to 30% DMI). Some varieties may have higher levels of mimosine and hence caution has to be exercised in feeding subabul. If it is fed at higher levels, hair loss occurs in the rabbits.

It is recommended to add 2-5% oil in the diet for non-lactating animals (Tobin, 1996). Pascual *et al.* (1999) found lactating does had higher milk yields, higher weight gains and lower mortality of young ones when fed diets containing 9.9% or 11.7% lipid compared to those fed a diet with 2.6% lipid.

Pelleted diets: Rabbits prefer a pelleted diet to that in a meal form. Some individuals may refuse to consume a nonpelleted diet while others adjust to a meal diet and accept it satisfactorily. But during the adjustment period feed intake is very low and feed wastage is much. Molasses or fat has to be added to the meal diet to reduce dustiness and to increase palatability. Growth rate and feed efficiency were significantly better with the pelleted diets. Molasses is added at 2-3% to 6% to improve palatability and to reduce dust.

Pellet Binders: The fibre content of rabbit rations is higher than in rations for most other livestock. When pelleted, high fibre rations are usually very friable and give rise to unacceptable wastage.

Calcium lignosulphonate, a byproduct from wood pulp manufacture, is widely used as pellet binder in animal foods. Calcium and sodium lignosulphonates in rabbit diets have been shown to be associated with a high incidence of ulceration of the colon and high mortality whereas magnesium lignosulphonate appears to have no harmful effect. But rabbits found to grow more slowly. Similar effects of lignosulphonates have been shown in the guinea pig.

So lignosulphonates are to be excluded and sodium bentonite is preferred. Concentrate feed pellets of 3-4 mm to 4-6 mm diameter and 10 -15 mm length are preferred.

Feeding Behaviour

Baby rabbits: Introduce creep feed from 16th day onwards. Baby rabbits start to leave the nest and eat small quantities of compound feed at about 21 days old. Caecotrophy starts early, probably at the time when intake of solid food begins and is well established by 4-6 weeks of age. Weaning is done at 3-5 weeks of age.

Feeding Strategies Around Weaning

Analysis of the literature shows that the nutritional requirements of the young rabbits and those of their mother are antagonistic: the former require a high dietary fibre and a low starch content, whereas the latter need a high-energy diet.

To reduce the stress of a sudden change in diet in the case of early weaning (going from a diet consisting, almost exclusively of milk to solid food), it is possible to stimulate the start of solid food ingestion in rabbits by means of progressive weaning. This can be done by leaving out some sucklings before weaning (for example on the 16th, 18th, 20th, and 22nd days of lactation, for a weaning at 23 days). It is of course necessary that the rabbits have access to water and solid food. This solution would have the dual advantage of progressively reducing the milk production of the mothers and reducing the risk of appearance of mastitis.

Experimental results indicated that the digestive capacity of young rabbits (25 days of age) for starch is limited, but the addition of enzymes (α-amylase, xylanase, β-glucanase and polygalacturanase) and heat treatment improved food digestion. As regards the source of the starch, the young rabbits grew better on wheat than on peas, whose starch is less easily digested. Early weaning (< 26 days) could be a promising way to provide adequate feeding for the young as soon as they begin to eat solid food.

Young growing rabbits: After weaning, food intake quickly increases until DM intake is about 5.5% of live weight and this level is maintained until maturity (Table 3).

Amounts of Food Eaten

Age	Weight of food (g/day)	
Birth-15 days	0	
15-21 days	0-20	Water consumption
21-35 days	10-50	is about twice the
35-42 days	40-80	weight of food DM
42-49 days	70-110	consumed
49-63 days	100-160	

Under Indian conditions the feed intakes reported are:

At 4 weeks of age	40 g
At 10 weeks of age	100 g and
Adults	120-160 g

Adult Doe: It is usually fed restricted quantity of food to prevent overfatness (Table 3). If fertility is poor in maiden does which have been on a restricted regime, "flushing ration" for 4 days before and one day after mating has been shown to improve fertility considerably.

A restricted (140 g/day-Californian does) level during pregnancy followed by unrestricted feeding during lactation resulted in a higher milk yield and better growth rate in their young in the first week of life. Food and water intakes usually decrease sharply on the last day before parturition. Soaked Bengal gram (50 g/day) can be given to lactating does for better performance. As lactation becomes established food intake increases to a maximum after 20-30 days.

The meat rabbit: The New Zealand White and the Californian are important examples.

Weight of foetus at day 16	1 g
Birth weight	60 g

Individual birth weight has been shown to decrease as litter size increases.

Age at slaughter :	8 - 10 weeks
Weight :	2.1 - 2.7 kg
Killing out percentage :	50 - 55
	Adult weight
The New Zealand White	4.0-5.5 kg
The Californian	3.5-4.8 kg

Feed conversion ratio (The NewZealand White)

2:1 at 3 weeks age (Two kg or food eaten per kg of weight gained)

3:1   at 8 weeks
4:1   at 10 weeks
5:1   at 12 weeks or more.

A meat rabbit should attain 2.4 kg live weight at about 10 weeks old. Since growth rate begins to diminish after 8 weeks, attainment of the desired market weight during or soon after the phase of rapid growth is therefore of paramount importance for economic production of rabbit meat.

Lactation: The rabbit is unusual among domestic mammals because the young are suckled only once per day usually in the early morning and is completed in 2-5 minutes. Occasionally some does will permit their young to suckle more than once in the first 2-3 days of life.

The doe's milk production follows a typical mammalian lactation curve, reaching a peak at 18-21 days and then decreasing rapidly until weaning takes place [(3 to 5 weeks under commercial conditions or natural weaning after 6 weeks of parturition (kindling)]. Peak yield is 280 g/day; six-week lactation yield is about 7 kg, 55% of it in the first 3-weeks/4 weeks.

The nutrients used by the lactating mammary gland resemble those of the ruminant; acetate is the most important precursor for milk fat synthesis.

Table 3   Feed Consumption of Rabbits as % of Live Weight (LW) during Different Physiological States.

Body Weight (kg)	Total daily feed (% of LW)
	Normal growth, Does or Bucks, av. 3 kg
1.5 - 4.0	5.8
	Normal growth and fattening, Does or Bucks
1.8	6.2
2.3	6.0
2.7	5.7
3.2	5.4
	Maintenance, Does or Bucks
2.3	4.0
4.5	3.3
6.8	3.0
	Pregnant Does
2.3	5.0
4.5	4.1
6.8	3.7

Example of a purified diet (Table 4) and complete diets for rabbits of different physiological stages (Table 5 and 6) are furnished for perusal and learning.

Table 4 Purified Diet for Rabbits.

Ingredient	% of Diet
Isolated soy protein	20.0
Purified cellulose	16.0
Corn oil	5.0
Mineral mixture[a]	6.6
Vitamin mixture[b]	0.2
Choline chloride (70%)	0.1
Antioxidant (Ethoxyquin)	0.025
DL-Methionine	0.2
Glucose monohydrate	15.0
Corn dextrin	5.0
Corn starch	27.4
Water (for pelleting)	5.0
α-Tocopherol acetate	50 IU/kg

(a) Composition (in mg/kg): $CoCl_2. 6H_2O$, 3.5; $CuSo_4. 5 H_2O$, 34.6; $MnSO_4. H_2O$, 81.1: $ZnSO_4$, 169; $FeC_6H_5O_4. 14H_2O$,706.3; $(NH_4)_6 MO_7O_{24}. 4H_2O$, 22.7; (in g/kg): K_2HPO_4, 10; $KHCO_3$, 10; $NaHCO_3$, 8; NaCl, 5; $CaCO_3$, 12.5; $CaHPO_4$, 10.

(b) Composition (in mg/kg): thiamin-HCl, 25; riboflavin, 16; Ca pantothenate, 20; pyridoxine-HCl, 6; biotin, 0.6; folic acid, 4; menadione, 5; vitamin B_{12}, 0.02; ascorbic acid, 250, niacin, 150; vitamin A, 10,000 IU; l vitamin D_3, 600 IU: a-tocopherol acetate, 10 IU.

Source: NRC, 1977.

Feeding of Angora Rabbits

The quantity of feed required by Angora rabbit depends upon the age, body weight, season and physiological status of the animal. Adult, non-breeding, non-lactating does, and non-breeding male rabbits can be fed concentrate at 120-150 g per day, preferably in the morning. This feed should contain about 14-16% DCP. Does in advanced pregnancy and lactating stages will need about 200 g of quality balanced concentrate feed containing 18-20% DCP and 12-16% of crude fibre. The growing young Angora should be given 80-100 g of good-quality feed.

The nutrition of Angora rabbit must be very good as the animal has to produce wool protein throughout the year. There is a higher requirement of sulphur-containing amino acids, e.g, methionine. Roughage supplement in the feed is highly desirable to avoid wool eating and formation of hair-balls in the stomach. Improper and inadequate nutrition of rabbits will lead to rough coats, poor wool production, lack of body growth, deformed skeletons,

Table 5 Examples of Adequate Diets for Commercial Production (suitable for pelleting).

Kind of animal	Ingredients	% of Total Diet*
Growth, 0.5 to 4 kg	Alfalfa hay	50
	Maize grain	23.5
	Barley grain	11
	Wheat bran	5
	Soybean meal	10
	Salt	0.5
Maintenance, does and bucks, av. 4.5 kg	Clover hay	70
	Oats grain	29.5
	Salt	0.5
Pregnant does av. 4.5 kg	Alfalfa hay	50
	Oats grain	45.5
	Soybean meal	4
	Salt	0.5
Lactating does, av. 4.5 kg	Alfalfa hay	40
	Wheat grain	25
	Sorghum grain	22.5
	Soybean meal	12
	Salt	0.5

*Composition given on as-fed basis.

Table 6 Examples of Complete Feeds for Rabbits.

Nutritive value (%)		Feedstuff	Grower diet	Maintenance diets		
TDN	CP			1	2	3
60	15	Cowpea hay	30	50	50	50
80	10	Maize grain	28	10	10	-
67	10	DORB	25	33	38	46
72	45	GNC (Exp)	15	5	-	2
-	-	Min. mixture	1.5	1.5	1.5	1.5
-	-	Salt	0.5	0.5	0.5	0.5
			100	100	100	100
		Crude Protein %	16.6	14	12.3	13.0
		Total digestible nutrients %	68.0	65	63.5	62.24

dull/watery eyes, poor reproductive efficiency and higher rate of mortality in the flock.

Commercial Rearing of Rabbits

Sheep Breeding Research Station, Sandynallah, Nilgiris district, Tamil Nadu produced crossbred rabbits using high yielding New Zealand White (NZW) and the local 'Nilgiri'. Weaning weight at 3 weeks of age are 250 g and 500 g in respect of crossbreds and NZD, respectively, while the weight at 12 weeks age are 1-1.5 kg and 2.5 kg. Litter size is 6 bunnies per litter. One commercial unit consists of one male buck and 10 does. Up to 4 litters a year are obtained; kits are weaned at 4-6 weeks of age; young reach sexual maturity in four months; age to breed is 6 months; there is no regular oestrus cycle observed in rabbits, and normally they are believed to come to heat once every five days. Mother doe can be allowed to mate leaving a week's rest after weaning. By adopting 10 + 2 units one can get 192 rabbits every year.

Under commercial system, rabbits can be fed with concentrate feed pellets of 4-6 mm diameter and 10-15 mm length along with 200 g of greens/day. Generally concentrate feeding precedes greens (grass + forages) feeding. Concentrate feed has to be given in two divided doses. Rabbits generally eat more during night in summer. With the onset of winter, the requirement increases and the feeding shift to day time. However, regular timetable for feeding is advisable so that rabbits do not feel any stress due to the change in their daily routine. Sudden changes in feeds and feeding systems should be avoided. The rabbits must be fed at the same time every day. While offering green grass, it should be wilted for one day. Providing adequate fibre in the ration is a must to prevent enteric diseases and fur chewing.

Fur chewing can be controlled by increasing the fibre and protein contents of the ration. Further addition of 200 grams of magnesium oxide per quintal of feed helps control fur chewing. Since weaners are more sensitive to change of feed, care must be taken to avoid carbohydrate overload. Clean potable water must be provided throughout the day.

Rabbits under backyard system can be raised on grain free diets comprising of forages, grain by-products, tree leaves, vegetable wastes, culled vegetables and kitchen wastes. Broiler type rabbits can be raised on sole feeding of mixed greens and vegetable wastes and the final bodyweight at 12 weeks and 24 weeks would be 1.0 kg and 2.0 kg respectively.

References

Gidenne, T. 2003. Fibres in rabbit feeding for digestive troubles prevention: respective role of low-digested and digestible fibre. Livestock Production Science 81, 105-117.

Gidenne, T., Arveux, P. and Madec, O. 2001. The effect of the quality of dietary lignocellulose on digestion, zootechnical performance and health of the growing rabbit. Animal Science 73, 97-104.

Gidenne, T. and Fortun-Lamothe, L. 2002. Feeding strategy for young rabbits around weaning: a review of digestive capacity and nutritional needs. Animal Science 75, 169-184.

Pascual, J.J, Cervea, C., Blas, E. and Fernandez-Carmona, J. 1999. Effect of high fat diets on performance and milk composition of mulltiparous rabbit does. Animal Science 68, 151-162.

Phull, A. and Phull, R.K. 2003. Rabbit farming and its economics. 2nd revised and enlarged edition, published by International Book Distributing Co. Lucknow.

Tobin, G. 1996. Small pets, food types, nutrient requirements and nutritional disorders. In: Kelly, N. and Wills, J. (eds) Manual of Companion Animal Nutrition and Feeding. British Small Animal Veterinary Association, Cheltenham, U.K., pp. 208-225.

15

Laboratory Animal Nutrition

Though the majority of animals used in biomedical research at present are mice and rats, a number of other species continue to serve as models in the effort to advance human and animal health. These include laboratory rabbit, guinea pig, hamster, chinchilla, gerbil, vole, degu (*Octodon degus*).

Guinea pigs first became popular as pets in the 16th century because of their size and docile nature. Since that time, they have contributed significantly to advancements in biomedical research in areas such as reproduction and respiratory physiology. A principal reason for the overall decline in their use is the increased use of mice as a favoured animal model. Guinea pigs remain a valuable model of several human disease conditions. Guinea pigs currently play a prominent role in hearing research, toxicology, and the study of allergic diseases, non-infectious pulmonary diseases, reproductive disorders, osteoarthritis, and atherosclerosis. They are also used routinely to study a wide variety of bacterial, viral, and fungal infections.

General Considerations for Feeding and Diet Formulation

A nutritionally balanced diet is important both for the welfare of laboratory animals and to ensure that experimental results are not biased by unintended nutritional factors. The nutritional status of the laboratory animal influences its general well-being and its ability to respond to pathogens and other environmental stresses.

It is important to recognize that the estimated requirements of the laboratory animals have been determined under specific restrictive conditions. The physicochemical characteristics of feeds such as physical form, sensory properties, naturally occurring refractory or antinutritive compounds, chemical contaminants, and conditions of storage affect feed palatability and intake, nutrient absorption and utilization, and excretion.

Domestic Guinea Pig

The domestic guinea pig (*Cavia porcellus*) has been bred in captivity for at least 400 years and probably originated in Peru, Argentina, or Brazil. In its natural habitat this herbivorous animal consumes large quantities of vegetation. The molar teeth are especially suited to grinding and, like other species of rodents, the guinea pig has open-rooted incisors that grow continuously throughout its life.

Like the rat, mouse, and rabbit, the guinea pig is simple stomached; but in contrast to these species, the entire stomach of guinea pig is lined with glandular epithelium. Intestine allows growth of gram positive bacterial flora, which may contribute to the nutritional requirements of the host perhaps through direct absorption of bacterial metabolites or digestion and absorption of intestinal bacteria and other materials following coprophagy. It has a large semicircular caecum with numerous lateral pouches. This organ resembles that of the rabbit and possibly has similar digestive functions, e.g. synthesis of B vitamins and indispensable amino acids by microorganisms and recycling of intestinal contents by coprophagy.

Few serious attempts have been made to determine the contribution of coprophagy to the nutrition of the guinea pig.

Some Data on Production

Male Guinea pig (Boar): one for every five females (Sows)
Female Guinea pig:
Average litter size = 3.5 (range 1-8)
Weight at birth = 85 to 100 g
Weaning age = 12 to 14 days or at 170 g weight
Age to breed = 2.5 to 3 months
Gestation period = 66 to 72 days (68 ± 2)
Breeding life = 4 to 6 months of age to 2 years
No. of litters/year = 3
Guinea pigs in advanced pregnancy are placed in hutches. Parturition takes place in hutches.
Average body weight of adult animal = 500 g
Adult animals consume diet at the rate of 7 to 8% of B.W.

Data on Feed Consumption

Growing guinea pigs	=	20-30 g/day
Adult guinea pigs	=	30-50 g/day

Pregnant and lactating guinea pigs $\quad = \quad$ 40-60 g
(depending upon the litter size and season)
Dry matter consumption is reduced during hot summer.

Table 1 Requirements for Compounded Feeds for Guinea Pigs (BIS Requirements).

Sl. No	Characteristics		Requirements	
1.	Moisture	, % by weight,	Max	10
2.	CP	, % by weight,	Min	22
3.	EE	, % by weight,	Min	4
4.	CF	, % by weight,		9-14
5.	Total ash	, % by weight,		9
6.	AIA	, % by weight,	Max	1.0
7.	Calcium	, % by weight,	Min	1.2
8.	P	, % by weight,	Min	0.6
9.	Vitamin C mg/kg		Min	200

Feeding of Guinea Pigs

In the laboratory, the guinea pig's diet is much higher in energy density and lower in fibre content than the diet of green vegetation and fruits it consumes in the wild. The guinea pig consumes many small meals throughout the day, is fastidious in choice of foods, and may resist abrupt changes in composition or form of the diet. Animals fed pelleted natural-ingredient diets often do not readily accept a powdered purified diet unless introduced gradually.

Newborn animals can consume semisolid and solid food immediately, although weaning is followed around 3 weeks of age. Guinea pigs normally gain as much as 5 to 7 g/day during the rapid growth period when allowed to eat good feed *ad libitum*. Growth slows after 2 months and maturity is reached at about 5 months. Weight gain can continue until 12 to 15 months of age and level off at 700 to 850 g for females and 950 to 1,200 g for males. Mating is most often successful when females are 450 to 600 g (2.5 to 3 months old).

Nutrient requirements (Tables 1 and 2) and examples of natural-ingredient diet (Table 3) and purified diets (Table 4) are presented for information. Maintenance energy requirement is 136 Kcal ME/BW $kg^{0.75}$.

The guinea pig is best known, from a nutritional standpoint, by its requirement for dietary vitamin C. This feature has made the guinea pig particularly useful in studies of collagen biosynthesis, wound healing, and bone growth.

Dietary fructooligosaccharides: The dietary fructooligosaccharides had no significant effects on body weight gain or N digestibility, but showed significantly lower value for the urinary N excretion and ADF digestibility and significantly higher N retention in the guinea pigs allowed caecotrophy (Kawasaki et al., 2013). In the guinea pigs prevented from caecotrophy, FOS had no effect on N retention. These results suggest that FOS stimulates caecal microbial proliferation, thereby improving nitrogen utilization in the guinea pigs.

Table 2   Estimated Nutrient Requirements for Growth for Guinea Pig*.

Nutrient	Unit	Amount per kg diet	Comments
Protein (28.6 g N × 6.25)	g	180.0	
Essential fatty acids (n-6)	g	1.33-4.0	10 g corn oil/kg diet is satisfactory
Fibre	g	150.0	Used cellulose and/or materials of low digestibility to supply bulk
Amino acids			
Arginine	g	12.0	
Histidine	g	3.0	
Isoleucine	g	6.0	
Leucine	g	10.8	
Lysine	g	8.4	
Methionine	g	6.0	
Phenylalanine	g	10.8	
Threonine	g	6.0	
Tryptophan	g	1.8	
Valine	g	8.4	
Dispensable nitrogen	g	16.9	
Minerals			
Calcium	g	8.0	Requirements for calcium,
Phosphorus	g	4.0	phosphorus, magnesium and
Magnesium	g	1.0	potassium seem to reflect
Potassium	g	5.0	interactions among them.
Chloride	g	0.5	From the estimate for
Sodium	g	0.5	rats fed purified diet
Copper	mg or ppm	6.0	
Iron	mg	50.0	Estimate

[Table Contd.]

[*Table Contd.*]

Manganese	mg	40.0	
Zinc	mg	20.0	
Iodine	μg or ppb	150.0	Based on rat requirement
Molybdenum	μg	150.0	Based on rat requirement
Selenium	μg	150.0	Based on rat requirement

Vitamins

A (retinol) or	mg	6.6	Equivalent to 21,960 IU/kg
(β-carotene)	mg	28.0	Used 40% as efficiently as preformed vitamin A
D₃ (cholecalciferol)	mg	0.025	Adequate; no quantitative data. Equivalent to 1000 IU/kg.
E (RRR-α-tocopherol)	mg	26.7	Adequate; Equivalent to 40 IU/kg. Higher concentrations may be required if high fat diets are used.
K (Phylloquinone)	mg	5.0	Adequate; dietary deficiency has not been produced
Ascorbic acid	mg	200.0	
Biotin (d-biotin)	mg	0.2	Adequate; Simple dietary deficiency has not been produced
Choline			
(Choline bitartrate)	mg	1,800	
Folic acid	mg	3.0-6.0	
Niacin	mg	10.0	
Pantothenic acid			
(Ca-d-pantothenate)	mg	20.0	
Pyridoxine	mg	2.0-3.0	
Riboflavin	mg	3.0	Estimated
Thiamin	mg	2.0	
(Thiamin - HCl)			

Note: Nutrient requirements are expressed on an as-fed basis for diets containing 10% moisture; 2.8-3.5 Kcal ME/g (11.7-14.6 KJ ME/g) and should be adjusted for diets of differing moisture and energy concentrations. Unless otherwise specified, the listed nutrient concentrations represent minimal requirements and do not include a margin of safety. Higher concentrations for many nutrients may be warranted in natural-ingredient diets.

Table 3   Example of a Natural-Ingredient Diet used for Guinea Pig Breeding Colonies at the National Institute of Health, USA.*

Ingredient	Amount (g/kg)
Alfalfa meal (17% protein)	350.0
Soybean meal (49% protein)	120.0
Ground whole oats	252.5
Ground whole wheat	236.0
Soybean oil	15.0
Dicalcium phosphate	5.0
Calcium carbonate	10.0
Salt	7.5
Mineral and vitamin premixes[a,b]	4.0

a Specifications for mineral premix provided by the manufacturer (mg/kg diet): cobalt 1.5 (as cobalt carbonate); copper, 6.6 (as copper sulfate); manganese, 39.7 (as manganese oxide); zinc, 19.8 (as zinc oxide); iodine, 1.1 (as calcium iodate).
b Specifications for vitamin premix provided by the manufacturer (IU/kg diet); vitamin A, 6,614 (from stabilized vitamin A palmitate or acetate); vitamin D_3, 2,200 (from d-activated animal sterols); and (mg/kg diet) vitamin E, 22 (from all-rac-α-tocopheryl acetate); vitamin K,5 (menadione activity); thiamin, 4.4 (thiamin mononitrate); riboflavin, 3.3; niacin, 11; pantothenic acid, 11 (from Ca-d-pantothenate); choline, 529 (from choline chloride); pyridoxine, 5 (from pyridoxine-HCl); folic acid, 4.8; biotin, 2.2; ascorbic acid, 992; methionine hydroxy analogue, 500; and vitamin B_{12} (11 μg/kg diet).
* Adapted from Nutrient Requirements of Laboratory Animals, 4th revised edition 1995.

Table 4   Examples of Four Satisfactory Purified Diets for Guinea Pigs.*

Nutrient	Amount, g/kg diet			
	Navia and Lopez, 1973	O'Dell et al., 1989	Typpo et al., 1985	Apgar and Everett, 1991 a, b
Casein	300.0[a]		300.0[a]	300.0 [a]
Other protein			200.0[b]	
Sucrose, granulated	431.4	488.0	50.0	
Sucrose, powdered			196.0	
Glucose monohydrate			150.0	310.0
Corn oil	40.0[c]	40.0	30.0	100.0
Fibre[d]	130.1	150.0	150.0	150.0
L-arginine			3.0	
DL-methionine	2.0	5.0[e]		

Mineral mixture	72.2^f	85.0^g	75.0^h	100.0^i
Vitamin mixture	3.3^j	30.0^k	42.0^l	40.0^m
Choline chloride	1.0	2.0	2.0	n
Myo-inositol			2.0	
Agar	20.0			o

Note: See each reference for special diet preparation. Nutrient requirements are expressed on an as-fed basis for diets containing 10 percent moisture. Diet used by Apgar and Everett (1991 a, b) is satisfactory for pregnant guinea pigs.

a   Vitamin-free casein. Apgar and Everett (1991 a, b) treated casein with EDTA primarily to remove zinc.

b   Isolated soybean protein or heat-treated casein, egg white or lactalbumin.

c   Cottonseed oil instead of corn oil.

d   Cellulose, except wood pulp (O'Dell *et al.*, 1989) and cellophane (Typpo *et al.*, 1985).

e   With isolated soybean protein only.

f   Mineral ingredients (g/kg diet): $CaHPO_4$, 8.30; $CaCO_3$, 14.50; $KC_2O_2H_3$, 27.00; KCl, 4.50; NaCl, 2.80; MgO,5.00; $MgSO_4$, 0.50; $MgCO_3$, 1.00; $Fe_3(PO_4)$, 1.60; $MnSO_4.H_2O$, 0.80; KIO_3, 0.038; $ZnSO_4.7H_2O$, 0.025; $CuSO_4$, 0.036; $CoCl_2.6H_2O$, 0.03; $AlK(SO_4)_2.12H_2O$, 0.007, NaF; 0.04.

g   Mineral ingredients (g/kg diet): $CaHPO_4.2H_2O$,25.4; $CaCO_3$,9.0; $NaHPO_4$,6.4; $KC_2O_2H_3$,25; NaCl,2.6; MgO,5.0; $MgSO_4$,3.0; $MnSO_4.H_2O$,0.61; Fecitrate, 0.36; $CuSO_4$,0.02; KIO_3,0.017. Diet supplemented with 100 mg Zn/kg as $ZnCO_3$.

h   Mineral ingredients (g/kg diet): $CaHPO_4$,34.92; $CaCO_3$,5.94; $KC_2O_2H_3$,24.93; KCl, 7.74; NaCl, 5.76; MgO, 4.96; $MgSO_4$, 4.59; Fecitrate, 0.64; $MnSO_4.H_2O$, 0.37; KIO_3, 0.015; $ZnCO_3$, 0.13; $CuSO_4$, 0.005; $KCr(SO_4)_2.12H_2O$, 0.010; $Na_2MoO_4.2H_2O$,0.0005; $NiCl_2.6H_2O$,0.0002; Na_2SeO_3,0.0002.

i   Mineral ingredients (g/kg diet): $CaHPO_4$, 7.4; $CaCO_3$, 12.9; $NaHPO_4.7H_2O$, 28; $KC_2O_2H_3$, 24; NaCl, 2.5; KCl, 4; $MgSO_4.7H_2O$, 4.9; MgO, 4.4; $MgCO_3$, 0.9; $FeSO_4.7H_2O$, 2.04; $MnSO_4.H_2O$, 0.71; KIO_3, 0.034; $CuSO_4.5H_2O$, 0.05; $CoCl_2.6H_2O$, 0.027. Zinc was supplied in drinking water at 15 mg/L (as Zn acetate).

j   Vitamin mixture supplied (mg/kg diet): ascorbic acid, 2,000; biotin, 0.2; folic acid, 10; inositol, 1,000; niacin, 50; Ca-pantothenate, 30; pyridoxine-HCl, 10; riboflavin, 10; thiamin, 10; vitamin B_{12} (triturated with mannitol at a concentration of 0.1 percent), 30; menadione, 10; (IU/kg diet): vitamin A, 28,500; vitamin D_2, 285; all-rac-α-tocopherol, 40.

k   Vitamin mixture in sucrose supplied (mg/kg diet): biotin, 0.2; folic acid, 6; niacin 50; Ca-pantothenate, 30; pyridoxine-HCl,10; riboflavin, 10; thiamin, 10; vitamin B_{12}, 0.03; menadione, 10; (IU/kg diet); retinyl acetate, 20,000; cholecalciferol, 2,800; α-tocopherol, 20. Ascorbic acid was given in 30 mg doses 6 days/week *per os*.

1 Vitamin mixture supplied (mg/kg diet): ascorbic acid, 2000; biotin, 0.5; folic acid, 10; niacinamide, 200, Ca-pantothenate, 40; pyridoxine-HCl,16; riboflavin, 16; thiamin- HCl,16; vitamin B_{12} (0.1% trituration in mannitol), 50; retinal palmitate in oil, 52 (5.200 IU); cholecalciferol, 0.04; DL-tocopherol acetate, 20; menadione, 2.

m Vitamin mixture supplied (mg/kg diet): ascorbic acid, 4,000; biotin, 12.6; choline, 3,100; folic acid, 12; myo-inositol, 4,000; niacin,400; Ca-pantothenate, 60; pyridoxine-HCl,13.5; riboflavin, 30; thiamin-HCl,30; vitamin B_{12},0.02; menadione, 4.6; (IU/kg diet): retinyl palmitate 45,000; ergocalciferol, 4,400; α-tocopheryl acetate, 198.

n Provided in vitamin mixture.

o The diet was mixed 1:1 with a 2 percent agar solution.

RAT

Breeds

The Black rat (*Rattus rattus*)
The Norway rat (*Rattus norvegicus*) $\Big\}$ Laboratory rat
The brown rat (*Rattus norvegicus*)

The laboratory rat (*Rattus norvegicus*) has long been favoured as an experimental animal for nutritional research because of its moderate size, profligate reproduction and adaptability to diverse diets. It is now the species of choice because of the large body of available data and the availability of strains with specific characteristics that facilitate the study of disease and other processes.

Females produce 1 to 12 litters per year, and those in a colony nurture their young collectively. The Norway rat is omnivorous, eating a wide variety of seeds, grains, and other plant matter as well as invertebrates and small vertebrates (Nowak, 1991). The rat's digestive tract resembles that of other omnivorous rodents (gall bladder is absent in the rat) in that the stomach contains both nonglandular and glandular regions, the small intestine is of moderate length, and the caecum is relatively well developed.

Some data on Production

1. Weight at birth : 4 to 5 g. May fall below 4 g if litter size is 10 to 12
2. The eyes are opened at 14 to 16 days of age.
3. Weaning age : 21 days
   Weight at weaning : 35 g
4. Gestation period : 21 days

5. Age at 1st litter : 93 to 111 days
6. Litter size : 4 to 8
7. Productive life in females : 480 to 512 days
8. Life span : 2.5 to 3 years
9. No. of litters in life time : 5-7/rat
10. Weight of adult rat at 1 year age
    Rattus rattus   Male : 203 g
                      Female : 193 g
11. Feed intake:
    Growing rats ⎫
    Adult rats at maintenance ⎭ 15 g/rat/day
    Pregnant rats : 15 to 20 g/rat/day
    Lactating rats 30 to 40 g/rat/day

Nutrient Requirements

Maintenance energy requirement of adult rat is 114 Kcal ME/BW kg $^{0.75}$. However, it has been reported that the requirement for fat rats (e.g. Obese zucker) is approximately 15% lower than the requirement for normal rats. How do you explain this difference in maintenance energy requirement between normal and obese adults ? It is well established that resting heat production per kg metabolic body size is greater in working and producing animals than in nonworking animals.

Energy requirement for growing, pregnant and lactating rats are higher proportionate to the productivity status.

Although no definite carbohydrate requirement has been established, rats perform best with glucose or glucose precursors (such as other sugars, glycerol, glucogenic amino acids) in their diets.

Table 5 Requirements for Compounded Feeds for Laboratory Mice and Rats (BIS).

Sl. No	Characteristics		Requirements
1.	Moisture, % by weight	Max	10
2.	CP, % by weight	Min	24
3.	EE, % by weight		5
4.	CF, % by weight	Max	6
5.	Total ash, % by weight	Max	9
6.	AIA, % by weight	Max	1
7.	Ca, % by weight	Min	0.6
8.	Available P, % by weight	Min	0.3
9.	Tryptophan, % by weight	Min	0.2

[Table Contd.]

[*Table Contd.*]

10.	L-Lysine , % by weight	Min	1.0
11.	Met + Cystine, % by weight	Min	0.8
12.	L-Arginine, % by weight	Min	0.2
13.	EFA, % by weight	Min	0.2
14.	Vitamin A, IU/kg	Min	2700
15.	Vitamin D, IU/kg	Min	200
16.	Vitamin E, mg/kg	Min	40
17.	Vitamin B_2 mg/kg	Min	6
18.	Calcium-d-pantothenate, mg/kg	Min	20
19.	Nicotinic acid, mg/kg	Min	60
20.	Vitamin B_{12}, μg/kg	Min	100
21.	Choline, mg/kg	Min	1100

Nutrient requirements of rats (Table 5 and 6), examples of natural-ingredient diets (Table 7) and purified diet (Table 8) are presented as a guide for ration formulation.

Table 6 Estimated Nutrient Requirements for Maintenance, Growth, and Reproduction of Rats*.

Nutrient	Unit	Amount per kg diet		
		Maintenance	Growth	Reproduction (Female)
Fat	g	50.0	50.0	50.0
Linoleic acid (n-6)	g	+	6.0[+]	3.0[+]
Linolenic acid (n-3)	g	R	R	R
Protein	g	50.0[a]	150.0[a]	150.0
Amino acids[b]				
Arginine	g	ND	4.3	4.3
Aromatic AAs[c]	g	1.9	10.2	10.2
Histidine	g	0.8	2.8	2.8
Isoleucine	g	3.1	6.2	6.2
Leucine	g	1.8	10.7	10.7
Lysine	g	1.1	9.2	9.2
Methionine + cystine[++]	g	2.3	9.8	9.8
Threonine	g	1.8	6.2	6.2
Tryptophan	g	0.5	2.0	2.0
Valine	g	2.3	7.4	7.4
Other (including nonessentials)	g	41.3	66.0	66.0
Minerals				
Calcium	g	d	5.0	6.3

[*Table Contd.*]

[*Table Contd.*]

Chloride	g	d	0.5	0.5
Magnesium	g	d	0.5	0.6
Phosphorus	g	d	3.0	3.7
Potassium	g	d	3.6	3.6
Sodium	g	d	0.5	0.5
Copper	mg	d	5	8.0
Iron	mg	d	35.0	75.0
Manganese	mg	d	10.0	10.0
Zinc[e]	mg	d	12.0	25.0
Iodine	μg	d	150.0	150.0
Molybdenum	μg	d	150.0	150.0
Selenium	μg	d	150.0	400.0
Vitamins				
A (retinol)[f]	mg	d	0.7	0.7
D (cholecalciferol)[g]	mg	d	0.025	0.025
E (RRR-alpha-tocopherol)[h]	mg	d	18.0	18.0
K (phylloquinone)	mg	d	1.0	1.0
Biotin (d-biotin)	mg	d	0.2	0.2
Choline (free base)	mg	d	750.0	750.0
Folic acid	mg	d	1.0	1.0
Niacin (nicotinic acid)	mg	d	15.0	15.0
Pantothenate (Ca-d pantothenate)	- mg	d	10.0	10.0
Riboflavin	mg	d	3.0	4.0
Thiamin (thiamin-HCl)[i]	mg	d	4.0	4.0
B$_6$ (pyridoxine)	mg	d	6.0	6.0
B$_{12}$	μg	d	50.0	50.0

Note: Nutrient requirements are expressed on an as-fed basis for diets containing 10% moisture and 3.8-4.1 Kcal ME/g (16-17 KJ ME/g) and should be adjusted for diets of differing moisture and energy concentrations. Unless otherwise specified, the listed nutrient concentrations represent minimal requirments and do not include a margin of safety. Higher concentrations for many nutrients may be warranted in natural-ingredient diets. R, required but no concentration determined; other long-chain n-3 polyunsaturated fatty acids may substitute for linolenic acid. ND, not determined.

a Estimates based on highly digestible protein of balanced amino acid composition (e.g. lactalbumin).

b Asparagine, glutamic acid, and proline may be required for very rapid growth.

c Phenylalanine plus tyrosine. Tyrosine may supply up to 50 percent of aromatic acid requirement.

d Separate requirements for maintenance have not been determined for minerals and vitamins. Requirements presented for growth will meet maintenance requirements.

e Higher concentration is required when ingredients that contain phytate (such as soybean meal) are included in the diet.

f Equivalent to 2,300 IU/g. Requirement may also be met by 1.3 mg β-carotene/kg diet. Higher vitamin A concentration is needed under conditions of stress (e.g. surgical recovery).

g   Equivalent to 1,000 IU/kg.

h   Equivalent to 27 IU/kg. Higher concentration may be required if high fat diets are fed.

i   Higher concentration may be required with low-protein, high-carbohydrate diets.

*   Adapted from "Nutrient requirements of Laboratory Animals", 4th revised edition 1995.

\+   Females require only 2 g/kg linoleate for growth. Separate requirements for maintenance have not been determined for linoleate. Requirements presented for growth will meet maintenance requirements.

\++ Cystine may supply up to 50% of the methionine plus cystine requirements on a weight basis.

Table 7   Examples of **Natural-ingredient Diets** used for Rat and Mouse Breeding Colonies at the National Institute of Health, USA*

Ingredient	Conventional (NIH-07)	Autoclavable (NIH-31)
Basic Diet, g/kg diet		
Dried skim milk	50.0	
Fish meal (60% protein)	100.0	90.0
Soybean meal (48% protein)	120.0	50.0
Alfalfa meal, dehydrated (17% protein)	40.0	20.0
Corn gluten meal (60% protein)	30.0	20.0
Ground #2 yellow shelled corn	245.0	210.0
Ground hard winter wheat	230.0	355.0
Ground whole oats		100
Wheat middlings	100.0	100.0
Brewer's dried yeast	20.0	10.0
Dry molasses	15.0	
Soybean oil	25.0	15.0
Salt	5.0	5.0
Dicalcium phosphate	12.5	15.0
Ground limestone	5.0	5.0
Mineral premix	1.2	2.5
Vitamin premix	1.3	2.5
Mineral Premix, mg/kg diet		
Cobalt (as cobalt carbonate)	0.44	0.44
Copper (as copper sulfate)	4.40	4.40
Iron (as iron sulfate)	132.30	66.20
Manganese (as manganous oxide)	66.20	110.0
Zinc (as zinc oxide)	17.60	11.00
Iodine (as calcium iodate)	1.54	1.65

[*Table Contd.*]

[*Table Contd.*]

Vitamin Premix, per kg diet

Stabilized vitamin A palmitate or stearate	6,060.00 IU	24,300.00 IU
Vitamin D_3 (D-activated animal sterol)	5,070.00 IU	4,190.00 IU
Vitamin K (menadione activity)	3.09 mg	22.10 mg
All-rac-α-tocopheryl acetate	22.10 mg	16.50 mg
Choline chloride	617.00 mg	772.00 mg
Folic acid	2.43 mg	1.10 mg
Niacin	33.10 mg	22.10 mg
Ca-d-pantothenate	19.80 mg	27.60 mg
Pyridoxine-HCl	1.87 mg	2.21 mg
Riboflavin supplement	3.75 mg	5.51 mg
Thiamin mononitrate	11.0 mg	71.7 mg
d-Biotin	0.15 mg	0.13 mg
Vitamin B_{12} supplement	0.004 mg	0.015 mg

Note: Amounts listed for mineral and vitamin premixes represent the mass or IU of the specific mineral element or vitamin rather than the added compound.

*   Nutrient Requirements of Laboratory Animals, 4th revised edition 1995.

Table 8   Example of a Commonly used **Purified Diet** (AIN-76A) for Rats*.

Ingredient	Amount, g/kg diet
Basic Diet	
Sucrose	500.0
Casein (≥ 85% protein)	200.0
Corn starch	150.0
Corn oil (including 0.01-0.02% antioxidant[a])	50.0
Fibre source (cellulose-type)	50.0
Mineral mix (listed below)	35.0
Vitamin mix (listed below)	10.0
DL-methionine	3.0
Choline bitartrate	2.0
Mineral Premix	
Calcium phosphate, dibasic ($CaHPO_4$)	500.00
Potassium citrate, monohydrate	220.00

[*Table Contd.*]

[*Table Contd.*]

($K_3C_6H_5O_7.H_2O$)	
Sodium chloride	74.00
Potassium sulfate	52.00
Magnesium oxide	24.00
Ferric citrate (16-17% Fe)	6.00
Manganous carbonate (43-48% Mn)	3.50
Zinc carbonate (70% ZnO)	1.60
Chromium potassium sulfate	0.55
[$CrK(SO_4)_2. 12H_2O$]	
Cupric carbonate (53-55% Cu)	0.30
Potassium iodate (KIO_3)	0.01
Sodium selenite ($Na_2SeO_3. 5H_2O$)	0.01
Sucrose, finely powdered	118.03

Vitamin Premix

Nicotinic acid or nicotinamide	3.000
Calcium d-pantothenate	1.600
Pyridoxine-HCl	0.700
Thiamin - HCl	0.600
Riboflavin	0.600
Folic acid	0.200
d-Biotin	0.020
Cyanocobalamin (vitamin B_{12})	0.001
Retinyl palmitate or acetate (vitamin A)	+[b]
α-Tocopheryl acetate (vitamin E)	+[c]
Cholecalciferol (vitamin D_3)	0.0025
Menaquinone (vitamin K)	0.005
Sucrose, finely powdered	To make < 1,000 g

[a] Betahydroxytoluene or Santoquin.
[b] As stabilized powder to provide 400,000 IU vitamin A activity (120,000 retinol equivalents).
[c] As stabilized powder to provide 5,000 IU vitamin E activity.
* Nutrient Requirements of Laboratory Animals, 4th Rev. edn. 1995.

Mouse

Mice (*Mus musculus*) have been used extensively as animal models for biomedical research because of its high fertility rate, short gestation period, small size, ease of maintenance, susceptibility or resistance to different infectious agents, and susceptibility to noninfectious or genetic diseases that afflict humans. Estimating the quantitative nutrient requirements for mice is particularly challenging because of the large genetic variation within the species and the different criteria used to assess nutritional adequacy of diets. Research to determine nutrient requirements for reproduction, lactation, and maintenance of mice has received relatively little attention.

Hamster

Hamsters are classified within *Rodentia*, the largest mammalian order. Rodents are classically divided into three suborders: *Sciuromorpha*, *Myomorpha*, and *Hystricomorpha*. *Muroidea*, a superfamily within the suborder *Myomorpha*, includes the closely related families *Muridae* and *Cricetidae*, murine rodents and hamsters, respectively. The natural habitat of Syrian hamsters is a small area in northwest Syria in the vicinity of Aleppo where they originated. Syrian hamsters construct deep, chambered burrows in which they store grain and other feedstuffs foraged from the fields. Their natural habitat is dry, rocky steppes, or brush slopes. They not only have a very narrow genetic base, but they have been domesticated for a relatively short time in comparison with mice, rats, and guinea pigs. With reference to coat colour and other coat characteristics, variants include white, cream, piebald, albino, hairless, and longhair.

An adult laboratory **golden Syrian hamster** (*Mesocricetus auratus*) is approximately 14-19 cm in length and weighs approximately 114-140 gm. Hamsters have thick compact bodies with short legs, a short tail, large cheek pouches, and excess loose skin. The free margins of the lips form a three-cornered flap, which seals the mouth opening when closed and aids in filling the cheek pouches.

Hamsters are generally housed in cages that are appropriate for housing other laboratory rodents. Contemporary cages are generally made of commercially manufactured rigid plastic materials (i.e., polycarbonate, polysulfone, and polypropylene) or stainless steel. Hamsters are generally provided commercially produced pelleted rodent diet intended for mice and rats, and animals raised on such diets show normal growth and reproduction.

They are not typical nocturnal rodents because they are active only during the dark cycle with limited or no seasonal differences in activity. The **European hamster** is not a widely used research laboratory animal.

The **Chinese hamster**, also known as the **striped-back or gray hamster**, is indigenous to Northern Asia. Its small size, polyestrous cycle,-short gestation period, and low chromosome number are among the biological attributes that have made it an invaluable laboratory animal for biomedical research. Other hamsters used for biomedical research are the *Phodopus sungorus* (Djungarian hamster), *mesocricetus brandti* (Turkish hamster), *cricetulus migratorius* (Armenian hamster), and the *mesocricetus newtoni* (Romanian hamster).

Hamsters are primarily granivorous, but also eat green plant parts and shoots, roots, insects, and fruits.

Digestive system: Unlike simple-stomached rats, mice, and guinea pigs, hamsters, like voles, have a stomach that consists of two distinct compartments: cardiac stomach (a keratinized, nonglandular forestomach) and pyloric stomach (glandular region) separated by sphincter-like muscular marginal folds that control movement of ingesta from esophagus to duodenum. The structure and function of the forestomach is similar to the rumen of herbivores. Ingesta enter the forestomach from the esophagus and pass into the glandular stomach in 10 to 60 minutes. The hamster caecum is a J-shaped structure with numerous lateral sacculations and has more volume than the stomach.

Reproduction: Sexual maturity in the hamster generally occurs at approximately 6 weeks (42 days) of age, although copulatory activity can begin as early as 4 weeks of age. Reproductive performance of the Syrian hamster is sensitive to length of the photoperiod and successful reproduction requires a long (i.e. 14-hour) light cycle. Specific nutritional requirements of hamsters have not been described. Hamsters show normal growth and reproduction when provided diets formulated for rats and mice. Feed is typically presented on the cage floor, as hamsters may experience difficulty accessing feed from traditional wire bar food hoppers used with the other rodents. Although aggressive, hamsters are successfully bred in a research setting. Female hamsters demonstrate a postovulatory vaginal discharge that is used to stage estrus and allows hand (timed) mating of the hamster.

Vole

It has been demonstrated that voles are useful as a small-animal model for testing the quality of forages and other agricultural crops (Keys and Van Soest, 1970).

In nature, voles rely on grasses both for shelter and as a primary food source (Getz, 1985). It seems that voles select food plant species on the basis of availability, composition (particularly nitrogen and fibre fractions), and deterrent secondary compounds such as phenolics and tannins (Batzli, 1985). Unlike many small rodents, voles remain active in winter months-tunneling under snow, if necessary, and feeding on senescent grasses, rhizomes, seeds, and other plant material. Ability to survive in cold conditions on foods of low digestible energy content appears to be a key adaptive feature of voles.

Rapid reproductive rates are also characteristic of voles when food is abundant. Because female voles typically enter into estrus and are inseminated shortly after giving birth, concurrent pregnancy and lactation are common, leading to the production of litters at about 3-week intervals (Kudo and Oki, 1984; Keller, 1985).

Gerbil

The gerbil is usually nonaggressive and is one of the easiest rodents to maintain and handle. **Mature gerbils** are smaller than rats, but larger than mice, Mongolian gerbils are attracted to saliva and use salivary cues to discriminate between siblings and nonsiblings, and females use oral cues in the selection of sociosexual partners. Gerbils have been used as experimental models in a number of areas of biomedical research. Gerbils are excellent subjects for laboratory animal research as they are susceptible to bacterial, viral, and parasitic pathogens that affect humans and other species.

The Mongolian gerbil, *Meriones unguiculatus*, is used in laboratories in the United States. The Mongolian gerbil is one of 13 similar species of gerbils and jirds of the genus *Meriones* distributed in North Africa, the Middle East, and central and eastern Asia. The gerbils as a group are typically arid-adapted inhabitants of deserts and dry steppes and they produce concentrated urine and have low water turnover rates.

The stomach of the gerbil is simple and the cecum and colon are not especially well developed, suggestive of a species that in nature consumes mostly low-fibre foods such as seeds. Gerbils generally have had acceptable growth and reproduction when fed pelleted natural-ingredient diets formulated for other rodent species such as rats, mice, and guinea pigs.

Chinchillas

Chinchillas (*Chinchilla laniger*) have proven to be a practical animal model because of their small size, ease of handling, long life span (12-20 years), and relative freedom from diseases that interfere with research. Chinchillas weigh an average of 400-600 gm and their bodies, about 12-14 inches long, are short, stocky, and compact. Chinchillas are described as gentle, docile, quiet, and timid. They use their mouths to explore, and may perform trial bites when exploring an object or person. They also gnaw regularly similar to other rodents. Chinchillas are naturally nocturnal, being active at dusk and at night in the wild, but in captivity they can adapt to a diurnal lifestyle. They are active and agile, and enjoy climbing and jumping.

Chinchillas are housed in either solid-bottom or suspended (metal or plastic) cages. Chinchillas consume between 4-5% of their body weight daily when offered a complete pelleted diet. Maintaining chinchillas in a laboratory setting is easily accomplished because their care and husbandry are similar to that of rabbits and other hystricomorph rodents.

Functional Foods

Fructans: Prebiotics and Immunomodulators

Fructans are natural fructose polymers that are used in functional foods for their prebiotic and health improving properties. It was found that inulin-type fructans act as signals in animals, stimulating immune cell activity through Toll Like Receptor (TLR)° mediated signaling. Fructans and their fermentation products (short chain fatty acids and hydrogen gas) lead to a more reduced cellular status and a modulation of the immune system, aiming at disease prevention. It may be concluded that fructans are of interest in functional foods because of their prebiotic, antioxidant and immunomodulatory properties (Daren Peshev and Wim Van den Ende, 2014).

Pineapple Peel - a Functional Ingredient

Water-insoluble fibre is high in pineapple peel (about 42%). It could be a promising candidate for a functional ingredient beneficial to intestinal function and health. Cellulose, hemicellulose (xylan and xyloglucan) and pectic substances are the major polysaccharides of pineapple peel. Water-insoluble fibre-rich fraction from pineapple peel was fed to male **Golden Syrian hamsters** at graded levels of 2.5, 5 or 10% (Huang et al., 2014). The supplementation at a level of 2.5% decreased the daily faecal ammonia output, shortened the gastrointestinal transit time, reduced the activities of β-D-glucosidase, β-D-glucuronidase, mucinase and urease in faeces; it also enhanced the total amounts of short-chain fatty acid in the caecal content and the growth of gut microflora such as *Lactobacillus spp* and *Bifidobacterium spp*. The results of the study indicate that pineapple peel could improve caecal ecosystem function of hamsters by reducing the toxic compounds excreted by intestinal microflora.

Different forms of Lab Animal Feeds

Commercially available lab animal diets are pelleted diets, extruded diets and irradiated diets. Readers may refer 'chapter on Feed Technology' in Principles of Animal Nutrition and Feed Technology textbook for more information.

Sterilized diets are required to feed the laboratory animals used in 'high end studies' like specific pathogen-free (SPF), germ-free and transgenic animals. Several methods are used to produce sterilized diets. These include application of heat by autoclave, ethylene oxide gas sterilization and gamma irradiation. Sterilization by gamma irradiation is preferred because it does not alter nutritive value, texture and appearance of feed.

References

AFRC, 1998. *The Nutrition of Goats*. CAB International, New York, NY, pp. 41-51. BAHS 2010. Basic Animal Husbandry Statistics. http://dahd.nic.in/dahd/upload/BAHS 2010.pdf.

Benchaar, C, Hassanat, F., Gervais, R., Chouinard, P.Y., 2013. Effects of increasing amounts of corn dried distillers grains with solubles in dairy cow diets on methane production, ruminal fermentation, digestion, N balance, and milk production. J. Dairy Sci. 96, 2413-2427.

Bhatia, S.S. 1996. AICRP on Pigs, Status Paper, IVRI, Izatnagar.

Cools, A., Maes, D., Buyse, J., Kalmar, I.D., Vandermeiren, J-A and Janssens, G.P.J., 2010. Effect of N,N-dimethylglycine supplementation in parturition feed for sows on metabolism, nutrient digestibility and reproductive performance, Animal 4:12, pp 2004-2011

Counotte G, Kampman, G and Hinnen, V (2014) Feeding magnesium to foals reduces osteochondrosis prevalence, Journal of Equine Veterinary Science, doi: 10.1016/j.jevs.2013.12.009.

Davis C L and Clark J H. 1981. Ruminant digestion and metabolism. *Developmental Microbiology*, 22: 247 - 259.

DePeters, E.J., and L.W. George (2014). Rumen transfaunation, Immunology Letters, 162, 69-76.

Dicks, L.M.T., M. Botha, E. Dicks, M. Botes (2014). The equine gastro-intestinal tract: An overview of the microbiota, disease and treatment. Livestock Science, 169: 69-81.

Eklund, M., Mosenthin, R and Piepho, H. P., 2006. Effects of betaine and condensed molasses solubles on ileal and total tract nutrient digestibilities in piglets. Acta Agriculturae Scandinavica, Section A-Animal Science 56. 83-90.

FAO. 2012. *Balanced feeding for improving livestock productivity – Increase in milk production and nutrient use efficiency and decrease in methane emission*, by M.R. Garg. FAO Animal Production and Health Paper No. 173. Rome, Italy.

FAO. 2013. *Enhancing animal welfare and farmer income through strategic animal feeding – Some case studies*, Edited by Harinder P.S.Makkar. FAO Animal Production and Health Paper No. 175. Rome, Italy.

Gerber, P.J., Steinfeld, H., Henderson, B., Mottet, A., Opio, C., Dijkman, J., Falcucci, A., Tempio, G., 2013. Tackling climate change through livestock – A global assessment of emissions and mitigation opportunities. Food and Agriculture Organization of the United Nations (FAO), Rome, Italy.

Haenlein, G.F.W. and M. Anke (2011). Mineral and trace element research in goats: A review, Small Ruminant Research, 95: 2-19.

Haque, M.N., C. Cornou, and J. Madsen 2014. Estimation of methane emission using the CO_2 method from dairy cows fed concentrate with different carbohydrate compositions in automatic milking system. Livestock Science, 164: 57-66

Hassanat, F., Gervais, R., Julien, C., Masse, D.I., 2013. Replacing alfalfa silage with corn silage in dairy cow diets: Effects on enteric methane production, ruminal fermentation, digestion, N balance, and milk production. J. Dairy Sci. 96, 4553-4567.

Havlik, P., Valin, H., Herrero, M., Obersteiner, M., Schmid, E., Rufino, M.C., Mosnier, A., Thornton, P.K., Bottcher, H., Conant, R.T., Frank, S., Fritz, S., Fuss, S., Kraxner, F. and Notenbaert, A. (2014). Climate change mitigation through livestock system transitions. Proc Natl Acad Sci USA 111, 10: 3709-3714.

Herrero M, et al. (2013a). The roles of livestock in developing countries. Animal 7 (Suppl 1):3-18.

Herrero, M., Havlik, P., Valin, H., Notenbaert, A., Rubino, M.C., Thornton, P.K., Blummel, M.. Weiss, F., Grace, D. and Obersteiner, M. (2013b). Biomass use, production, feed efficiencies, and greenhouse gas emissions from global livestock systems. Proc Natl Acad Sci USA 110, 52: 20888-20893.

Hristov, A.N., Oh, J., Lee, C, Meinen, R., Montes, F., Ott, T., Firkins, J., Rotz, A., Dell, C, Adesogan,A., Yang, W., Tricarico, J., Kebreab, E., Waghorn, G., Dijkstra, J and Oosting, S. 2013. Mitigation of greenhouse gas emissions in livestock production - A review of technical options for non-C02 emissions. Edited by Pierre J. Gerber, Benjamin Hernderson and Harinder P.S.Makkar. FAO Animal Production and Health Paper No. 177. FAO, Rome, Italy.

ICAR 1998. *Nutritional Requirements of Domestic Animals*. Indian Council of Agricultural Research, New Delhi, pi 1.

Jiang (2014). Heat stress impairs the nutritional metabolism and reduces the productivity of egg-laying ducks. Animal Reproduction Science, <doi> http://dx.doi.org/10.1016/j .anireprosci.2014.01.002</doi>

Kalmar, I.D., Verstegen, M.W.A., Maenner, K., Zentek, J., Meulemans, G., Janssens, G;P.J., 2012. Tolerance and safety evaluation of N,N-dimethylglycine (DMG), a naturally occurring organic compound, as a feed additive in broiler diets. Br. J. Nutr. 107, 1635-1644.

Kalmar, I.D., Verstegen, M.W.A., Vanrompay, D., Maenner, K., Zentek, J., Iben, C, Leitgeb, R., Schiavone, A., Prola, L. and Janssens, G.P.J., 2014 Efficacy of dimethylglycine as a feed additive to improve broiler production. Livestock Science 164, 81-86.

Kearl, L.C. 1982. *Nutrient requirements of Ruminants in Developing Countries.* International Feedstuffs Institute, Utah Agricultural Experimental Station, Utah State University, Logon, Utah-84322, USA.

Klemashevich, C, Wu, C, Howsmon, D., Alaniz, R.C., Lee, K and Jayaraman, A., 2014. Rational identification of diet-derived postbiotics for improving intestinal microbiota function. Current Opinion in Biotechnology, 26: 85-90.

Luo J, Goetsch A L, Sahlu T, Nsahlai I V, Johnson Z B, Moore J E, Galyen M L, Owens F N and Ferrell C L. 2004. Prediction of metabolizable energy requirements for maintenance and gain of preweaning, growing and mature goats. *Small Ruminant Research* 58: 201-217.

Mandal, A.B., Elangovan, A.V. and Tyagi, P.K. 2005a. Poultry production for economic egg and meat production: A review. Indian Journal of Animal Sciences 75: 1215-1226.

Mandal A B, Paul S S, Mandal G P, Kannan A and Pathak N N. 2005. Deriving nutrient requirements of growing Indian goats under tropical condition. Small Ruminant Research 58: 201-217.

NRC, 1981. Nutrient requirements of goats: Angora, dairy and meat goats in temperate and tropical countries. National Academy of Sciences, National Research Council, Washington DC, pp 2-53.

NRC, 2012. Nutrient requirements of swine 11th Ed. National Academy Press, Washington, DC.

Nutrient Requirement of Animals - Cattle and Buffalo (ICAR-NIANP). 2013

Nutrient Requirement of Animals – Equines (ICAR-NIANP), 2013

Nutrient Requirement of Animals – Pigs (ICAR-NIANP), 2013

Nutrient Requirement of Animals – Poultry (ICAR-NIANP), 2013

Nutrient Requirement of Animals – Sheep, Goat and Rabbit (ICAR-NIANP), 2013

Paul S S and Lal D. 2010. Nutrient Requirement of Buffaloes. Satish Serial Publishing House. New Delhi.

Paul, S.S., Mandal, A.B., Chatterjee, P.N., Bhar, R. and Pathak, N.N. 2007.Determination of nutrient requirements for growth and maintenance of growing pigs under tropical condition, Animal 1: 269-282.

Rao S B N, Suresh K P and Tripathi P. 2011. Effect of feeding levels on nutrient utilization and prediction of nutrient requirements for Indian goats. *Indian Journal of Animal Nutrition.* 28: 149-152.

Reddy, D.V. 1981:."Effect of protein - energy relationships on performance and prediction of body composition of Large White Yorkshire pigs" MVSc thesis submitted to Andhra Pradesh Agricultural University, Hyderabad, AP, India.

Reddy, D.V. (2011). Precision Animal Nutrition for Pigs: A tool for Economic and Eco-friendly Animal Production ppl63-1 84, IN: 'Animal Nutrition Advances & Developments' published by Satish Serial Publishing House, Delhi-110033 [Editors: Dr U.R.Mehra (Chief Editor), Putan Singh and A.K.Verma; ISBN 81-89304-89-5; xiv plus 810 pages]

Reddy, D.V. (2011). Precision Animal Nutrition for Efficient and Economical Milk Production pp657-668, IN: 'Veterinary Nutrition and Health' published by Satish Serial Publishing House, Delhi-110033 [Editors: Dr.S.P.Tiwari and P.K.Sanyal; ISBN 978-93-81226-06-3; xii plus 723 pages]

Reddy D.V. and Krishna N (2009): Precision animal nutrition: A tool for economic and eco-friendly animal production in ruminants. *Livestock Research for Rural Development. Volume 21, 23 pages Article #36.* Retrieved from http://www.lrrd.orR/lrrd21/3/redd21036.htm

Reddy, D.V. and Prasad, D. A. 1985: Effect of protein-energy relationships on performance and body composition of growing and finishing large White Yorkshire pigs. Indian J. Anim. Sci. **55**, 468-476.

Reddy, D.V., Prasad, D. A., Charyulu, E. K., Reddy, M. R. N. and Audeyya, P. 1985: Effect of replacing maize with bagasse and molasses mixture (W/W) on growth and digestibility coefficients in desi pigs. Cheiron **14**, 1-7.

Reddy. D.V., Prasad, D. A., Charyulu, E. K., Audeyya, P. and Reddy, M. R. N., 1986 Effect of different levels of protein and energy on the performance and utilization of nutrients in growing desi pigs. Indian J. Anim. Sci. **56**, 105-109.

Reddy, D. V.; Prasad, D. A.; Reddy, B. S.; Charyulu, E. K., 1986 b: Effect of replacing maize with tamarind seed or rice polish on the performance characteristics and nutrient utilization by desi pigs. Indian J. Anim. Sci. 56, 1094-98.

Reddy, V.R.I996. Nutrient requirements of chicken-work done in India. Proceedings of World Poultry Congress, 2-5 September, New Delhi, Vol2, pp75-92.

Sampath K T, Prasad C S, Walli T K and Shivaramaiah M T. 1994. Methods to assess the protein value of feeds of ruminants - A Review. *Indian Journal of Dairy Science* 47 (5): 361 - 367.

SCA. Standing committee on Agriculture. 1990. Feeding standards for Australian livestock and ruminants. East Melbourne, Australia, CSRIO Publication.

Sengar OPS 1980. Indian Research on Protein and Energy Requirements of Goats. Journal of Dairy Science. 63 (10): 1655-1670.

Sumithra, T.G., V.K. Chaturvedi, S.J. Siju, C. Susan, M. Rawat, A.K. Rai, S.C. Sunita (2013). Enterotoxaemia in goats—A review of current knowledge. Small Ruminant Research, 114: 1-9.

Surai, P.F., 2002a. Selenium in poultry nutrition: a new look at an old element. 1. Antioxidant properties, deficiency and toxicity. Worlds Poultry Science Journal 58, 333-347.

Surai, P.F., 2002b. Selenium in poultry nutrition: a new look at an old element. 2. Reproduction, egg and meat quality and practical applications. Worlds Poultry Science Journal 58, 431^150.

Surai, P.F., 2006. Selenium in Nutrition and Health. Nottingham University Press, Nottingham, UK.

Surai, P.F and Fisinin, V.I., 2014. Selenium in poultry breeder nutrition: An update. Animal Feed Science Technology 191, 1-15.

Swiatkiewicz, A. Arczewska-Wlosek and D. Jozefiak (2014) Chitosan and its oligosaccharide derivatives (chito-oligosaccharides) as feed supplements in poultry and swine nutrition Journal of Animal Physiology and Animal Nutrition. DOI: 10.1111/jpn. 12222

Walli T K, 2005. Bypass protein technology and impact of feeding bypass protein to dairy \ animals in tropics: a review. Indian Journal of Animal Science, 75(1): 135 - 142

Xianyong Ma, Yingcai Lina, Hanxing Zhang, Wei Chen, Shang Wang, Dong Ruan, Zongyong

Zuidhof, M.J., B.L.Schneider, V.L.Carney, D.R.Korver and F.E.Robinson (2014) Growth, efficiency,a nd yireld of commercial broilers from 1957, 1978, and 2005. Poultry Science 93:2970-2982.

Appendix I

Table 1 Metabolic Size for Live Body Weight ($W_{kg}^{0.75}$).

W	$W^{0.75}$	W	$W^{0.75}$	W	$W^{0.75}$
0.5	0.60	130	38.50	480	102.55
1.0	1.00	140	40.70	490	104.15
1.5	1.36	150	42.86	500	105.74
2.0	1.68	160	44.99	510	107.32
2.5	1.99	170	47.08	520	108.89
3.0	2.28	180	49.14	530	110.47
3.5	2.56	190	51.17	540	112.02
4.0	2.83	200	53.18	550	113.57
4.5	3.09	210	55.16	560	115.12
5.0	3.34	220	57.12	570	116.65
5.5	3.59	230	59.06	580	118.19
6.0	3.83	240	60.98	590	119.71
6.5	4.07	250	62.87	600	121.23
7.0	4.30	260	64.75	620	124.2
7.5	4.53	270	66.61	640	127.2
8.0	4.76	280	68.45	660	130.2
8.5	4.98	290	70.28	680	133.2
9.0	5.20	300	72.08	700	136.1
9.5	5.41	310	73.88	720	139.0
10.	5.62	320	75.66	740	141.9
15.0	7.62	330	77.42	760	144.7
20.0	9.46	340	79.18	780	147.6
25.0	11.18	350	80.92	800	150.4
30.0	12.82	360	82.65	820	153.2
35.0	14.39	370	84.36	840	156.0
40.0	15.91	380	86.07	860	158.8

[*Table Contd.*]

[*Table Contd.*]

45.0	17.37	390	87.76	880	161.6
50.0	18.80	400	89.44	900	164.3
60.0	21.56	410	91.11	920	167.0
70.0	24.20	420	92.78	940	169.8
80.0	26.75	430	94.43	960	172.5
90.0	29.22	440	96.07	980	175.2
100	31.62	450	97.70	1000	177.8
110	33.97	460	99.33		
120	36.26	470	100.94		

Table 2 Conversion Factors.

Unit given	Unit wanted	Multiply by
lb (pound)	g	453.6
lb	kg	0.4536
oz (ounce, avdp)	g	28.35
kg	lb	2.2046
ppm	μg/g	1.0
ppm	mg/kg	1.0
mg/kg	%	0.0001
ppm	%	0.0001
mg/g	%	0.1
g/kg	%	0.1
Atmosphere	Bar	1.01325
Atmosphere	mm of Hg (0ºC)	760
Atmosphere	lb / sq. inch	14.6960
Kcal (Calorie)	joule	4.184
cft (cubic foot)	m^3 (cubic meter)	0.028316847
m^3 (cubic metre)	cft	35.314667
Litre	cu centimetre	1000.027
lb/cft	kg/m^3	16.018463
Sq foot	Sq metre	0.09290304
Sq foot	Sq yard	0.111111
Sq metre	Sq foot	10.763910
Sq metre	Sq yard	1.19599
Sq yard	Sq foot	9
Ton (long)	kg	1016.0469
Ton (metric)	kg	1000
Ton (short)	kg	907.18474
Yard	ft	3
	metre	0.9144

[*Table Contd.*]

[Table Contd.]

mg%	μg%	1000
	mg/litre	10
	m Eq/litre	10/eq.wt
mEq/litre	mg%	0.1 × eq.wt
	μg%	100 × eq.wt
	mg/litre	eq.wt

avdp - Avoirdupois weight; one litre is the volume of pure water at 4°C and 760 mm
    pressure which weighs 1 kg.

To convert Fahrenheit temperature into Celsius: subtract 32 and multiply by 5/9. To
    convert Celsius temperature into Fahrenheit: multiply by 9/5 and add 32.

Table 3 Prefix Names of Multiples and Submultiples of Units.

Decimal equivalent	Prefix	Symbol	Exponential expression
1, 000, 000, 000, 000	TERA	T	10^{12}
1, 000, 000, 000	GIGA	G	10^9
1, 000, 000	MEGA	M	10^6
1, 000	KILO	K	10^3
100	HECTO	h	10^2
10	DEKA	da	10
0.1	DECI	d	10^{-1}
0.01	CENTI	c	10^{-2}
0.001	MILLI	m	10^{-3}
0.000 001	MICRO	μ	10^{-6}
0.000 000 001	NANO	n	10^{-9}
0.000 000 000 001	PICO	p	10^{-12}
0.000 000 000 000 001	femto	f	10^{-15}
0.000 000 000 000 000 001	ATTO	a	10^{-18}

Table 4 Ready reckoner for calculation of animal's body weight (BW) from body
    measurement

Heart Girth (inches)	Length (inches)	B W (Seer*)	BW (Kg)
35	28	109	101
37	30	123	115
39	32	139	129
42	34	159	148
43	36	172	160
45	39	195	181

[Table Contd.]

[*Table Contd.*]

47	40	209	194
49	43	234	218
51	45	255	237
53	46	271	252
56	46	286	266
58	49	316	294
60	50	333	310
62	54	372	346
64	55	391	364
66	56	435	404
68	58	464	432
70	60	494	460
73	63	541	503
75	65	574	533
80	65	612	569
82	67	687	639
84	68	714	664
86	68	731	680
88	69	759	706
90	72	810	753

Reference: Thomas, C.K., and Sastry N.S.R. (2009) Dairy Bovine Production, Kalyani Publication, New Delhi; Aggarwal's modified Shaeffers formula (Seer) = Girth (inches) X length (inches) / Y

* 1 Seer = 0.933 kg; Y = 9 if girth is less than 65*; Y = 8.5 if girth is 65-80*; Y = 8 if girth is over 80*

Table 5   Minimum and maximum concentrations of total and forage NDF and NFC of diets (% DM) of lactating cows, fed on a total mixed ration*

Minimum forage NDF	Minimum dietary NDF	Maximum dietary NFC	Minimum dietary ADF
19	25	44	17
18	27	42	18
17	29	40	19
16	31	38	20
15	33	36	21

* Source: Adapted from NRC (2001) Nutrient Requirement of Dairy Cattle, National Research Council, Washington D.C.

Table 6 Macro mineral requirements (g/d) for maintenance of cattle and buffalo*

BW (Kg)	Ca[a] Dry	Ca[a] Lactating	P[b]	Na[c] Dry	Na[c] Lactating	Cl[d] Dry	Cl[d] Lactating	K[e]	Mg[f]	S[g]
200	8	9	4	3	7	5	20	36	4	1
250	10	11	5	4	9	6	25	44	5	1
300	12	14	6	5	10	8	30	53	6	1
350	14	16	7	6	12	9	35	62	7	1
400	16	18	8	7	14	10	40	71	8	2
450	18	20	9	8	15	11	45	80	8	2
500	20	23	10	8	17	13	50	89	9	2
550	22	25	11	9	19	14	55	98	10	2
600	24	27	12	10	21	15	60	107	11	2
650	26	30	13	11	22	16.	65	116	12	3
700	28	32	14	12	24	18	70	124	13	3
750	30	34	15	13	26	19	75	133	14	3
800	32	36	16	13	27	20	80	142	15	3

*Adapted from "NRC (2001) Nutrient Requirement of Dairy Cattle. National Research Council, Washington D; Source: ICAR (2013)

[a] Ca   Absorption coefficient of roughages and concentrates was taken as 30 and 60, respectively. Assuming roughage: concentrate to be 70:30, the absorption coefficient was calculated to be 0.42, but considering the poor quality of roughages absorption coefficient is taken as 0.38 as per NRC, 1989. Net requirement for maintenance of non-lactating animals (0.0154 g/kg BW) was calculated as per the NRC (1989, 2001) and corresponding value i.e. 0.031 g/kg BW was taken for lactating animals.

[b] P   Assuming 2% DMI, the requirement was calculated on the basis of 1 g P/kg DMI as suggested by AFRC (1991).

[c] Na   Net requirement calculated as per NRC (2001) using value of 1.5 g/100 kg BW for non lactating and 3.8 g/100 kg BW for lactating cattle. The absorption coefficient was taken as 0.9. During summer season, when the temperature is > 30°C: additional dietary Na @ 0.44 g/l00kg BW to be added.

[d] Cl   Net requirement was calculated using the value of 2.25 g/100 kg BW and absorption coefficient as 0.9 (NRC, 2001)

[e] K   Requirements was calculated using the factor 3.8 g/100 kg BW and in addition to this 2.6 and 6.1 g/kg DMI were added for non-lactating and lactating animals, respectively (NRC, 2001). Absorption coefficient was taken as 0.9. During summer months when the temperature is > 30°C: additional dietary K @ 0.44 g K/100 kg BW should be added in the diet (NRC, 2001).

[f] Mg   Net requirement, i.e. 0.3 g/100 kg BW and absorption coefficient was taken as 0.16 as per NRC (2001).

[g] S   Calculated on the basis of at 0.2% of DMI.

Table 7 Trace mineral requirements for maintenance*

Mineral	Requirement
Cobalt	0.11 mg/kg DMI
Copper	10 mg/kg DMI
Iron	50 mg/kg DMI
Manganese	15 mg/kg DMI
Selenium	0.25 mg/kg DMI
Zinc	40 mg/kg DMI and 80 mg/kg DMI during summer and transitional animals, respectively
Iodine	0.25 mg/kg DMI (in extreme summers, reduce the content to 0.15 mg/kg DMI)

*ICAR (2013)

Table 8 Requirement of major minerals g per kg milk production*

	[a]Ca	[b]P	[c]Na	[d]Cl	[e]K	[f]Mg
Cattle	3.2	1.8	0.7	1.3	1.7	0.7
Buffalo	4.8	1.8	0.5	0.8	1.2	1.2

Adapted from "NRC (2001) Nutrient Requirement of Dairy Cattle, National Research Council, Washington D

[a] Considering Ca content 1.23 and 1.84 g/1 in cow and buffalo milk; [b]P content 0.9 g/1 milk and absorption coefficient 0.5; [c]Na content is 0.6 and 0.45 g/kg milk in cattle and buffalo milk; [d]Cl content average values i.e. 1.15 and 0.68 g/kg milk in cattle and buffalo milk; [e]K based on 1.5 and 1.1 g/kg milk in cow and buffalo milk; [f]Mg based on 0.12 and 0.19 g/kg milk in cow and buffalo milk. * Source: ICAR (2013)

Table 9 Trace minerals requirement mg per kg milk production

	[a]Co	[b]Cu	Zn	Mn	[e]I	[f]Fe
Cattle	0.006	3.75	26.67	3.0	5 to 50	2.25
Buffalo	0.012	3.75	33.33	3.0	8.5 to 19.5	5.0

Adapted from "NRC (2001) Nutrient Requirement of Dairy Cattle, National Research Council, Washington D C

[a] net content in milk; [b]Cu content in milk, 0.15 mg/lt for cattle and buffalo; [e]I net content in milk; [f]Fe is 0.45 and 1.0 mg/kg milk in cattle and buffalo milk

Transfaunation: Transfaunation is transfer of rumen fluid from rumen of a donor to the rumen of a recipient. Rumen fluid contains a broad spectrum of microorganisms including bacteria, protozoa, fungi, and archaea. Defaunation of the rumen referred to elimination of protozoa. Rumen transfaunation using the cud from a healthy donor animal to treat a sick recipient animal was practiced long before our understanding of rumen microorganisms (DePeters and George, 2014).

Rumen transfaunation is a common practice to treat digestive disorders such as simple indigestion. The clinical sign of simple indigestion is anorexia (reduction in appetite) with lesser ruminal movements (hypomotility) to ruminal atony or stasis. Collection of large volumes of rumen fluid is most easily accomplished using a rumen fistulated animal or else rumen fluid may be collected by stomach tubing a non-fistulated donor. Volume transferred ranges from 1 L for calves to 8-16 L for adult cattle, while for small ruminants 1 L may be used. Rumen fluid should be transferred as soon as possible post-collection. Some researchers suggested that the rumen fluid can be stored for up to 9 h at room temperature and for 24h at refrigeration temperature (DePeters and George, 2014).

Appendix II

1. Calculation of digestibility coefficients of groundnut cake nutrients by difference method

Experimental animals: Adult cattle

Oat hay is the basal feed and groundnut cake is the test feed.

I trial: Oat hay digestibility is determined

II trial: Oat hay and groundnut cake is fed at 10 kg and 1 kg, respectively.

Digestion trial is conducted and dung is collected.

Feeds and dung (3.3 kg DM) are analysed and the calculations are furnished in the Table.

% Chemical composition on DMB

	CP	EE	CF	NFE
Oat hay	5.0	1.0	35.0	47.0
Groundnut cake	50.0	4.0	4.0	35.0
Dung	10.0	1.0	37.0	46.0 1

% Digestibility of nutrient calculation

	CP	EE	CF	NFE
Intake from oat hay, kg	0.5	0.1	3.5	4.7
Intake from groundnut cake, kg	0.5	0.04	0.04	0.35
Total intake, kg	1.0	1.04	3.54	5.05
Total voided in dung, kg	0.33	0.033	1.22	1.52
Total digested, kg	0.67	0.107	2.32	3.53
Digested from hay as found in a separate experiment, *kg*	0.23	0.076	2.30	3.35
Digested from groundnut cake, kg	0.44	0.031	0.02	51.4
Digestibility coefficients of nutrients of GNC	88.0	77.5	50.0	51.4

2. Calculation of DCP and TDN

Proximate principle	%	Digestibility coefficient	Digestible nutrients	TDN
Crude protein	14.95	66.93	DCP 10.00	10.00
Ether extract	02.26	54.85	DEE 1.24	1.24 x 2.25 = 2.76
Crude fibre	43.36	72.20	DCF 31.30	31.30
Nitrogen free extract	24.08	50.43	DNFE 12.14	12. 14; Total = 56.20

The experimental ration has DCP 10% and TDN 56.20%.

Conversion of TDN to DE and ME

1 kg TDN = 4.409 Mcal DE or 3.616 Mcal ME; ME = 0.82 DE

562 g TDN = 4.409 x 562 ÷ 1000 = 2.48 Mcal DE

562 g TDN = 3.616 x 562 ÷ 1000 = 2.03 Mcal ME

3. Analysed mineral composition (g/kg) of feedstuffs and supplements*

Feedstuff/Supplement	Calcium	Total P	Phytin P	Fluorine
Yellow maize	2.02	2.67	1.96	—
Soybean meal	4.41	5.10	4.02	—
Sunflower meal	5.95	7.85	4.92	—
Dicalcium phosphate	210.1	193.1	—	0.0
Bone meal	120.3	63.1	—	0.81
Low fluorine rock phosphate	255.4	121.4	—	11.3
Commercial mineral mixture	162.2	109.8	—	18.3
High fluorine rock phosphate	216.0	98.4	—	36.3
Oyster shell grit	330.0	—	—	—

* S.V. Rama Rao and V. Ramasubba Reddy (2005) Livestock and Feed Trends CLFMA of India 3 (6) 7-12.

4. Acidifying rations and alkalizing rations: Dietary bases

Common animal feeds do not contain significant amounts of free acids. However, plant cells contain dissolved anions of organic acids such as citric acid, oxalic acid, malonic acid and fumaric acid. The balancing cation is mainly K^+. During metabolism (via the citric acid cycle), these dietary organic anions are converted to their corresponding acids. Consequently HCO_3 is produced.

$$CO_2 + H_2O \leftrightarrow H_2CO_3 \leftrightarrow H^+ + HCO_3^-$$

This is balanced by predominantly K^+. Both the organic anion and HCO_3^- can bind H^+ and are therefore bases. The influence of a feed on the acid-base status of the body depends on the balance between dietary bases and components that give rise to non-volatile acids when the feed is absorbed and metabolized. By manipulating the feed composition, it is possible to obtain both acidifying and alkalizing rations.

Dietary Cation–Anion Balance (DCAB)

Dietary cation-anion balance is the difference between the concentrations of inorganic cations and anions in the feed, and reflects the tendency for a feed, or a whole ration, to change the normal acid-base balance of the body.

DCAB Calculation in herbivorous diets: In herbivorous diets, where the protein concentration is low compared to carnivorous animals, DCAB is calculated according to the formula

DCAB (moles / kg) = Na / 23 + K / 39 – Cl / 35.5

The symbols of the elements represent their concentrations in grams per kg of feed, and the denominators are their respective atomic weights in daltons. Ca or Mg is present in much lower concentration; furthermore Ca and Mg are absorbed to a much smaller extent and hence are not included.

- **When DCAB is zero,** no effect on the acid-base balance of the animal is to be expected from the diet.
- **When DCAB is positive,** there is surplus of inorganic cations (K^+, Na^+) relative to inorganic anions (Cl^-). This surplus will be compensated by organic anions in the feed, since the feed always contains equal amounts of positive and negative ionic charge. When these organic anions are oxidized they will give rise to HCO_3^-, which produces alkaline urine when subsequently excreted.
- **When DCAB is negative:** A negative DCAB shows that the feed or diet contains a deficit of K^+ and Na^+ relative to the concentration of inorganic anions. For example, this is the case when the diet contains a strong mineral acid like HC1. The H^+ that is absorbed together with the inorganic anions is buffered in the body, but will acidify the urine when excreted.

DCAB Calculation in Carnivorous and Omnivorous Diets

In carnivorous and omnivorous diets, the content of proteins are usually much higher than in the diets of herbivores. When oxidized, the amino acids cysteine and methionine give rise to CO_2, H^+ and SO_4^{2-}. The sulphuric acid thus produced will have an acidifying effect on the organism, and the concentration of sulphur in the diet should be added.

DCAB (moles / kg) = Na / 23 + K / 39 − Cl / 35.5 −2 S/32.1

In the formula for DCAB, the concentration of sulphur in the feed is multiplied by two, because each sulphate ion carries two unit charges.

5. Nutritive Value Index (NVI) for forages

Crampton *et al* (1960) formulated a numerical NVI for forages which took into consideration both voluntary (relative) intake and gross energy digestibility measurement while calculating it. Their hypothesis concerning the effective feeding value of forages can be summarized as follows:

1. The feeding value of a forage depends on its voluntary intake by the animal.
2. Voluntary intake of a forage is limited primarily by the rate of digestion of its cellulose.
3. The rate of rumen digestion is retarded by factors which interfere with the activity of rumen microbes. These include lignification of the forage, deficiency of nitrogen and minerals to microbes and the presence of bacteriostatic agents.
4. The effective feeding value of a forage depends jointly on how much of it an animal will voluntarily consume and the completeness of its energy digestibility.

Crampton *et al* (1962) recommended the following formula to calculate NVI for sheep and cattle.

For sheep NVI

$$= \frac{100 \times \text{g daily forage intake}}{80 \text{ g per kg metabolic body weight}} \times \text{digestibility of energy}$$

For cattle NVI

$$= \frac{100 \times \text{g daily forage intake}}{140 \text{ g per kg metabolic body weight}} \times \text{digestibility of energy}$$

NVI could be expressed:

NVI = Relative daily intake x digestibility of energy

Standard forage = a leafy legume hay, cut during early bloom, field chopped and dehydrated by aeration; apparent energy digestibility = 70%.

Relative daily intake $= 100 \times \dfrac{\text{Observed intake of the test forage}}{\text{Expected intake of standard forage}}$

Problem

A sheep weighing 50 kg eats 1100 g of the test forage (energy digestibility = 60%) in 24 hours. The expected intake of the standard forage would be $50^{\circ 75} \times 80 = 18.8 \times 80 = 1504$ g.

The relative intake of this forage is then

RI=100 x 1100-1504 = 73

NVI of test forage = Relative daily intake x digestibility of energy

= 73 x 60 = 43.8

NVI of standard forage = 100 x 70 = 0.70

Effective feeding value of test forage = 43.8 ÷ 0.70 = 62.5%.

It is as good as standard forage.

6. **Ratio between n-6 Fatty Acid and n-3 Fatty Acid**

Diets have changed with the advent of civilization. Now humans eat less roughage (fibre) and more processed foods. It is recommended that ratio between n-6 FA and n-3 FA is as close to 1:1 as possible, which is of prehistoric man's diet. Now it is as bad as 13:1 in some countries to 20 to 30: 1 in several others. Considering this, WHO recommends that the ratio between n-6 FA and n-3 FA be as 6:1.

The n-6 and n-3 fatty acid contents (%) and n6:n3 of certain oils are furnished here: canola oil 20.0, 9.3 and 2.2; corn oil 59.5, 1.0 and 59.5; fish oil 1.5, 21.4 and 0.1; linseed oil 12.7, 53.3 and 0.2; olive oil 9.6, 1.0 and 9.6; peanut oil 33.0, 0.5 and 66.0; sunflower oil 67.3, 1.1 and 61.2 and soybean oil 54.2, 7.7 and 7.0.

Because algae synthesize high amounts of omega-3 fatty acids, most marine animals contain relatively high amounts omega-3 fatty acids. Hence omega 3 fat enriched eggs and meat are to be produced.

7. **In defense of meat**

Positive points: Meat eating can pose a threat to healthy living, but there are a number of plus points as well. Meat is an excellent source of quality protein: 17-20% in chicken, mutton and beef; 11-15% in pork. Meat is a rich source of easily available iron: The iron in vegetables and cereals is inorganic and is available to a lesser extent due to the presence of phytates, phosphates and oxalic acids, which combine with iron and form insoluble salts. Meat is a good source of phosphorus: Phosphorus present in animal foods is absorbed to a greater extent than that present in cereals and legumes. Meat is a fairly good source of vitamin A:

Vitamin A occurs only in foods of animal origin. Organ meats are rich sources of vitamin A. Meat is a rich source of vitamin B_{12}: This vitamin is present only in foods of animal origin and cannot be obtained from any plant source. Liver is the richest source.

Negative points: Meat lacks fibre and it is very high in saturated fats (3% in chicken to 20% in red meats). This high fat content leads to increased synthesis of cholesterol and bile acids by the liver. This excess is then converted into potential carcinogens by intestinal bacteria. In addition, excess cholesterol clogs up the arteries paving the way for heart disease. Since meat has no fibre, the transit time of faecal matter in the intestines is increased leading to altered bacterial flora.

Overcoming the negative aspects of meat: Remove skin in case of chicken meat; trim away all excess fat; pressure cooking / microwaving; eat plenty of vegetables, fruits, whole grains to obtain fibre and vitamin C; limit consumption to 60-75 g /day for 3 days in a week. Meat is good if eaten in moderation and cooked rightly.

8. Energy and protein content of common foodstuffs

Energy and Protein Content of Common Foodstuffs
(per 100 g of Edible Portion)*.

Foodstuff	Energy (Kcal)	Protein (g)
Rice, raw, milled	345	6.8
Wheat, whole	346	11.8
Cereals, average	345	9.8
Bengalgram dhal	372	20.8
Blackgram dhal	347	24.0
Greengram dhal	348	24.5
Redgram dhal	335	22.3
Peas, dry	315	19.7
Rajmah	346	22.9
Soybean	432	43.2
Green leafy vegetables		
Amaranth group (Amaranth, Coriander, Fenugreek, Mint)	50	4.3
Drumstick leaves, Agathi, Ponnaganti,	86	6.7
Cabbage	27	1.8

[Table Contd.]

454

Roots & tubers		
Potato	97	1.6
Onion	50	1.2
Carrot	48	0.9
Radish	17	0.7
Other vegetables		
Beans (average)	49	4.7
Brinjal, (egg plant)	24	1.4
Ladies finger, (okra)	35	1.9
Drumstick	26	2.5
Plantain green	64	1.2
Plantain stem	42	0.5
Average for gourds	18	0.7
Nuts & oilseeds		
Cashewnut	596	21.2
Groundnut	567	25.3
Coconut, fresh	444	4.5
Gingilly seeds	563	18.3
Mustard seeds	541	20.0
Fruits		
Apple	59	0.2
Banana	116	1.2
Grapes	71	0.5
Orange	48	0.7
Papaya	32	0.6
Tomato, ripe	20	0.9
Guava	51	0.9
Lemon	57	1.0
Milk (4.1% fat)	67	3.2
Curd	60	3.1
Egg	143	11.3
Fish (Seer)	126	22.5
Mutton, muscle	194	18.5
Cheese (40.3% moisture)	348	24.1
Butter (19% moisture)	729	-
Sugar	400	0.1
Jaggery	383	0.4
Chillies, green	29	2.9

[*Table Contd.*]

[*Table Contd.*]

Chillies, dry	246	15.9
Coriander	288	14.1
Fenugreek seeds	333	26.2
Garlic, dry	145	6.3
Pepper, dry	304	11.5
Tamarind pulp	283	3.1
Turmeric	349	6.3

* Adapted from "Nutritive value of Indian Foods "1989, NIN, Hyderabad

9. Chemical composition of common foodstuffs

Chemical Composition of Common Foodstuffs
(All values are per 100 g of Edible Portion)*.

Name of the foodstuff	1 Moisture g	2 Protein g	3 Fat g	4 Fibre g	5 Energy Kcal	6 Ca mg	7 P mg	8 Fe mg
1. Cereals (Bajra, Jowar, Maize, Ragi, Rice, Wheat)	13.2	9.8	2.3	1.8	345	79	269	4.0
* exclusive of Ragi						26*		
2. Dhals (Bengalgram, blackgram, green-gram, redgram)	11.8	22.9	2.5	1.1	351	90	356	3.9
3. Peas, dry	16.0	19.7	1.1	4.5	315	75	298	7.1
4. Rajmah	12.0	22.9	1.3	(4.8)	346	260	410	5.1
5. Soybean	8.1	43.2	19.5	3.7	432	240	690	10.4
6. GLV: Amaranth group (Amaranth, Coriander, Fenugreek, Mint)								
	84.5	4.3	0.7	1.5	50	275	64	9.2
7. Agathi group (Agathi, drumstick, Ponnaganti)								
	75.5	6.7	1.3	2.0	86	690	70	2.1
8. Cabbage	91.9	1.8	0.1	1.0	27	39	44	0.8
Root & tubers								
9. Potato	74.7	1.6	0.1	0.4	97	10	40	0.5
10. Onion	86.6	1.2	0.1	0.6	50	47	50	0.6
11. Carrot	86.0	0.9	0.2	1.2	48	80	530	1.0
12. Radish, white	94.4	0.7	0.1	0.8	17	35	22	0.4
Other vegetables								
13. Brinjal	92.7	1.4	0.3	1.3	24	18	47	0.4
14. Beans	82.0	4.7	0.4	2.8	49	113	81	1.7
15. Drumstick	86.9	2.5	0.1	4.8	26	30	110	0.2

[*Table Contd.*]

[*Table Contd.*]

16.	Ladies finger	89.0	1.9	0.2	1.2	35	66	56	0.35
17.	Plantain green	83.2	1.4	0.2	0.7	64	10	29	6.3
18.	Plantain stem	88.3	0.5	0.1	0.8	42	10	10	0.1
19.	Gourds (bitter gourd, bottle gourd, ridge gourd, snake gourd)								
		95.0	0.7	1.8	0.7	18	22	32	0.7
20.	Groundnut kernel	3.0	25.3	40.1	3.1	567	90	350	2.5
21.	Gingilly seeds	5.3	18.3	43.3	2.9	563	1450	570	9.3
22.	Banana, ripe	70.1	1.2	0.3	0.4	116	17	36	0.4
23.	Grapes	79.2	0.5	0.3	2.9	71	20	30	0.5
24.	Guava	81.7	0.9	0.3	5.2	51	10	28	0.3
25.	Tomato, ripe	94.0	0.9	0.2	0.8	20	48	20	0.6
26.	Fish (Seer)	72.7	22.5	4.0	-	126	71	572	5.4
27.	Egg	73.7	11.3	10.2	-	143	60	220	2.1
28.	Mutton, muscle	71.5	18.5	13.3	-	194	150	150	2.5
29.	Milk	87.5	3.2	4.1	-	67	120	90	0.2
30.	Jaggery	3.9	0.4	0.1	-	383	80	40	2.6

* Adapted from "Nutritive Value of Indian Foods" 1989, NIN, Hydrabad.

10. Rations for ducks, turkeys, Japanese quails, Emus, Vanaraja, Gramapriya and Guinea

A. Ration for Ducks

Ingredients	Starter (0-8 weeks)	Grower (8-16weeks)	Rearer (16-20 weeks)	Layers (>20 weeks)
Maize	30	40	25	52.6
Jowar	15	0	0	0
Bajra	0	10	0	0
Rice broken	0	0	20	0
DORB	6	25.8	35	10
Rice polish	14.3	0	0	5
SBM	25	16	10	18
GNC-Ext.	5	0	0	4
SFOC	0	4	5.9	0
DCP	1.3	1	0.8	1
Calcite	1.8	1.8	1.9	8
Lysine	0.15	0.06	0.06	0.06
Methionine	0.15	0.07	0.07	0.07
Salt	0.4	0.4	0.4	0.4
Feed additives*	0.9	0.9	0.9	0.9
	100	100	100	100

B. Ration for turkeys

Ingredients	0-6 weeks	6-12 weeks	12-18 weeks	18 weeks pre-laying	Breeder
Maize	30	43.2	30	30	30
Jowar	6.5	10	20	0	20
Rice broken	0	0	0	20	0
DORB	0	0	18.2	29.6	26.1
Rice polish	14.1	5	0	0	0
SBM	35	32	20	11	12
GNC-Ext.	8	5	0	0	4
Oil	1.5	0	0	0	0
SFOC	0	0	8	6.5	0
DCP	1.3	1.9	1	0.3	0.6
Calcite	1.8	1.4	1.4	1.3	6
Lysine	0.35	0.1	0.1	0.05	0
Methionine	0.16	0.11	0.05	0	0
Salt	0.4	0.4	0.4	0.4	0.4
Feed additives*	0.9	0.9	0.9	0.9	0.9
	100	100	100	100	100

C. Ration for Japanese quails

Ingredients	Growing		Breeder/ layer (5-30 weeks)	
	0-3 week	3-5 week	Meat line	Egg line
Maize	35	40.7	40	30
Jowar	5	0	0	15
Bajra	0	10	0	0
Rice broken	0	0	12	0
Rice polish	4	5	0	15
SBM	39.7	30	27.7	23.5
GNC-Ext.	7	6	0	5
Oil	4.5	3.5	5.5	2.5
SFOC	0	0	10	0
DCP	1.35	1.85	1.85	0.6
Calcite	1.8	1.4	1.4	6.9
Lysine	0.15	0.1	0.12	0.1
Methionine	0.2	0.15	0.13	0.1
Salt	0.4	0.4	0.4	0.4
Feed additives*	0.9	0.9	0.9	0.9
	100	100	100	100

D. Ration for Emus

Ingredients	Starter (0-14 wks/ up to 10kg body weight)	Grower (15-34 wks/10-25 kg body weight)	Finisher (25-40 kg body weight)	Breeder (4-5 wk before breeding)	Maintenance (non-breeding)
Maize	30	40	40	26	25
Jowar	15	0	0	15	0
Bajra	0	10	10	0	0
Rice broken	0	0	0	0	15
DORB	10	16	24.2	10	34
Rice polish	8.6	0	0	8.6	0
SBM	25	20	16	25	10
GNC-Ext.	5	0	0	6.5	0
SFOC	0	8	4	0	10
DCP	1.9	1.5	1	1.1	0.8
Calcite	3	3.1	3.5	6.4	3.9
Lysine	0	0	0	0	0
Methionine	0.2	0.1	0.06	0.1	0
Salt	0.4	0.4	0.4	0.4	0.4
Feed additives*	0.9	0.9	0.9	0.9	0.9
	100	100	100	100	100

E. Ration for Vanaraja (egg and meat type breeders)

Ingredients	Chicks (0-6 wks)	Grower (7-16 wks)	Pre-breeder (17-23 wks)	Breeder (>23 wks)	Male breeders (>23 wks)
Maize	30	49	35	40	40
Jowar	15	0	0	15	0
Bajra	0	10	0	0	10
Rice broken	0	0	5	0	0
DORB	0	9.4	17.2	4	14
Rice polish	16.1	0	15	9.7	14
SBM	25	23	15	15	0
GNC-Ext.	9	0	0	6	5
SFOC	0	4	7	0	13.3
DCP	1.4	1.5	0.7	0.7	0.7
Calcite	1.95	1.7	3.7	8.2	1.62
Lysine	0.1	0	0.05	0	0
Methionine	0.15	0.1	0.08	0.1	0.08
Salt	0.4	0.4	0.4	0.4	0.4
Feed additives*	0.9	0.9	0.9	0.9	0.9
	100	100	100	100	100

F. Ration for Gramapriya breeders

Ingredients	Chicks (0-6 wks)	Grower (7-16 wks)	Pre-breeder (17-23 wks)	Breeder (>23 wks)	Male (>23 wks)
Maize	30	494	35	40	40
Jowar	15	0	0	15	0
Bajra	0	10	0	0	10
Rice broken	0	5	5	0	0
DORB	0	9.4	17.2	4	14
Rice polish	16.1	0	15	9.7	14
SBM	25	23	15	15	0
GNC-Ext.	9	0	0	6	5
SFOC	0	4	7	0	13.3
DCP	1.4	1.5	0.7	0.7	0.7
Calcite	1.95	1.7	3.7	8.2	1.62
Lysine	0.1	0	0.05	0	0
Methionine	0.15	0.1	0.08	0.1	0.08
Salt	0.4	0.4	0.4	0.4	0.4
Feed additives*	0.9	0.9	0.9	0.9	0.9
	100	100	100	100	100

G. Ration for Guinea keets (hot season in tropics)

Ingredients	Starter (0-4 wks)	Grower (5-8 wks)	Finisher (9-12 wks)
Maize	41.7	50	45
Jowar	10	0	10
Bajra	0	5	0
DORB	6.2	0	0
Rice polish	0	9.5	14.9
SBM	32	26	16
GNC-Ext.	5	5	10
DCP	2.7	2.4	2.1
Calcite	1	0.8	0.7
Lysine	0	0	0
Methionine	0.1	0.06	0.02
Salt	0.4	0.4	0.4
Feed additives*	0.9	0.9	0.9
	100	100	100

H. Ration for Guinea keets (cold season in tropics)

Ingredients	Starter (0-4 wks)	Grower (5-8 wks)	Finisher (9-12 wks)
Maize	30	47.5	42
Jowar	11	0	10
Bajra	0	4.5	0
Rice polish	5	9	15.9
SBM	34	26	15.8
GNC-Ext.	10.4	5.8	10
Oil	4.5	3	2
DCP	2.7	2.1	2.1
Calcite	1	0.72	0.83
Lysine	0	0	0
Methionine	0.1	0.08	0.07
Salt	0.4	0.4	0.4
Feed additives*	0.9	0.9	0.9
	100	100	100

I. Ration for Guinea fowl

Ingredients	AMEn (kcal/kg, DM)		
	2800	2900	3000
Maize	40.7	31	30
Jowar	11	11	0
Bajra	0	0	10
DORB	10	0	0
Rice polish	5	20	17.1
SBM	8.5	11.3	12.8
GNC-Ext.	8	8	8
Oil	4	5	8
DCP	2.5	2.9	3
Calcite	9	9.5	9.8
Lysine	0	0	0
Methionine	0	0	0
Salt	0.4	0.4	0.4
Feed additives*	0.9	0.9	0.9
	100	100	100

List of feed additives*	(common for all the rations)
	%
Trace mineral mixture	0.10
Vitamin AB$_2$D$_3$K	0.0125
B- Complex vitamins	0.075
Choline chloride	0.10
Enzymes	0.10
Probiotic	0.10
Antibiotic	0.10
Toxin binder	0.25
Antioxidant	0.0125
Coccidiostat	0.05
	0.90

11. Vitamins and Minerals along with their sources

Nutrient	Sources
Vitamin A	Retinal: egg, liver, cheese, cream, butter, fortified margarine and milk. Beta-carotene: coloured vegetables and fruits
Vitamin D	Synthesized in the body with the help of sunlight; egg yolk, liver, fatty fish, fortified milk and margarine.
Vitamin E	Polyunsaturated plant oils, fish oils, green leafy vegetables (GLV), wheat germ, whole-grain products, nuts, sunflower seeds, pumpkin seeds, liver, egg yolks.
Vitamin K	Bacterial synthesis in the digestive tract (vitamin K needs can not be met from bacterial synthesis alone; however, it is a potentially important source in the jejunum and ileum, where absorption efficiency ranges from 40 to 70%); liver, GLV, cabbage-type vegetables, milk.
Thiamin	Pork, ham, bacon, liver, whole-grain or enriched breads and cereals, legumes (black beans, green peas), nuts.
Riboflavin	Milk, yoghurt, cottage cheese, meat, GLV (spinach), whole-grain or enriched breads and cereals.
Niacin	Milk, eggs, meat, fish, whole-grain and enriched breads and cereals, nuts, and all protein-containing foods.
Vitamin B$_6$	GLV, meats, fish, shellfish, legumes, fruits, whole grains
Folate	GLV, legumes, sunflower seed, oranges, liver
Pantothenic acid	Widespread in foods
Biotin	Widespread in foods
Vitamin B$_{12}$	Animal products: meat, fish, poultry, shellfish, milk, cheese, eggs.

Vitamin C	Citrus fruits: orange (kamala), mosambi (sathkudi); cabbage-type vegetables, dark green vegetables, tomatoes, potatoes with skin, fruits: papayas, guava, mango
Calcium	Milk and milk products, small fish with bones, legumes, tofu (soybean curd), broccoli, cauliflower.
Phosphorus	All animal tissues: meat, fish, poultry, eggs, milk; plant protein supplements, cereal brans
Magnesium	Nuts, legumes, whole grains, dark green vegetables, carrots, seafood, chocolate, cocoa
Sodium and chloride	Table salt, soy sauce, moderate amounts in meats, milk, vegetables; large amounts in many processed foods
Potassium	All whole foods; meats, milks, fruits: banana, vegetables, grains, legumes
Sulphur	All protein-containing foods: meats, fish, eggs, milk, legumes, nuts
Iodine	Indized salt, seafood
Iron	Red meats, fish, poultry, shellfish, eggs, legumes, dried fruits
Zinc	Protein-containing foods: meats, fish, whole grains, pulses, vegetables; oysters, crab meat
Copper	Meats, drinking water
Fluoride	Seafood, drinking water
Selenium	Seafood, meat, grains
Chromium	Meats, unrefined foods, fats, vegetables oils
Cobalt	Foods of animal origin: meats, milk and milk products
Molybdenum	Legumes, cereals, organ meats
Manganese	Widespread in foods

Index